In A Page
Signs & Symptoms

Scott Kahan, MD
Intern, Franklin Square Hospital
Baltimore, Maryland

Ellen G. Smith, MD, FAAFP
Director of Education,
Harrisburg Family Practice Residency Program,
PinnacleHealth Hospitals
Harrisburg, Pennsylvania

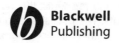
Blackwell
Publishing

© 2004 by Blackwell Publishing

Blackwell Publishing, Inc., 350 Main Street, Malden, Massachusetts 02148-5018, USA
Blackwell Publishing Ltd, 9600 Garsington Road, Oxford OX4 2DQ, UK
Blackwell Science Asia Pty Ltd, 550 Swanston Street, Carlton, Victoria 3053, Australia

04 05 06 07 5 4 3 2

ISBN: 1-4051-0368-X

Library of Congress Cataloging-in-Publication Data

In a page. Signs & symptoms / [edited by] Scott Kahan, Ellen G. Smith.
    p. cm.
    Includes index.
    ISBN 1-4051-0368-X
    1. Diagnosis, Differential—Handbooks, manuals, etc.   2. Symptoms—Handbooks, manuals, etc.
    I. Title: Signs & symptoms.   II. Title: Signs and symptoms.   III. Kahan, Scott.   IV. Smith, Ellen G.

    RC71.5.I5 2004
    616.07'5—dc22

                                                                    2003063939

A catalogue record for this title is available from the British Library

Acquisitions: Beverly Copland
Development: Kate Heinle
Production: Debra Murphy
Cover design: Gary Ragaglia
Interior design: Meral Dabcovich
Typesetter: Techbooks in New Delhi, India
Printed and bound by Sheridan Books in Ann Arbor, MI

For further information on Blackwell Publishing, visit our website:
www.blackwellmedstudent.com

Notice: The indications and dosages of all drugs in this book have been recommended in the
medical literature and conform to the practices of the general community. The medications
described and treatment prescriptions suggested do not necessarily have specific approval by
the Food and Drug Administration for use in the diseases and dosages for which they are
recommended. The package insert for each drug should be consulted for use and dosage as
approved by the FDA. Because standards for usage change, it is advisable to keep abreast of
revised recommendations, particularly those concerning new drugs. This book is intended solely
as a review book for medical students and residents. It is not written as a guide for the intricate
clinical management of medical patients. The publisher and editor cannot accept any legal
responsibility for the content contained within this book nor any omitted information.

Table of Contents

Table of Contents

Table of Contents

Table of Contents

Table of Contents

Abbreviations

5-FU	5-Fluorouracil		CA	Cancer
$5\text{-}HT_1$	5-Hydroxytryptamine$_1$		Ca	Calcium
β-hCG	Human Chorionic Gonadotropin		CABG	Coronary Artery Bypass Grafting
A-a	Alveolar-Arterial Oxygen Gradient		CAD	Coronary Artery Disease
AAA	Abdominal Aortic Aneurysm		CAH	Congenital Adrenal Hyperplasia
ABG	Arterial Blood Gas		CBC	Complete Blood Count
ABI	Ankle-Brachial Index		CDC	Centers for Disease Control
AC	Acromioclavicular		CGD	Chronic Granulomatous Disease
ACE	Angiotensin Converting Enzyme		CHF	Congestive Heart Failure
ACL	Anterior Cruciate Ligament		CIDP	Chronic Inflammatory
ACLS	Advanced Cardiac Life Support			Demyelinating Polyneuropathy
ACTH	Adrenocorticotropin Hormone		CMT	Charcot-Marie-Tooth Disease
ADH	Antidiuretic Hormone		CMV	Cytomegalovirus
AFB	Acid Fast Bacilli		CN	Cranial Nerve
AFP	Alpha Fetoprotein		CNS	Central Nervous System
AIDS	Acquired Immunodeficiency		CO	Carbon Monoxide
	Syndrome		CO_2	Carbon Dioxide
ALS	Amyotrophic Lateral Sclerosis		COP	Cryptogenic Organizing
ALT	Alanine Aminotransferase			Pneumonia
ANA	Anti-nuclear Antibody		COPD	Chronic Obstructive Pulmonary
ANCA	Antineutrophil Cytoplasmic			Disease
	Antibodies		COX	Cyclooxygenase
A/P or AP	Anterior/Posterior		CP	Cerebral Palsy
AR	Aortic Regurgitation		CP	Cerebellar-Pontine
ARB	Angiotensin Receptor Blocker		CPAP	Continuous Positive Airway
ARDS	Acute Respiratory Distress			Pressure
	Syndrome		CPEO	Chronic Progressive External
AS	Aortic Stenosis			Ophthalmoplegia
ASD	Atrial Septal Defect		CRI	Chronic Renal Insufficiency
ASO	Antistreptolysin O antibodies		CPK	Creatine Phosphokinase
AST	Aspartate Aminotransferase		CREST	Calcinosis, Raynaud's
ATP	Adenosine Triphosphate			Phenomenon, Esophageal
AV	Arteriovenous			Dysmotility, Sclerodactyly,
AV	Atrioventricular			Telangiectasia
AVM	Arterovenous Malformation		CRP	C-Reactive Protein
AVNRT	AV Nodal Re-entrant Tachycardia		CSF	Cerebrospinal Fluid
AVRT	AV Re-entrant Tachycardia		CT	Computerized Tomography
AZT	Zidovudine or Azidothymidine		CTA	Computerized Tomographic
BAPS	Biomechanical Ankle Platform			Angiography
	System		CVA	Cerebrovascular Accident
BID	Twice a Day		CVA	Costovertebral Angle
BiPAP	Bilevel Positive Airway Pressure		CXR	Chest X-ray
BM	Bowel Movement		D_5	5% Dextrose Solution
BNP	Brain or B-Type Natriuretic Peptide		D_5W	5% Dextrose Solution in Water
BOOP	Bronchiolitis Obliterans Organizing		D_{50}	50% Dextrose Solution
	Pneumonia		DASH	Dietary Approaches to Stop
BP	Blood Pressure			Hypertension
BPH	Benign Prostatic Hypertrophy		DC	Direct Current
Bpm	Beats Per Minute		DDAVP	Desmopressin Acetate
BPV	Benign Positional Vertigo		DES	Diethylstilbestrol
BS	Breath Sounds		DHEA-S	Dehydroepiandrosterone-sulfate
BUN	Blood Urea Nitrogen		DI	Diabetes Insipidus
BV	Bacterial Vaginosis		DIC	Disseminated Intravascular
C1	Complement Factor 1			Coagulation

Abbreviations

DJD	Degenerative Joint Disease	ICP	Intracranial Pressure
DKA	Diabetic Ketoacidosis	ICU	Intensive Care Unit
DLE	Discoid Lupus Erythematosus	IFG	Impaired Fasting Glucose
DM	Diabetes Mellitus	IgE	Immunoglobulin E
DNA	Deoxyribonucleic Acid	IgG	Immunoglobulin G
DRPLA	Dentatorubropallidoluysian Atrophy	IgM	Immunoglobulin M
		IJ	Intrajugular
DSM-IV	Diagnostic Statistical Manual IV	IM	Intramuscular
DUB	Dysfunctional Uterine Bleeding	INH	Isoniazid
EBV	Epstein-Barr Virus	INR	International Normalized Ratio
ECF	Extracellular Fluid	ITP	Idiopathic Thrombocytopenic Purpura
ECG	Electrocardiogram		
ECT	Electroconvulsive Therapy	IUD	Intrauterine Device
EEG	Electroencephalogram	IV	Intravenous
EGD	Esophagogastroduodenoscopy	IVIG	Intravenous Immunoglobulin
EMG	Electromyogram	IVP	Intravenous Pyelogram (Urogram)
ENT	Otolaryngology (Ear, Nose, and Throat)	K	Potassium
		KOH	Potassium Hydroxide
EOM	Extraocular Muscles	KUB	Kidney, Ureters, and Bladder (X-ray)
ERCP	Endoscopic Retrograde Cholangiopancreatography		
		JVD	Jugular Venous Distension
ESR	Erythrocyte Sedimentation Rate	JVP	Jugular Venous Pressure
FH	Family History	LBP	Low Back Pain
FSH	Follicle Stimulating Hormone	LCL	Lateral Collateral Ligament
FTA	Fluorescent Treponemal Antibody	LCV	Leukocytoclastic Vasculitis
GBM	Glomerular Basement Membranes	LDH	Lactate Dehydrogenase
GBS	Guillain-Barré Syndrome	LES	Lower Esophageal Sphincter
GC	Gonococcal (Gonorrhea)	LH	Lactate Dehydrogenase
GERD	Gastroesophageal Reflux Disease	LH	Luteinizing Hormone
GGTP	Gammaglutamyl Transpeptidase	LFT	Liver Function Test
GI	Gastrointestinal	LP	Lumbar Puncture
GnRH	Gonadotropin-Releasing Hormone	LSD	Lysergic Acid Diethylamide
GU	Genitourinary	LV	Left Ventricular
H	Hydrogen	LVH	Left Ventricular Hypertrophy
H_2O	Water	MAO	Monoamine Oxidase
Hb or Hgb	Hemoglobin	MAT	Multifocal Atrial Tachycardia
HEENT	Head, Eyes, Ears, Nose, and Throat	MCH	Mean Corpuscular Hemoglobin
		MCHC	Mean Corpuscular Hemoglobin Concentration
Hb_{A1C}	Glycohemoglobin		
HIT	Heparin-Induced Thrombocytopenia	MCL	Medial Collateral Ligament
		MCP	Metacarpophalangeal
HIV	Human Immunodeficiency Virus	MCTD	Mixed Connective Tissue Disease
HLA	Human Leukocyte Antigen	MCV	Mean Corpuscular Volume
HPV	Human Papilloma Virus	Mg	Magnesium
HRT	Hormone Replacement Therapy	MGUS	Monoclonal Gammopathy of Uncertain Significance
HSP	Henoch-Schönlein Purpura		
HSV	Herpes Simplex Virus	MI	Myocardial Infarction
HTLV	Human T Cell Lymphotropic Virus	MPTP	1-Methyl-4-Phenyl-1,2,3,6-Tetrahydropyridine
HTN	Hypertension		
HUS	Hemolytic Uremic Syndrome	MR	Mitral Regurgitation
HZV	Herpes Zoster Virus	MRA	Magnetic Resonance Angiography
IBD	Inflammatory Bowel Disease	MRI	Magnetic Resonance Imaging
IBS	Irritable Bowel Syndrome	MRV	Magnetic Resonance Venography
ICD	Implantable Cardiac Defibrillator	MS	Multiple Sclerosis

Abbreviations

MTX	Methotrexate	PTH	Parathyroid Hormone
MVA	Motor Vehicle Accident	PTT	Partial Thromboplastin Time
MVP	Mitral Valve Prolapse	PTU	Propylthiouracil
Na	Sodium	PUD	Peptic Ulcer Disease
NaCl	Sodium Chloride	PUVA	Psoralen with Ultraviolet A
NARES	Nonallergic Rhinitis with		Phototherapy
	Eosinophilia	PVD	Peripheral Vascular Disease
NASH	Nonalcoholic Steatohepatitis	QD	Once a Day
NBT	Nitroblue Tetrazolium	QID	Four Times a Day
NCT	Nerve Conduction Test	RA	Rheumatoid Arthritis
NG	Nasogastric	RBC	Red Blood Cell
NPO	Nil Per Os (Nothing By Mouth)	RDW	Red Cell Distribution Width
NSAID	Nonsteroidal Anti-inflammatory	REM	Rapid Eye Movement
	Drug	RF	Rheumatoid Factor
NSS	Normal Saline Solution	RIND	Reversible Ischemic Neurologic
	(0.9% NaCl)		Deficits
O_2	Oxygen	RLS	Restless Legs Syndrome
OA	Osteoarthritis	RMSF	Rocky Mountain Spotted Fever
OCD	Obsessive-Compulsive Disorder	R/O	Rule Out
OCD	Osteochrondritis Dissecans	ROM	Range of Motion
OCP	Oral Contraceptive Pill	RPR	Rapid Plasma Reagin
OE	Otitis Externa	RSV	Respiratory Syncytial Virus
OM	Otitis Media	RUQ	Right Upper Quadrant
Osm	Osmolality	RV	Right Ventricular
PA	Pulmonary Artery	S1 or S_1	First Heart Sound
PAN	Polyarteritis Nodosa	S2 or S_2	Second Heart Sound
PAP	Papanicolaou	S3 or S_3	Third Heart Sound
PAS	Periodic Acid Schiff	S4 or S_4	Fourth Heart Sound
PCL	Posterior Cruciate Ligament	SAH	Subarachnoid Hemorrhage
PCOS	Polycystic Ovarian Syndrome	SBE	Subacute Bacterial Endocarditis
PCP	*Pneumocystis carinii* Pneumonia	SBP	Systolic Blood Pressure
PCP	Primary Care Physician/Provider	SBP	Spontaneous Bacterial Peritonitis
PCP	Phencyclidine	SCA	Spinocerebellar ataxia
PCT	Porphyria Cutanea Tarda	SCIWORA	Spinal Cord Injury Without
PDA	Patent Ductus Arteriosis		Radiographic Abnormality
PE	Pulmonary Embolus	SIADH	Syndrome of Inappropriate
PEEP	Positive End-Expiratory Pressure		Antidiuretic Hormone Secretion
PET	Positron Emission Tomography	SJS	Stevens Johnson Syndrome
PID	Pelvic Inflammatory Disease	SLE	Systemic Lupus Erythematosus
PMH	Past Medical History	SOB	Short of Breath
PMI	Point of Maximal Impulse	SPEP	Serum Protein Electrophoresis
PMLE	Polymorphous Light Eruption	SQ	Subcutaneous
PMN	Polymorphonuclear Cell	SSRI	Selective Serotonin Reuptake
PND	Paroxysmal Nocturnal Dyspnea		Inhibitor
P_{osm}	Plasma Osmolality	SSS	Sick Sinus Syndrome
PPD	Purified Protein Derivative	STD	Sexually Transmitted Disease
	(TB Test)	T_3	Tri-iodothyronine
PPI	Proton Pump Inhibitor	T_4	Thyroxine
PR	Pityriasis Rosea	TAO	Thyroid-Associated Orbitopathy
PRP	Pityriasis Rubra Pilaris	TB	Tuberculosis
PSA	Prostate Specific Antigen	TEE	Transesophageal Echocardiogram
PT	Prothrombin Time	TEN	Toxic Epidermal Necrolysis
PTCA	Percutaneous Transluminal	TFT	Thyroid Function Test
	Coronary Angioplasty	TIA	Transient Ischemic Attack

Abbreviations

TIBC	Total Iron Binding Capacity	UOP	Urine Output
TIPS	Transjugular Intrahepatic Portosystemic Shunt	U_{osm}	Urine Osmolality
		UPEP	Urine Protein Electrophoresis
TM	Tympanic Membrane	URI	Upper Respiratory Infection
TMJ	Temporomandibular Joint Dysfunction	UTI	Urinary Tract Infection
		UVA	Ultraviolet A
TNF	Tumor Necrosis Factor	UVB	Ultraviolet B
TORCH	Toxoplasmosis, Rubella, Cytomegalovirus, Herpes Simplex	VCUG	Voiding Cystourethrogram
		VDRL	Venereal Disease Research Laboratory
TSH	Thyroid Stimulating Hormone		
TSS	Toxic Shock Syndrome	VEP	Visual Evoked Potential
TTKG	Transtubular Potassium Gradient (in Kidney)	Vfib	Ventricular Fibrillation
		VIP	Vasoactive Intestinal Polypeptide
TTP	Thrombotic Thrombocytopenic Purpura	VMA	Vanillylmandelic Acid
		VQ or V/Q	Ventilation-Perfusion (Scan)
TURP	Transurethral Resection of the Prostate	VSD	Ventricular Septal Defect
		VT	Ventricular Tachycardia
UA	Urinalysis	VZV	Varicella Zoster Virus
UC	Ulcerative Colitis	WBC	White Blood Cell
UGI	Upper Gastrointestinal	WPW	Wolff-Parkinson-White Syndrome

Associate Editor

Ronald J. Williams, MD, FAAP, FACP
Associate Professor of Pediatrics
Assistant Professor of Internal Medicine
Director, Combined Internal Medicine/Pediatrics Residency Program
Pennsylvania State University
Milton S. Hershey Medical Center
Hershey, Pennsylvania

Contributors

Heidi Alexandra Baer
Class of 2005
Drexel Medical School
Philadelphia, Pennsylvania

Melissa Beagle, MD
Resident, Department of Family Medicine
University of Colorado Health Sciences Center
Denver, Colorado

Nicole Garofola Bentze, DO
Faculty Physician
Harrisburg Family Practice Residency
PinnacleHealth Hospital System
Harrisburg, Pennsylvania

Caryn Brenner-Williams, MD
Faculty Physician
Department of Family Practice
PinnacleHealth
Harrisburg, Pennsylvania

Christian Caicedo, MD
Resident, Family Practice
PinnacleHealth
Harrisburg Hospital
Harrisburg, Pennsylvania

Timothy D. Carter, MD
Associate Professor of Neurology
Medical University of South Carolina
Attending Neurologist
Medical University of South Carolina Medical Center
Charleston, South Carolina

Douglas A. Chen, MD
Clinical Associate Professor
University of Pittsburgh
Pittsburgh, Pennsylvania

Contributors

Stefan O. Ciurea, MD
Chief Medical Resident
PinnacleHealth System
Harrisburg, Pennsylvania

Harold V. Cohen, DDS
Professor, Division of Oral Medicine, Department of Diagnostic Sciences
University of Medicine and Dentistry of New Jersey-New Jersey Dental School
Attending, Department of Dental Medicine-Hospital Dentistry
University of Medicine and Dentistry of New Jersey-The University Hospital
Newark, New Jersey
Staff-Dental Department
Robert Wood Johnson University Hospital
New Brunswick, New Jersey

Peter Foster Cronholm, MD
Clinical Instructor, Department of Family Practice and Community Medicine
University of Pennsylvania
Attending Family Practitioner
Hospital of the University of Pennsylvania
Philadelphia, Pennsylvania

Augusta Czysz
Class of 2004
Pennsylvania State University College of Medicine
Hershey, Pennsylvania

Michael DiLorenzo
Class of 2005
Columbia University
New York, New York

Emmy M. Fernandez, MD
Resident, Department of Dermatology
Pennsylvania State University College of Medicine
Milton S. Hershey Medical Center
Hershey, Pennsylvania

John G. Fernandez, MD
Resident, Department of Surgery
St. Luke's – Roosevelt Hospital Center
New York, New York

Michael Fernandez, MD
Resident, Department of Orthopedics
Pennsylvania State University College of Medicine
The Milton S. Hershey Medical Center
Hershey, Pennsylvania

Contributors

Kara Garcia
Medical Student
Pennsylvania State University College of Medicine
Hershey, Pennsylvania

Dennis Gingrich, MD
Associate Professor Department of Family and Community Medicine
Pennsylvania State University College of Medicine
Hershey, Pennsylvania

Andrea Gordon, MD
Faculty
Harrisburg Family Practice Residency Program
Harrisburg Hospital
Harrisburg, Pennsylvania

Joseph W. Gravel, Jr, MD
Assistant Clinical Professor Family Medicine and Community Health
Tufts University School of Medicine
Boston, Massachusetts
Program Director
Tufts University Family Practice Residency
Malden, Massachusetts

Faina Gurevich
Medical Student
Pennsylvania State University College of Medicine
Hershey, Pennsylvania

Cynthia Haensel
Class of 2004
Pennsylvania State College of Medicine
Hershey, Pennsylvania

Sang H. Hong, MD
Assistant Professor
Orbital & Ophthalmic Plastic Surgery
Neuro-Ophthalmology
Department of Ophthalmology
The Eye Institute
Medical College of Wisconsin
Milwaukee, Wisconsin

Jessica Inwood
Class of 2004
Pennsylvania State University College of Medicine
Hershey, Pennsylvania

Contributors

Marc S. Itskowitz, MD
Assistant Professor of Medicine
Drexel University College of Medicine
Associate Program Director
Internal Medicine Residency Program
Allegheny General Hospital
Pittsburgh, Pennsylvania

Jacquelyn Leung, MD
Resident Physician
Family Medicine
Tufts School of Medicine
New England Medical Center
Boston, Massachusetts

Jennifer L. Lewis, MD
Third Year Medicine Clerkship Director
Assistant Professor of Medicine
Drexel University College of Medicine
Attending Physician
Allegheny General Hospital
Pittsburgh, Pennsylvania

Gary Luttermoser, MD
Attending Physician
Harrisburg Family Practice Residency
Harrisburg Hospital
PinnacleHealth
Harrisburg, Pennsylvania

Geoffrey M. Margo, MD, PhD
Clinical Associate Professor of Psychiatry
University of Pennsylvania
Director, Consultation/Liaison Psychiatry
Pennsylvania Hospital
Philadelphia, Pennsylvania

Katherine Margo, MD
Assistant Professor
Predoctoral Director
Department of Family Practice and Community Medicine
University of Pennsylvania School of Medicine
Philadelphia Pennsylvania

Melanie Maytin, MD
Teaching Fellow in Medicine, Cardiology
Boston University School of Medicine
Fellow, Cardiology
Boston University Medical Center
Boston, Massachusetts

Contributors

Nathan W. Mick, MD
Clinical Fellow, Pediatric Emergency Medicine
Children's Hospital of Boston
Boston, Massachusetts

Rupa Mokkapatti, MD, PhD
Attending Physician
Drexel University School of Medicine
Allegheny General Hospital
Pittsburgh, Pennsylvania

Glenn Nordehn, DO
Assistant Professor
University of Minnesota School of Medicine Duluth
Duluth, Minnesota

Soheila Nouri, MD
Clinical Instructor of Medicine
University of Arizona – Tucson Hospital
Internal Medicine/Medical Staff Member
Tucson Medical Center Hospital
Tucson, Arizona

Richard Prensner, MD
Associate Program Director
Harrisburg Family Residency Program/Pinnacle Health
Pennsylvania State University
Hershey, Pennsylvania
Drexel University
Philadelphia, Pennsylvania

Hisana Qamar, MD
Resident, Family Practice
Harrisburg Family Practice Residency Program
Harrisburg, Pennsylvania

Abigail M. Rattin, BS
Medical Student
Pennsylvania State College of Medicine
Hershey Medical Center
Hershey, Pennsylvania

Richard M. Rayner, MD
Medical Director
Harrisburg Family Practice Residency Program
PinnacleHealth System
Harrisburg, Pennsylvania

Contributors

Maria Rosa Robinson
Class of 2003
Pennsylvania State University
Hershey, Pennsylvania

Neil Romberg
Medical Student
Pennsylvania State University College of Medicine
Hershey, Pennsylvania

David Sachs, MD
Resident, Department of Ophthalmology
Nassau University Hospital
Hempstead, New York

Dean Thomas Scow, MD
Faculty Physician
Harrisburg Family Practice Residency Program
PinnacleHealth
Harrisburg, Pennsylvania

James Shaffer, MD
Resident, Orthopaedic Surgery
San Francisco Orthopaedic Residency Program
San Francisco, California

Naureen A. Shaikh, MD
Tamalpais Family Practice
Marin General Hospital
Larkspur, California

Serene Shereef
Class of 2005
Pennsylvania State University College of Medicine
Hershey, Pennsylvania

George A. Small, MD
Assistant Professor of Neurology
Program Director, Clinical Neurophysiology Fellowship
Drexel University School of Medicine
Director, Neuromuscular Division
Allegheny General Hospital
Pittsburgh, Pennsylvania

Ryan J. Smith, MD
Resident, Department of Medicine
Lehigh Valley Hospital
Allentown, Pennsylvania

Contributors

Thomas W. Stein, Jr., MD
Harrisburg Family Practice
Pinnacle Health System
Harrisburg, Pennsylvania

Joseph B. Straton, MD, MSCE
Assistant Professor
Department of Family Practice and Community Medicine
University of Pennsylvania
Philadelphia, Pennsylvania

Mark Su, MD
Clinical Instructor
Tufts University Department of Family Medicine
Malden, Massachusetts
Private Practice, Cornerstone Family Practice
Rowley, Massachusetts

Parra Tomkins, MD
Assistant Clinical Professor
Tufts University School of Medicine
Boston, Massachusetts
Attending Faculty
Lawrence Memorial Hospital
Medford, Massachusetts

Serv Wahan, DMD, MD
Resident, Oral and Maxillofacial Surgery
Allegheny General Hospital
Pittsburgh, Pennsylvania

Cecily Wang, MD
Resident, General Surgery
Union Memorial Hospital
Baltimore, Maryland

Ronald J. Williams, MD, FAAP, FACP
Associate Professor of Pediatrics
Assistant Professor of Internal Medicine
Director, Combined Internal Medicine/Pediatrics Residency Program
Pennsylvania State University
Milton S. Hershey Medical Center
Hershey, Pennsylvania

Steven H. Williams, PhD
Director of Behavioral Medicine
Harrisburg Family Practice Residency Program
PinnacleHealth System
Harrisburg, Pennsylvania

Contributors

Donald E. Yarbrough, MD
Resident, Department of Surgery
Mayo Clinic College of Medicine
Rochester, Minnesota

Jane Yu, MD
Resident, Family Practice
Tufts University Family Practice Residency Program
Malden, Massachusetts

Jennifer C. Zampogna, MD, FAAD, FASMS
Board Certified Dermatologist
Advanced Dermatology and Skin Surgery
Mechanicsburg, Pennsylvania

Melissa Zerr
Class of 2005
Pennsylvania State College of Medicine
Hershey, Pennsylvania

Consultants

Geoffrey J. Brent, MD
Premier Eye Care, Inc.
Camp Hill, Pennsylvania

Jon Brillman, MD
Chairman of Neurology
Allegheny General Hospital, Pittsburgh, PA
Professor of Neurology
Drexel University College of Medicine
Philadelphia, Pennsylvania

Richard Evans, DO
Pulmonary and Critical Care Medicine Associates
Harrisburg, Pennsylvania

Dennis Gingrich, MD
Associate Professor Department of Family and Community Medicine
Pennsylvania State University College of Medicine
Hershey, Pennsylvania

Jean Hauser, MD, FACOG
Resident Director and Director of Medical Education
Department of Obstetrics and Gynecology
PinnacleHealth System
Harrisburg, Pennsylvania

Michelle Huston, MD
Department of Emergency Medicine
Franklin Square Hospital
Baltimore, Maryland

Robert Loeb, MD
Clinical Assistant Professor of Ophthalmology
University of Maryland School of Medicine
Baltimore, Maryland

Paula Mackrides, DO
Faculty Physician
Harrisburg Family Practice Program
Harrisburg, Pennsylvania

Rajnish Prasad, MD
Director, Cardiac Care Unit
University of Maryland Medical Center
Assistant Professor of Medicine
University of Maryland School of Medicine
Baltimore, Maryland

Consultants

John J. Raves, MD
Senior Attending Staff
Division of General Surgery
Allegheny General Hospital
Pittsburgh, Pennsylvania
Assistant Professor of Surgery
Drexel University
Pittsburgh, Pennsylvania

Richard M. Rayner, MD
Medical Director
Harrisburg Family Practice Residency Program
PinnacleHealth System
Harrisburg, Pennsylvania

Preface

The *In A Page* series was designed to streamline the vast amount of material that saturates the study of medicine, providing students, residents, and health professionals a high-yield, big-picture overview of the most important clinical medical topics. We expect this book to be especially useful for medical students, interns, physician assistants, nurse practitioners, and other health professionals.

In A Page Signs & Symptoms is the sixth handbook of this series. Whereas previous books have been organized by a disease per page, this book is organized by a sign or symptom per page. Thus, it is essentially a handbook of differential diagnoses. The format we use is especially effective for use in clinical settings, where knowledge of a quick, thorough list of differential diagnoses and a simple diagnostic scheme are necessary to work up the patient.

As in the initial books of the series, we were constrained by the size of the template and the need to keep each sign or symptom within a single page. We had to be quite succinct in our explanations and descriptions and we sacrificed details in some cases, such as drug dosages. Furthermore, we abbreviated liberally.

We are certain that the final product will be a very effective resource. Reviews from medical students and residents have been very positive. We anticipate that this book will be a valuable tool in clinical settings, board review, and for independent study. We welcome any comments, questions, or suggestions. Please address correspondence to drkahan@yahoo.com.

Scott and Ellen

Acknowledgments

I must extend our heartfelt gratitude to all contributors and consultants of this book. This was a group of advanced medical students who have recently sat for the boards, residents who have experienced medicine from the viewpoints of both students and physicians, and experienced faculty physicians. Special thanks to Ron Williams, Associate Editor, and the faculty of Harrisburg Family Practice. All our thanks to the staff at Blackwell Publishing, especially Bev Copland, Kate Heinle, Deb Murphy, and Laura DeYoung. Finally, I thank Ellen Smith, my co-editor and friend, for a job well done.

—Scott

I take this opportunity to express love and gratitude to the three most important people in the world to me; my dear husband, John, and my children, David and Kelly. The pages of this book came out of their generous support and giving of their personal time. I also thank my parents, Ruth George and John and Jean George, who have taught me that "It is better to do your best and fail, than to never have tried at all," and my siblings, David, John, and Diane. Hopefully, this book succeeds in helping medical students and residents everywhere to succeed. I also thank each member of the faculty at Harrisburg Family Practice Residency, as well as Dana Kellis, MD, who have been very supportive throughout the yearlong process of editing. In addition, I offer my utmost appreciation and thanks to my residency staff, Carole Harmon, Lisa Dininni, Jan Patton, and Jean Mackey, who encouraged me while I edited this book.

—Ellen

1. Abdominal Bruit

An abdominal bruit is a murmur that corresponds to the cardiac cycle. It is heard best with the diaphragm of the stethoscope, usually over the abdominal aorta, renal arteries, or spleen. It can be a sign of atherosclerosis or fibromuscular hyperplasia. However, it may also be heard over a large, highly vascular tumor, or as a result of partial occlusion of a vessel, secondary to external compression (e.g., due to extreme pressure by stethoscope or a mass).

Differential Diagnosis

- Abdominal aortic aneurysm
- Hepatocellular carcinoma (hepatoma)
- Cirrhosis
- Liver hemangioma
- Arteriovenous malformation
- Renal artery stenosis
- Celiac artery stenosis
- Superior mesenteric artery stenosis
- Tricuspid regurgitation
- Turbulence of the splenic artery
- Hepatic venous hum
    - High-pitched continuous murmur that decreases with forced held expiration
- Cruveilhier-Baumgarten murmur
    - High-pitched venous hum of portal hypertension that becomes louder with forced expiration
- Abdominal friction rub
    - Associated with hepatoma, cholangiocarcinoma, liver metastases, inflammatory processes
- Takayasu's arteritis

Workup and Diagnosis

- History and physical exam with focus on abdominal exam (may have palpable thrill), cardiac exam, four extremity pulses, and blood pressure
- Ultrasound is often the initial test and is diagnostic for AAA, liver metastases, and liver and spleen sizes
- Abdominal CT will demonstrate abdominal pathology and is useful to better delineate anatomy
- Arterial Doppler ultrasound
- Angiography is diagnostic for stenosis
- Measuring renal vein renin levels following a captopril challenge is diagnostic for renal artery stenosis
- Radionuclide nephrograms or IV urography will demonstrate differences in perfusion of kidneys with stenotic artery
- Echocardiogram may be indicated to evaluate for valvular dysfunction
- Laboratory studies may include a lipid panel to evaluate for arteriosclerosis; CBC and ESR if inflammatory processes are suspected; liver function tests to evaluate for liver dysfunction; and electrolytes and renal function tests if renal artery stenosis is suspected

Treatment

- Initial treatment is to stabilize and resuscitate the patient as needed
    - Attention to airway, breathing, and circulation
    - Immediate repair of ruptured abdominal aneurysm
- Treat the underlying etiology
- Vascular surgical consultation may be necessary for severely stenotic and/or symptomatic vessels
- Nephrology consult may be needed for renal insufficiency or to help with appropriate medication choices
- Treat hypertension if present
    - Always avoid ACE inhibitors in patients with bilateral renal artery stenosis

2. Abdominal Distension

Abdominal distension is a common complaint that must be evaluated carefully and systematically to expediently rule out serious and life-threatening diagnoses and evaluate for mundane diagnoses, such as swallowing air or overeating, without embarking upon unnecessary testing. A careful history and physical examination are necessary to develop an appropriate differential upon which to base a diagnostic plan.

Differential Diagnosis

- Functional gas/constipation
- Bladder distension
- Overeating
- Lactose intolerance
- Air swallowing (nervous habit)
- Ascites
  - Portal hypertension (e.g., cirrhosis)
  - Congestive heart failure
  - Nephrotic syndrome
  - Hypoalbuminemia (e.g., malnutrition, liver failure)
  - Metastatic cancer (e.g., colon, ovarian)
- Irritable bowel syndrome
- Ovarian cancer
- Leukemia
- Lymphoma
- Spontaneous bacterial peritonitis (SBP)
- Umbilical or ventral hernia
- Obesity
- Bowel obstruction
- Abdominal aneurysm
- Paralytic ileus (postsurgical; secondary to infection or other illness)
- Pancreatitis and complications (pseudocyst)
- Pregnancy
- Infectious diarrhea
- Abdominal trauma with intra-abdominal bleeding
- Toxic megacolon
- Colonic pseudo-obstruction (Ogilvie's syndrome)

Workup and Diagnosis

- History should include duration, weight gain, bloating, flatus, reflux, last bowel movement, diarrhea, last menstrual period, sexual history, and presence of fever and constitutional symptoms
- Physical exam should include full abdominal exam, including palpation for hernias and masses, pelvic exam in women, signs of cirrhosis and portal hypertension, abdominal tenderness, and fluid wave
- Initial laboratory testing may include CBC, ESR (malignancies, SBP), stool cultures, workup for liver disease (liver function tests, hepatitis panel, liver biopsy), and pregnancy testing
- Biopsy may be indicated for masses and suspected tumors
- Plain KUB X-rays may reveal bowel obstruction (distended proximal bowel loops), constipation, air swallowing, paralytic ileus
- Abdominal and pelvic CT scans may reveal pancreatic pseudocyst, ovarian masses, cirrhosis, and/or aneurysm
- Abdominal and pelvic ultrasound may reveal ovarian mass, ascites, liver disease, and/or pregnancy
- Paracentesis is diagnostic for SBP and malignant ascites and may provide symptomatic relief
- Lower GI endoscopy may be indicated to rule out organic pathology before diagnosing irritable bowel syndrome

Treatment

- Identify, treat, and/or refer based on underlying causes
- Nasogastric tube decompression and bowel rest may be indicated (e.g., bowel obstruction, pancreatitis)
- Laxatives for constipation
- Antibiotics for SBP
- Treat underlying liver diseases (and manage complications)
- For distension from swallowing air, awareness can lead to self-control: Eat slowly; avoid carbonated drinks, chewing gum or sucking on candies, drinking through a straw, or sipping hot drinks
- Change diets or reduce milk intake for malabsorption
- Irritable bowel syndrome is treated with increased dietary fiber, stress reduction, and antispasmodics
- Surgical referral for hernias when appropriate

3. Abdominal Guarding

Abdominal guarding refers to muscular rigidity of the abdomen upon palpation. It may be involuntary or voluntary. The examiner may try to limit the voluntary guarding during the physical examination by having the patient bend both knees and/or rest the head on a pillow, and asking the patient to voluntarily relax the abdominal muscles. Involuntary guarding may be an early sign of peritonitis.

Differential Diagnosis

- Appendicitis
- Pancreatitis
- Diverticulitis
- Abdominal wall strain/injury
- Pelvic inflammatory disease
- Ectopic pregnancy
- Bowel obstruction
- Ileus
- Pneumonia
- Dyspepsia
- Nephrolithiasis
- Peptic ulcer disease
- Abdominal aortic aneurysm
- Anxiety
- Malingering
- Spontaneous bacterial peritonitis (SBP)
- Mesenteric ischemia
- GERD
- Ovarian cyst
- Hepatic or splenic contusion/laceration
- Pneumoperitoneum secondary to trauma
- Urinary tract infection/pyelonephritis
- Zoster
  - –Skin lesions may not be visible until another day or two
- Insect toxins (e.g., black widow spider)
- Abscess (e.g., iliopsoas)
- Incarcerated hernia
- Abdominal migraine
- Intussusception
- Volvulus

Workup and Diagnosis

- History and physical examination
- Initial laboratory studies may include CBC, electrolytes, BUN/creatinine, glucose, liver function tests, amylase/lipase, β-hCG, urinalysis, and urine culture
- CT scan is often indicated to diagnose appendicitis, diverticulitis, aneurysm, organ contusion or lacerations, and bowel obstruction
- Abdominal, pelvic, and/or transvaginal ultrasound may be diagnostic for appendicitis, aneurysm, peritonitis, ectopic pregnancy, ovarian cysts, and fluid/blood secondary to trauma
- Plain KUB X-rays may reveal bowel gas pattern and nephrolithiasis
- Paracentesis is diagnostic for spontaneous bacterial peritonitis and may provide symptomatic relief
- Empiric trial of medications may be useful for diagnosis and treatment of GERD/dyspepsia (H2 blocker or proton pump inhibitor), zoster (acyclovir), anxiety (lorazepam), and abdominal wall strain (NSAIDs)
- Cervical cultures to diagnose pelvic inflammatory disease
- *Helicobacter pylori* testing and upper GI endoscopy may be indicated for suspected cases of peptic ulcer disease

Treatment

- Immediate attention to hemodynamic status and life-threatening disease
  - –Replace volume with normal saline and possibly a blood transfusion
  - –Evidence of hemorrhage (e.g., ruptured AAA, ruptured ectopic pregnancy) or early sepsis (e.g., perforated diverticulitis, perforated bowel) may be a life-threatening emergency that requires urgent surgical intervention
- Place NG tube for obstruction or persistent vomiting
- Administer broad-spectrum empiric antibiodics if a perforated viscus or intra-abdominal infection is suspected
- Direct treatment toward the specific condition

4. Abdominal Masses

Many disease processes, including malignancies, infections, and bowel obstruction, present with abdominal masses. The most serious and dramatic etiology is an abdominal aortic aneurysm, which is responsible for 15,000 deaths per year. More frequently, abdominal masses are due to constipation and other non-emergent etiologies.

Differential Diagnosis

- Constipation/inability to pass stool
  - Most commonly due to dehydration and/or low dietary fiber intake
  - Hirschsprung's disease (congenital aganglionic megacolon)
  - Medications: Narcotics, opiates, or anticholinergic medications
  - Ogilvie's syndrome (colonic pseudo-obstruction)
- Ascites
  - May be due to malignancy, nephrotic syndrome, liver disease, or congestive heart failure
- Large or small bowel obstruction
- Soft tissue mass
  - Tumor (e.g., ovarian, uterine, bowel, liver)
  - Uterine fibroids
  - Lipoma: Soft, fleshy, mobile, and contained in the subcutaneous tissue of the abdominal wall
  - Hernia: Bowel sounds may be audible over the mass; incarceration causes pain; strangulation leads to bowel death
  - Pyloric stenosis: Seen primarily in infants; palpable pyloric olive-shaped mass
  - Pregnancy
  - Massive lymphadenopathy (e.g., lymphoma)
  - Organomegaly (e.g., hepatomegaly, splenomegaly)
  - Infection: Intra-abdominal or tubo-ovarian abscess
  - Abdominal aortic aneurysm: Associated with pulsatile mass and hypotension
- Cyst
  - Mesenteric cysts: Fluid collections in the mesentery; typically benign
  - Hydatid cyst: Caused by larval form of *Echinococcus granulosus;* typically found in the liver in patients with history of travel to tropical areas
  - Dermoid cyst: May be massive due to delayed presentation
- Palpable gallbladder (Courvoisier's sign): Associated with common bile duct obstruction and a distended gallbladder

Workup and Diagnosis

- History and physical examination
  - Note associated symptoms (especially fever, changes in bowel habits, weight change, urinary symptoms, and rectal bleeding)
  - Abdominal and pelvic examinations to localize areas of tenderness
- Initial laboratory studies may include CBC, electrolytes, BUN/creatinine, liver function tests, urinalysis, and β-hCG
- Tumor markers (if malignancy is a concern), blood cultures (if infection is suspected), and toxicology screen may be indicated
- Plain KUB X-rays may reveal constipation, obstruction, or free intraperitoneal air
- Abdominal CT scan with IV and oral contrast will evaluate for abscess, bowel pathology, and hepatosplenomegaly
- Barium enema may reveal abnormal bowel in cases of malignancy
- Colonoscopy is useful for diagnosis of bowel pathology
- Laparoscopy allows direct visualization of the intra-abdominal cavity
- Paracentesis with fluid evaluation

Treatment

- Immediate attention to life-threatening causes (e.g., ruptured abdominal aortic aneurysm)
- Most cases of abdominal masses are treatable once the etiology is identified
- Many malignant and benign masses (e.g., fibroids, hernia) require surgical intervention
- Infectious causes require antibiotics and may require operative intervention (e.g., abscess drainage)
- Constipation is typically treated with laxatives, enemas, and increased dietary fiber and fluids; manual disimpaction is reserved for fecal impaction; discontinue offending medications (e.g., narcotics)
- Hirschsprung's disease may require operative treatment
- Ogilvie's syndrome responds to decompression by rectal tube or IV neostigmine
- Organomegaly typically resolves once the underlying process is treated (e.g., mononucleosis resulting in splenomegaly)

5. Abdominal Pain in Lower Quadrants

Lower abdominal pain is a common complaint that must be evaluated carefully and systematically to reach the appropriate diagnosis in timely manner. All diagnoses must be considered, with the most emergent etiologies rapidly ruled out, followed by a careful evaluation and treatment for the most common diagnoses, and followed, if necessary, by a search for less common etiologies.

Differential Diagnosis

Right lower quadrant
• Appendicitis
• Diverticulitis
• Salpingitis/Pelvic inflammatory disease
• Endometritis
• Endometriosis
• Ectopic pregnancy
• Hemorrhage or rupture of ovarian cyst
• Renal calculus
• Intussusception

Pelvic/hypogastric region
• Cystitis
• Salpingitis/Pelvic inflammatory disease
• Ectopic pregnancy
• Diverticulitis
• Strangulated hernia
• Endometriosis
• Appendicitis
• Ovarian cyst
• Ovarian torsion
• Testicular torsion
• Bladder distension
• Nephrolithiasis
• Prostatitis
• Malignancy
• Abdominal aortic aneurysm

Left lower quadrant
• Diverticulitis
• Intestinal obstruction
• Colitis
• Strangulated hernia
• Inflammatory bowel disease
• Gastroenteritis
• Pyelonephritis
• Nephrolithiasis
• Mesenteric lymphadenitis or thrombosis
• Aortic aneurysm
• Volvulus
• Salpingitis/Pelvic inflammatory disease

Workup and Diagnosis

• Complete history and examination
  –Note progression of symptoms (duration, rapidity of onset, intensity), associated complaints (e.g., anorexia, diarrhea, fever), urinary complaints, exposure to illness and medication, and past medical history including prior episodes
  –Note body positioning that tends to relieve pain; signs of dehydration or fever
  –Vitals and full pulmonary, cardiac, abdominal, back, pelvic, and rectal examinations
  –Abdominal examination should include bowel sounds, distension, tympany, tenderness, palpation for masses and organomegaly, rebound tenderness, and guarding
• Initial evaluation includes CBC with differential cell counts, electrolytes, BUN/creatinine, glucose, calcium, urinalysis, urine culture, and β-hCG level
• Abdominal/pelvic ultrasound and/or CT, obstructive series, and KUB may be indicated
• Consider endocervical gonorrhea/chlamydia cultures in sexually active females, laparoscopy, barium enema, intravenous pyelogram, stool cultures, and/or fecal fat

Treatment

• Hemodynamically unstable patients require immediate resuscitation
  –Replace volume with normal saline and possibly a blood transfusion
  –Evidence of hemorrhage (e.g., ruptured AAA, ruptured ectopic pregnancy) or early sepsis (e.g., perforated diverticulitis, perforated bowel) may be a life-threatening emergency that requires urgent surgical intervention
• Place nasogastric tube for obstruction or persistent vomiting
• Administer broad-spectrum empiric antibiotics if a perforated viscus or intra-abdominal infection is suspected
• Direct treatment toward the specific condition
• Consider gynecology or surgery referral

6. Abdominal Pain in Upper Quadrants

Upper abdominal pain is a common presenting symptom. A complete differential diagnosis should be developed based on the organs in the upper abdomen in addition to the associated history and physical examination. Gallbladder disease and gastritis are two of the most common causes of upper abdominal pain. Be sure to consider nonabdominal etiologies in the differential of abdominal pain (e.g., pulmonary embolus, pneumonia, myocardial ischemia)

Differential Diagnosis

Right upper quadrant pain
- Cholecystitis
- Fatty liver or NASH
- Congested liver (e.g., secondary to heart failure)
- Cholangitis
- Hepatitis
- Gastritis or pancreatitis (see below)
- Pneumonia
- Fitz-Hugh-Curtis syndrome (gonococcal perihepatitis secondary to pelvic inflammatory disease)

Epigastric pain
- Gastritis
- PUD
- Pancreatitis
- Gastroenteritis
- Intestinal obstruction
- Myocardial infarction
- Aortic aneurysm

Left upper quadrant pain
- Peptic ulcer disease
- Gastritis
- GERD
- Splenic infarct
- Pulmonary embolism
- Pancreatitis
- Acute splenomegaly (e.g., mononucleosis)
- Left lower lobe pneumonia

Nonfocal pain
- Herpes
- Sickle cell crisis
- Irritable bowel
- Mesenteric ischemia
- Peritonitis
- Pleurisy
- Uremia
- Lead poisoning
- Porphyria
- Toxin ingestion

Workup and Diagnosis

- History of associated symptoms; relation of pain to eating; anorexia; alcohol use; and location, quality, and intensity of pain
- Physical exam should focus on heart, lungs, abdomen, and back examinations
- Initial laboratory tests may include CBC with differential, electrolytes, urinalysis, BUN/creatinine, liver function tests, LDH, amylase/lipase, magnesium, and PT/PTT/INR
- Chest and abdominal X-rays
- Abdominal ultrasound and/or CT scan
- Hepatitis viral serology
- Percutaneous transhepatic cholangiography (PTCA) and/or ERCP
- Upper GI endoscopy (EGD) or upper GI series with barium swallow
- Cultures of blood, urine, and trachea/gastric aspirates
- Evaluation of possible cardiac and pulmonary etiologies may require ECG (pulmonary embolus may show S in I, Q in III, inverted T in III), cardiac isoenzymes, pleural tap, echocardiogram, and stress test

Treatment

- Rule out or treat serious causes of pain (e.g., bowel obstruction, cholangitis, MI, PE)
- Urgent surgical intervention may be indicated for aortic aneurysm, splenic infarct, perforated viscus, and intestinal obstruction or infarct
- Esophagitis, gastritis, PUD, and GERD are primarily treated with lifestyle changes (e.g., avoid causative foods or medications) and PPIs or H2 blockers
    –Rule out malignancies in older patients or those with suggestive histories
- Pancreatitis: Aggressive IV hydration for lost fluids and third spacing; antibiotics; nasogastric tube insertion if vomiting; bowel rest; and narcotics for pain
- Gastroenteritis: Rehydration, correct electrolytes
- Intestinal obstruction: Bowel rest, surgery
- Cardiac and pulmonary etiologies are treated per protocols (e.g., supplemental O_2, aspirin, β-blocker, nitrates for MI; O_2, heparin and/or thrombolytics for PE; O_2, appropriate antibiotics for pneumonia)

7. Abdominal Pain with Rebound Tenderness

In evaluating an acute abdomen, rebound tenderness is one of the most important signs of peritonitis. It is elicited by pressing deeply on the abdomen and then suddenly releasing pressure, which stretches the peritoneum and causes increased abdominal pain. Guarding and rebound often indicate immediate surgical evaluation, as delay can be life threatening. Children, elderly patients, and immunocompromised patients may have atypical presentations and are less likely to show peritoneal signs.

Differential Diagnosis

- Appendicitis is the most common etiology
- Cholecystitis
- Diverticulitis
- Gastroenteritis
- Pancreatitis
- Perforated duodenal ulcer
- Gastritis
- Biliary or renal colic
- Mesenteric ischemia
- Ruptured abdominal aortic aneurysm
- Bowel obstruction
- Bacterial peritonitis
- Intra-abdominal or pelvic abscess
- Colitis
- Urinary tract infection or pyelonephritis
- Perforated viscus
- Sickle cell crisis
- Gynecologic etiologies
  - Pelvic inflammatory disease
  - Tubo-ovarian abscess
  - Ruptured ectopic pregnancy
  - Ovarian cyst rupture or torsion
- Intussusception
- Nonabdominal causes of pain that mimic an acute abdomen are numerous and may include myocardial infarction, atypical angina, pericarditis, pneumonia, pulmonary embolus, and pelvic pathology (e.g., pelvic inflammatory disease, ovarian torsion)

Workup and Diagnosis

- Distinguish etiologies requiring emergent or urgent surgical intervention (e.g., ruptured aortic aneurysm, perforated viscus, appendicitis, intestinal obstruction, ischemic bowel, ruptured ectopic pregnancy) from non-emergent causes
- History and physical examination
  - Nature of pain, location, onset, duration, intensity, similarity to past episodes, aggravating and alleviating factors, guarding, bowel sounds, distension, presence of a mass, blood on rectal exam, and cervical or adnexal tenderness
  - In general, patients who present with extremely severe pain of immediate onset require surgical intervention
  - Crampy, colicky pain that occurs in waves implies distension of a hollow viscus (e.g., renal colic, intestinal obstruction)
  - Constant, localized pain implies inflammation (e.g., appendicitis, diverticulitis, cholecystitis)
  - Hypotension and shock may be present
- Initial tests include CBC, electrolytes, BUN/creatinine, LFTs, amylase/lipase, urinalysis, and pregnancy test
- Plain abdominal X-rays may reveal obstruction, perforation (free air), or other pathology
- Ultrasound is a quick, inexpensive test for biliary tract disease, AAA, ectopic pregnancy, or peritoneal fluid
- Abdominal CT will often establish the diagnosis for appendicitis, aortic aneurysm, and diverticulitis
- Diagnostic peritoneal lavage may be indicated in cases of suspected trauma, bowel perforation, or peritonitis

Treatment

- Hemodynamically unstable patients require immediate resuscitation
  - Replace volume with normal saline and/or blood transfusion
  - Evidence of hemorrhage (e.g., ruptured AAA, ruptured ectopic pregnancy) or early sepsis (e.g., perforated diverticulitis, perforated bowel) may represent a life-threatening emergency that requires urgent surgical intervention
- Place nasogastric tube for obstruction or persistent vomiting
- Administer broad-spectrum empiric antibiotics if a perforated viscus or intra-abdominal infection is suspected
- Direct treatment toward the underlying condition
  - Definitive surgical repair of ruptured aneurysm, bowel perforation, ectopic pregnancy, or other pathology
  - Bowel rest and possible colon resection for diverticulitis or bowel obstruction

8. Abnormal Uterine Bleeding

Uterine bleeding is abnormal when the pattern (amount and/or duration) is irregular. Menorrhagia indicates regular but excessive uterine bleeding; metrorrhagia indicates irregular and, often, more frequent uterine bleeding; and menometrorrhagia indicates irregular and excessive uterine bleeding during menstruation and between cycles.

Differential Diagnosis

- Endometrial hyperplasia
  - Endogenous estrogen excess (e.g., obesity, tumor)
  - Exogenous estrogen
  - DUB is a diagnosis of exclusion (usually not cyclic, occurs irregularly throughout the menstrual cycle)
- Polycystic ovarian syndrome
- Hypo- or hyperthyroidism
- Endometrial atrophy
  - Caused by long-term progestin or oral contraceptive use
- Anatomic or structural lesions
  - Uterine leiomyoma (fibroids)
  - Foreign body (often intrauterine device)
  - Cervical or uterine polyps
- Pelvic infection (cervicitis, pelvic inflammatory disease)
- Hypothalamic lesion
- Hyperprolactinemia
- Medications (e.g., exogenous estrogen, phenothiazines, reserpine)
- Coagulation disorders
  - Platelet dysfunction: Thrombocytopenia, leukemia, medications (e.g., aspirin, NSAIDs)
  - Clotting factor abnormality: Von Willebrand's disease, hemophilia, hepatic or renal disease, anticoagulant use
- Complications of pregnancy
  - Spontaneous abortion (miscarriage)
  - Ectopic pregnancy
  - Placenta previa
  - Placental abruption
- Endometrial cancer
  - Risk factors include older age, chronic anovulation, obesity, hypertension, DM, and unopposed estrogen
- Systemic disease (e.g., HIV, hepatic disease, renal disease)
- Nonuterine bleeding
  - Vaginal (tear, trauma, or cancer)
  - Cervical (trauma or cancer)
  - Urinary (UTI or cancer)
  - Rectal (bleeding, trauma, fissure, or cancer)
- Other malignancy (ovarian or uterine tumor, sarcoma)
- Endometrioma

Workup and Diagnosis

- History, physical, pelvic, and rectal examinations
- Pap smear
- Initial labs may include β-hCG (qualitative and, if positive, quantitative); CBC with differential; TSH, LH, FSH, estradiol, testosterone, prolactin, and DHEA-S levels
- Consider PT/PTT, peripheral smear, clotting factor assays, liver function tests, serum progesterone, and BUN/creatinine to evaluate for coagulopathy, hepatic, or renal disease
- Pelvic ultrasound may reveal adnexal or uterine masses or other pathology
- Transvaginal ultrasound is more accurate than pelvic ultrasound in evaluating the endometrium
- Endometrial biopsy and progesterone challenge test are helpful in the evaluation of estrogen excess
  - Administration of medroxyprogesterone for 10 days results in withdrawal bleeding if adequate estrogen is present
- CT scan may be helpful if malignancy is suspected
- Hysteroscopy for evaluation of endometrium and uterine cavity
- Diagnostic dilatation and curettage is more invasive but offers more information than endometrial biopsy

Treatment

- Acute life-threatening bleeding must be treated emergently with IV estrogen, IV fluids and/or blood replacement, curettage, and possible ligation of uterine artery or hysterectomy
- Nonacute bleeding is often treated with oral contraceptives to regulate bleeding; consider dosage change if already on oral contraceptives
  - Estrogen/progesterone (avoid if contraindicated)
  - Cyclic progesterone (will not prevent pregnancy)
  - Other medications include tranexamic acid, danazol, GnRH agonists, megestrol, intrauterine progesterone, and fibrinolytic agents
- Surgery may be indicated for anatomic causes and/or if fertility is not desired
  - Endometrial ablation
  - Hysterectomy
- Treat underlying etiologies (e.g. thyroid hormones for hypothyroidism, chemotherapy for leukemia, withdraw offending medications)

9. Acne

Acne, the most common of all skin disorders, is a disease of pilosebaceous follicles. It affects 17 million people in the U.S., including 85% of adolescents and young adults. A genetic predisposition exists, but the pathogenesis is multifactorial and includes sebum secretion and retention under androgen stimulus, overgrowth of *Propionibacterium acnes* bacteria, and obstruction of epithelial cells within follicles.

Differential Diagnosis

• Acne vulgaris
  – Common in adolescents, especially boys
  – Most common on face, chest, and upper back
  – Due to hormones, *P. acnes,* and comedogenic cosmetics
  – May be secondary to or exacerbated by medications (e.g., corticosteroids, phenytoin, lithium, isoniazid) and polycystic ovarian syndrome
• Rosacea
  – Middle-aged to older adults
  – Papules and pustules in middle third of face, telangiectasia, flushing, erythema
  – No comedones
  – Often associated with ingestion of hot beverages, alcohol, or vasodilating medications
• Miliaria ("heat rash")
  – Burning, pruritic vesicles, papules, or pustules on covered areas, usually trunk and intertriginous areas
• Gram-negative folliculitis
  – *Klebsiella, Enterobacter, E. coli*
  – May develop during antibiotic treatment of acne
• Acne conglobata
  – Most severe form of acne
  – Deep nodules, cysts, ulcers, abscesses, sinus tracks, scars
  – Causes severe scarring and keloid formation if untreated
• Acne fulminans
  – Severely destructive form of acne
  – Ulcerations, fever, arthralgia
• Pyoderma faciale
  – Affects only adult women
  – Severe cysts and sinus tracks
• Hidradenitis suppurativa
  – Pustules and cysts, often draining and very painful
  – Especially in axilla, groin
• *Malassezia* folliculitis
  – Fungal infection
  – Occurs on back
  – No response to acne therapy

Workup and Diagnosis

• History and physical examination
  – Examination should include the face, chest, and back
  – Comedones are the hallmark of acne: Open comedones (blackheads) are follicles with dilated, black orifice; closed comedones (whiteheads) are white papules without surrounding erythema
  – Look for evidence of severe acne: Inflammatory papules, pustules, cysts, nodules, scars, pits
  – Document the number of comedones, inflammatory lesions, scars, and cysts
  – Assess acne severity (mild/moderate/severe) based on number, size, and extent of lesions and the presence/absence of scarring
• Measurement of androgen levels (testosterone, DHEA-S, 17-hydroxyprogesterone) for females with resistant acne and evidence of androgen excess (e.g., irregular menses, hirsutism, clitoromegaly)
• *Malassezia* infection may require biopsy for diagnosis
• Bacterial culture may be necessary to rule out folliculitis

Treatment

• Patient education: Dispel common myths (e.g., acne is not caused by dirt or diet); counsel against behaviors that may worsen acne (e.g., picking at lesions, using oil-containing cosmetics/moisturizers); assess level of psychological distress
• Topical therapies include benzoyl peroxide, antibiotics, retinoids, and salicylic acid
• Intralesional steroids may be used to transiently decrease inflammation in severe acne
• Systemic therapies include oral antibiotics and hormonal therapy (low-dose oral contraceptives)
• Isotretinoin (Accutane[R]) may be used for severe cystic acne unresponsive to conventional therapy
  – Highly teratogenic; *absolutely contraindicated* in pregnancy
• Dermatologist referral for disease that is refractory despite appropriate therapy; consideration of isotretinoin treatment; management of acne scars

10. Alopecia

Loss of hair is termed effluvium, and the resulting condition is alopecia. Alopecia is characterized as scarring (cicatricial) or non-scarring; non-scarring alopecia is the more common form. It is differentiated from scarring alopecia by the absence of visible inflammation of the involved skin. Scarring alopecias are caused by several dermatological conditions that also affect glabrous (non-hairy) skin. Scarring hair loss is often very difficult to diagnose correctly and is a challenge to manage. Be sure to rule out neoplastic and autoimmune processes.

Differential Diagnosis

Non-scarring alopecia
• Androgenetic alopecia (male pattern baldness, hereditary thinning)
    –After puberty in males, later in females
    –Presents as gradually thinning hair at the hairline or on vertex
• Telogen effluvium (telogen=resting hair)
    –Diffuse scalp hair loss following pregnancy, crash diets, change in birth control pills, stress, medications (e.g., ACE inhibitors, β-blockers, CNS agents)
• Anagen effluvium (anagen=growing hair)
    –Diffuse hair loss, as in telogen effluvium, but more rapid and pronounced
    –Usually caused by antineoplastic agents
• Alopecia areata
    –Loss of hair in localized rounded patches
    –May be associated with autoimmune disease (e.g., vitiligo, endocrine)
• Metabolic causes of diffuse hair thinning (e.g., thyroid disease)

Scarring (cicatricial) alopecia
• Tinea capitis/kerion
• Discoid lupus erythematosus
• Acne keloidalis
    –Hypertrophic scars are characteristic
    –Often in black men at the nape of the neck after a chronic papulopustular eruption
• Pseudopelade of Brocq
    –Primary or end stage of inflammatory diseases (e.g., lichen planus, SLE)
    –Presents with smooth, shiny, hairless scalp patches with absent hair follicles
• Folliculitis decalvans
    –Occurs in the beard or scalp area
    –Due to merging of pustular hair follicles
• Pseudofolliculitis barbae
    –Inflammatory response to ingrown beard and/or neck hairs
    –Secondary infection with gram-positives (e.g., S. aureus) may cause scarring
• Dissecting cellulitis
    –Boggy subcutaneous chronic scalp inflammation and/or infection
    –More common in blacks
• Lichen planopilaris
• Various neoplasms and infections
• Scleroderma, morphea, amyloidosis, lymphoma, and sarcoidosis may manifest as a scarring hair loss, but most often with other skin findings

Workup and Diagnosis

• History and physical examination
    –Note history of the hair loss (duration, tenderness, pruritus), past medical history (e.g., lupus, sarcoidosis, internal malignancies), and medications
    –Evaluate for presence or absence of scarring (loss of hair follicles, ablation of the follicular orifice), hair loss elsewhere on the body (lichen planopilaris, some autoimmune diseases, and some lymphomas may manifest with scarring alopecia not limited to the scalp), and rashes or plaques on any part of the body (e.g., scleroderma and sarcoidosis often have skin findings beyond the scalp)
    –Subcutaneous masses, bogginess of the scalp, and cervical lymphadenopathy may suggest infection
• Trichogram (forcible hair pluck) to evaluate hair phase [normally, 80–90% of hairs are in anagen (growth, translucent hair shaft, and deeply pigmented matrix) phase; in androgenetic alopecia and telogen effluvium, telogen (resting, large bulb, transparent hair shaft) hairs are increased]
• Perform a 4 mm punch biopsy of a hairless area; if there is any redness or scale, include that area in the biopsy so that the primary pathologic process can be examined
• Labs may include free and total testosterone, DHEA-S, prolactin, thyroid function tests, iron studies, RPR, ANA, ESR
• Obtain viral and bacterial cultures of any pustules

Treatment

• Once an area of scarring alopecia has developed, no hair will ever regrow in that area; the goal of treatment is to make the diagnosis and treat to avoid further hair loss
• Wigs and/or hair transplants (punch grafts of follicles from androgen-insensitive areas to androgen-sensitive bald areas)
• Androgenetic alopecia: Oral finasteride is currently approved for men only; visible results take 3–4 months; topical minoxidil provides moderate growth within 4–12 months; in women, use antiandrogens (e.g., spironolactone, cimetidine, flutamide) if adrenal androgens are increased
• Telogen effluvium: Reassure that recovery is the norm
• Anagen effluvium: Withdraw drug or treat illness
• Alopecia areata: Superpotent steroids, intralesional steroid injections, cyclosporine, glucocorticoids, PUVA
• Tinea capitis/kerion: Oral antifungals
• Treat the inciting causes of scarring alopecia (e.g., folliculitis, lupus; prevent ingrown follicles)

11. Amenorrhea

Amenorrhea (absence of menses) can be transient, intermittent, or permanent. It may result from dysfunction of the hypothalamus, pituitary, ovaries, uterus, or vagina. Primary amenorrhea is the absence of menarche by age 16; secondary amenorrhea is the absence of menses in women previously menstruating for at least three cycles or 6 months. Differentiate amenorrhea from oligomenorrhea, in which menses are less frequent than normal.

Differential Diagnosis

Secondary amenorrhea
- More common than primary
- Hypothyroidism
- Pregnancy
- Polycystic ovarian syndrome
  - Peripubertal onset of menstrual irregularities with hyperandrogenism (hirsutism) and obesity
- Functional hypothalamic amenorrhea due to stress, eating disorders, weight loss, or excessive exercise
- Hyperprolactinemia
  - Galactorrhea
  - Secondary to medications (e.g., OCP, phenothiazines) or primary due to pituitary adenoma

Primary amenorrhea
- Constitutional delay of puberty
  - Family history of late puberty
  - Normal development at later age
- Outflow tract disorders
  - Transverse vaginal septum
  - Imperforate hymen
  - Pelvic or lower abdominal pain are common presenting symptoms
- Complete androgen insensitivity syndrome
  - X-linked recessive disorder (46,XY)
  - Resistance to testosterone due to a defect in the androgen receptor
  - Testes may be palpable in labia or inguinal area
- Müllerian agenesis (Mayer-Rokitansky-Hauser syndrome)
  - Agenesis of fallopian tubes, uterus, vagina
  - Normally functioning ovaries

Less common etiologies
- Turner's syndrome
  - 45,X gonadal dysgenesis
  - Ovaries replaced with fibrous tissue
- Ovarian failure (autoimmune oophoritis or secondary to chemotherapy or radiation injury)
- 5-α reductase deficiency
- 17-α hydroxylase deficiency
- Craniopharyngioma
- Hypopituitarism
- Congenital GnRH deficiency (Kallman's syndrome if associated with anosmia)
- Cushing's syndrome

Workup and Diagnosis

- Complete history, physical, and pelvic examination
- All patients require an initial pregnancy test—*any woman with amenorrhea is considered pregnant until proven otherwise*
- Anatomic abnormalities should be excluded before performing an endocrine evaluation
  - Pelvic ultrasound will evaluate for the presence or absence of müllerian structures
- Endocrine evaluation may include LH, FSH, estradiol, testosterone, prolactin, TSH, 17-hydroxyprogesterone, and DHEA-S levels
  - Elevated gonadotropins suggest ovarian failure
  - Elevated FSH indicates primary ovarian failure
  - Low FSH suggests functional hypothalamic amenorrhea or congenital GnRH deficiency
  - Elevated DHEA-S suggests adrenal insufficiency or tumor
- Diagnostic administration of medroxyprogesterone acetate ("progesterone challenge test") may be used; if estrogen levels are adequate, menstrual bleeding should occur within a week and diagnosis is chronic anovulation
- Head MRI (or CT) is indicated if primary hypogonadotropic hypogonadism, elevated prolactin, visual field defects, or headaches are present
- Karyotype analysis is diagnostic in some cases (e.g., Turner's syndrome)

Treatment

- Imperforate hymen requires surgical correction
- Androgen insensitivity syndrome: Excise testes after puberty because of increased risk of testicular cancer
- Absent müllerian structure or presence of Y chromosome: Psychological counseling
- Ovarian failure: Consider hormone replacement therapy
- Polycystic ovarian syndrome
  - Oral contraceptives decrease ovarian androgen secretion
  - Weight reduction decreases peripheral estrogen
  - Clomiphene to enhance fertility
  - Cyclic progesterone prevents endometrial hyperplasia
- Functional hypothalamic amenorrhea
  - Weight gain and reduction in intensity of exercise
  - Consider oral contraceptives to prevent osteoporosis
  - Exogenous gonadotropins or pulsatile GnRH may be necessary

12. Amnesia

Amnesia is an inability to remember prior events and process new information despite a normal level of consciousness. The memory center in the brain is housed in the temporal lobes; thus, the development of true amnesia requires pathology of both temporal lobes. The most common cause of transient amnesia is acute head trauma with concussion. Alzheimer's disease is the most common nontransient cause of amnesia. Anterograde amnesia is defined as an inability to remember events that follow the onset of the amnesia, whereas retrograde amnesia is an inability to remember events that occurred before the onset of the amnesia.

Differential Diagnosis

- Head trauma (e.g., concussion, hemorrhage)
  –Usually results in transient retrograde and anterograde amnesia
- Alzheimer's disease
  –Most common cause of chronic amnesia
- Infection
  –Herpes simplex encephalitis is a particularly common cause of infectious amnesia, because it has a predilection for the temporal lobes
- Seizure disorders
  –Retrograde amnesia is most common after a generalized tonic-clonic seizure during the postictal period
  –Some complex partial seizure foci (particularly temporal lobe epilepsy) can also produce "blank" periods of memory
- Toxicologic insults
  –Binge alcohol consumption
  –Benzodiazepine use (e.g., "date rape" drug flunitrazepam, also known as Rohypnol)
- Psychogenic causes are relatively common, but should be a diagnosis of exclusion
- Korsakoff's syndrome
- Transient global amnesia
  –A rare, transient, ischemic attack-like condition of proposed vascular etiology
  –Causes abrupt onset of short-term memory loss for minutes to hours
  –Typically occurs in patients older than 50
  –Seen in patients with migraines

Workup and Diagnosis

- History and physical examination
  –Special attention to neurologic and head examination
  –Life-threatening head trauma and CNS infection should be considered initially in patients with altered mental status and amnesia
- Initial labs may include CBC, electrolytes, glucose, calcium, magnesium, phosphorus, coagulation studies, and serum and urine toxicology screens
- Lumbar puncture with CSF analysis should be considered early if CNS infection is suspected
  –Test for opening pressure, appearance (e.g., clear, cloudy, bloody), protein, glucose, CSF-to-serum glucose ratio, Gram stain, culture
  –Cryptococcal antigen and acid-fast bacilli smear and culture in patients in endemic areas or with HIV
  –If there is a delay in initiating lumbar puncture due to a need for imaging (e.g., head CT to rule out increased intracranial pressure), empiric antibiotics should be administered immediately
- Head CT without contrast may be needed to exclude bleeding in cases of head trauma, and may also identify structural lesions
- MRI of the head with diffusion-weighted imaging is more sensitive for diagnosing stroke, tumor, and the subtle white matter changes associated with vascular disease
- EEG to rule out seizure disorder

Treatment

- Immediate attention to airway, breathing, and circulation
- Prompt treatment of suspected infections and trauma
  –CNS infections: Antibiotic and/or antiviral therapy
  –Head trauma: Surgical intervention may be necessary to evacuate space-occupying traumatic lesions; concussions are treated symptomatically, and patients should refrain from contact sports until symptoms resolve; control elevated intracranial pressure with head elevation, moderate hyperventilation, mannitol administration, and/or surgical drainage
- Alzheimer's disease: Anticholinesterase medications (e.g., tacrine, donepezil) may improve cognitive function
- Seizure disorders: Anticonvulsant agents (e.g., phenytoin, carbamazepine, valproate)

13. Anemia

Anemia is defined as a hemoglobin <13.5 g/dL in men or <12.0 g/dL in women. Etiologies are categorized by decreased RBC production, increased RBC destruction, and/or blood loss. Evaluation of anemia begins with an assessment of the MCV to distinguish microcytic (MCV <80), normocytic (MCV 80–100), and macrocytic (MCV >100) anemias. MCHC is used to distinguish hypochromic (<33), normochromic (33–35), and hyperchromic (>35) anemia.

Differential Diagnosis

Microcytic
• Iron deficiency
  –Most common cause of anemia
  –Due to chronic blood loss (e.g., menstrual, GI bleeding, frequent blood donation)
• Sideroblastic anemia
• Lead poisoning
• Thalassemia
• Anemia of chronic disease (often late)

Macrocytic
• Vitamin B_{12} or folate deficiency
  –Malabsorption
  –Poor dietary intake
  –Pernicious anemia
  –Alcohol abuse
• Liver disease
• Alcohol and medications (e.g., chemotherapeutics, HIV medications)
• Hypothyroidism
• HIV
• Myelodysplastic syndrome
• Acute leukemia
• Reticulocytosis (e.g., hemolytic anemia, production of RBCs in response to blood loss and/or vitamin B_{12} or iron repletion)

Normocytic
• Hemorrhage, blood loss
• Anemia of chronic disease
  –Renal disease (due to decreased erythropoietin production)
  –Hypometabolic states (e.g., protein malnutrition, hypothyroidism)
• Infection
• Hemolysis (drug-induced, autoimmune, SLE, G-6PD deficiency)
• Bone marrow disease
  –Aplastic anemia
  –Bone marrow invasion (e.g., malignancy)
• Hypothyroidism
• Renal insufficiency
• Sickle cell disease
• Microangiopathy
• Membrane defects (e.g., hereditary spherocytosis)
• Disseminated intravascular coagulation
• Thrombotic thrombocytopenic purpura

Workup and Diagnosis

• Detailed history and physical examination
  –History of bleeding, past history of anemia, family history
  –Vital signs, including orthostatic blood pressure/pulse
  –Include rectal and stool guaiac
• Initial laboratory studies include CBC with red cell indices (MCV, MCHC, RDW), peripheral smear (may show characteristic cell types such as spherocytes, schistocytes, multinucleated cells), and reticulocyte count (increased if anemia is due to blood loss or RBC destruction; decreased if due to marrow failure)
• Further studies may include iron panel (iron, ferritin, transferrin saturation, TIBC), haptoglobin, vitamin B_{12} and folate levels, bilirubin, LDH, LFTs, TSH, renal function, hemoglobin electrophoresis, bone marrow aspirate, GI workup
• Etiology may be classified based on laboratory results
  –Iron deficiency: Decreased ferritin, reticulocytes, MCV, and MCH; increased TIBC
  –Chronic disease: Decreased reticulocytes and TIBC; normal MCV and MCH
  –B_{12} and/or folate deficiency: Decreased reticulocytes; increased MCV
  –Marrow failure: Decreased reticulocytes; may involve other cell lines
  –Hemolysis: Increased reticulocytes, bilirubin, and LDH; decreased haptoglobin in cases of intravascular hemolysis

Treatment

• Severe cases of anemia require immediate intervention if hemodynamic compromise occurs
• Administer supplemental O_2 as needed
• In cases of ongoing acute blood loss, establish two large-bore IVs; monitor and send for blood type and cross
• IV fluids as necessary to maintain blood pressure
• Blood transfusion is generally indicated for Hb <8
  –Young, healthy patients should only be transfused if symptomatic or have ongoing acute blood losses
  –Cardiac patients may require transfusion at Hb <10
  –Avoid transfusing beyond Hb >12, as this may increase blood viscosity and impair O_2 delivery
• Supplement vitamin B_{12}, folate, and iron as necessary
• Patients with primary marrow disorders require transfusions, further evaluation, and possibly a bone marrow transplant
• Treat underlying disease according to established protocols

14. Ankle Pain/Swelling

Ankle pain is a common problem that generally occurs secondary to acute or chronic injury or degenerative joint disease. Ankle sprains, most commonly due to traumatic inversion injury, are the most common cause of ankle pain. In cases of trauma, the Ottawa rules are used to decide whether X-rays are indicated and have been shown to improve the cost effectiveness of radiologic evaluation without compromising quality of care. Bilateral ankle swelling suggests cardiac or vascular etiologies (e.g., CHF) rather than intrinsic foot/ankle disease.

Differential Diagnosis

- Inversion sprain (85% of ankle sprains)
  - Results in pain, swelling, and ecchymosis of the lateral malleolar area
  - Damage occurs to the three ligaments of inferior fibula (anterior and posterior talofibular and calcaneofibular ligaments) and peroneal muscle
- Degenerative joint disease
  - Pain is present upon waking in the morning; relieved by mild activity
  - Grinding/popping occurs with motion
- Inversion/eversion injury of subtalar joint
  - Results in pain while walking on uneven ground
- Syndesmosis injury ("high ankle sprain")
  - Stretching of the interosseous membrane
  - Results in pain at the lower leg
- Avulsion fracture of the distal fibula
  - Results in persisting lateral malleolar pain
  - Difficult to differentiate from the epiphyseal line on X-ray
- Repetitive injury with disruption of the ankle retinaculum
  - Results in chronic pain of the posterior aspect of the ankle
- Poor shoe alignment
- Bimalleolar fracture
- Trimalleolar fracture: Bimalleolar fracture plus a fracture of the lateral aspect of the distal tibia
- Neoplasm
- Peroneal nerve entrapment
- Diabetic (Charcot's) arthropathy

Workup and Diagnosis

- History and physical examination
  - Ankle, foot, and lower leg examination
  - Always evaluate neurovascular status, including pulses, color, and capillary refill
  - Observation of bones and soft tissues, color, swelling
  - Anterior/posterior drawer test: Ankle is held in one hand and the lower tibia is pushed and pulled to evaluate for instability
  - Range of motion should be evaluate both actively and passively (grinding or popping suggests DJD)
- Ottawa ankle rules are used to determine whether an X-ray of the ankle is necessary following trauma
  - Tenderness of the distal 6 cm of the fibula or tibia
  - Tender navicular area
  - Tender proximal fifth metatarsal
  - Cannot bear weight (at least four steps)
- Standard three-view ankle X-rays, stress views (inversion or eversion), and consider foot series or lower leg series
- Lateral X-rays in plantar- or dorsiflexion may help evaluate for anterior or posterior impingement
- CT or MRI may be indicated to clarify findings on plain films and to evaluate cartilage, nerves, tendons, ligaments
- Muscle strength and range of motion testing

Treatment

- PRICE
  - Protection from additional strain/injury
  - Relative rest (stretching is okay) ± crutches
  - Ice for initial 24–48 hours after trauma
  - Compression (elastic wrap or ankle support)
  - Elevation of foot (higher than the pelvis)
- Casting is often indicated for fractures and significant ankle sprains
- Short-term bracing may reduce risk of reinjury
- Surgery may be indicated (e.g., bimalleolar fracture, trimalleolar fracture)
- Physical therapy referral to improve strength, range of motion, and proprioception
- NSAIDs or other analgesic

15. Anosmia

More than 2 million people in the U.S. (1–2% of the population) suffer from anosmia, an absent sense of smell. Temporary anosmia may result from any condition that irritates the nasal mucosa to cause swelling and obstruction of the nasal passages and sinuses. Permanent anosmia is commonly associated with damage and destruction of the olfactory neuroepithelium or a part of the olfactory nerve.

Differential Diagnosis

- Nasal and sinus disease
  - Most common cause of anosmia
  - Allergic or vasomotor rhinitis and sinusitis result in temporary anosmia: Associated with chronic nasal congestion, rhinorrhea, postnasal drip, pale/boggy nasal mucosa, sinus swelling/tenderness, and headaches
  - Intranasal polyposis may occur, resulting in obstruction of nasal passages with temporary anosmia
- Head/facial trauma
  - Second most common cause of anosmia
  - Permanent anosmia may result
  - CNS rhinorrhea may occur
- Post-upper respiratory viral infection
  - Accounts for 20–30% of cases of anosmia
- Iatrogenic
  - Amphetamines, certain antibiotics, nasal steroids, antithyroid agents, radiation
- Poisoning
  - Chemical pollutants, heavy metals (lead), organic/inorganic compounds
- Illicit drugs (e.g., intranasal cocaine)
- CNS disorders (e.g., Alzheimer's disease, Parkinson's disease, anxiety disorders)
- Neoplasms (e.g., nasal cavity, brain)
- Endocrine disorders (e.g., diabetes mellitus, hypothyroidism, adrenal insufficiency)
- Congenital disorders (e.g., Kallman's and Turner's syndromes)
- Sjögren's syndrome
- Vitamin deficiencies (e.g., vitamin B_{12}, zinc)

Workup and Diagnosis

- History and physical should include a complete head and neck exam and full neurologic exam
- Several types of smell tests are available
  - Olfactory threshold and odor identification test
  - University of Pennsylvania scratch and sniff test
  - Alcohol sniff test
- Initial labs may include CBC, electrolytes, glucose, BUN/creatinine, calcium, ESR, thyroid profile, liver function tests, and vitamin B_{12} level
- Blood and/or urine toxicology screen if drug use or poisoning is suspected
- Nasal discharge testing β-transferrin in CSF rhinorrhea of post-traumatic patients
- Allergy testing
- Head CT scan may be indicated to evaluate the skull base, brain, nasal cavity, and sinuses
- MRI may be indicated to evaluate the brain and soft facial tissues
- Antibodies to Ro/SSA and LA/SSB are positive in Sjögren's syndrome

Treatment

- Temporary anosmia due to nasal and/or sinus disease is usually successfully treated medically
  - Systemic and/or intranasal corticosteroids
  - Antibiotics if coexisting bacterial infection
  - Antihistamines and avoidance measures if allergic component
  - Decongestants and/or saline lavage for nasal congestion
  - Polypectomy and sinus surgery if initial therapy is ineffective
- No cure is available for permanent anosmia (e.g., due to postviral infections, trauma, congenital disorders); however, regeneration of neural elements may occur over a period of days to years
- Anosmia due to CNS and endocrine diseases require treatment of the underlying illness
- Vitamin supplementation in cases of vitamin deficiency

16. Anxiety

Anxiety includes symptoms of physiologic arousal (e.g., autonomic hyperactivity, increased motor tension) and psychological arousal (e.g., excessive worry, increased vigilance). It may present as a primary psychiatric condition or secondary to a broad variety of medical and psychiatric diseases.

Differential Diagnosis

- Generalized anxiety disorder
    - Excessive worry associated with at least three symptoms, including restlessness or edgy feeling, fatigue, difficulty concentrating, irritability, muscle tension, sleep disturbance
    - The most common anxiety disorder in primary care
- Panic disorder
    - Recurrent, unpredictable panic attacks with intense apprehension, fear or terror, and somatic symptoms (e.g., tachycardia)
    - May present with or without agoraphobia
- Depression: Anxiety often presents in a mixed state with depression
- Medications (e.g., bronchodilators, steroids, antidepressants, antihypertensives)
- Substance use, including drugs (e.g., alcohol, caffeine, cocaine, cannabis)
- Obsessive-compulsive disorder
    - Obsessions are persistent ideas, images, or impulses that generate anxiety
    - Compulsions are intentional repetitive behaviors or mental acts aimed at reducing the distress of obsessions
- Anxiety disorder due to a general medical condition
    - Cardiovascular etiologies include MI, angina, arrhythmias, CAD, CHF, MVP
    - Respiratory etiologies include asthma, COPD, and pulmonary embolism
    - Endocrine etiologies include hyper- or hypothyroidism, hypoglycemia, and Cushing's syndrome
    - Neurological etiologies include Parkinson's disease and epilepsy
    - Cancer
- Pheochromocytoma: Adrenal tumor that usually presents with hypertension and increased heart rate and sometimes with fright reaction of sweating, headache, and pale facial appearance
- Parkinson's disease: Presents with tremor at rest, usually in one hand (as opposed to the more generalized essential tremor in anxiety)
- Post-traumatic or acute stress disorder
- Social anxiety disorder
- Specific phobia
- Bipolar disorder (especially manic stage)

Workup and Diagnosis

- Detailed history of onset, duration, and type of anxiety symptoms as well as specific events, stressors, or medical illnesses that produce anxiety
    - Complete drug and medication history, including caffeine, alcohol, over-the-counter preparations, herbals, illicit drugs, and prescription drugs
    - Physical exam should be directed toward ruling out organic medical diseases that may present with anxiety, including cardiovascular, pulmonary, endocrine, and neurologic disorders
    - A complete psychiatric examination is indicated for all patients (e.g., appearance, sleep evaluation, mini-mental status exam, affect)
- DSM-IV criteria are used to determine the specific psychiatric disorders
- No diagnostic tests are indicated except those that may determine underlying medical disorders (e.g., thyroid function tests, ECG, urine catecholamines)

Treatment

- Patient education regarding available treatment and reassurance often has a calming effect
- Treatment usually combines pharmacologic and nonpharmacologic approaches, including cognitive-behavioral therapy, relaxation training, and biofeedback
- General anxiety disorder: Cognitive therapy has been proven to be beneficial; benzodiazepines, buspirone, and antidepressants (tricyclic antidepressants, SSRIs) are all effective; however, concern over dependence sometimes limits the use of benzodiazepines
- Panic disorder: SSRIs, tricyclic antidepressants, benzodiazepines, and cognitive-behavioral therapy are equivalently effective
- Obsessive-compulsive disorder: High-dose SSRIs and cognitive-behavioral therapy are effective

17. Aphasia

Aphasia refers to the inability to understand or express written or spoken words, despite preservation of the mechanical or visual means to do so; thus, facial weakness, oropharyngeal paresis, or primary disturbances of vision and hearing do not constitute aphasia. To localize the lesion within the cerebrum, aphasias are generally separated into receptive (Wernicke's aphasia) or expressive (Broca's aphasia) types. Further subgroups include anomic, conduction, and transcortical sensory, and transcortical motor.

Differential Diagnosis

- Stroke is the most common cause of aphasia
  - Sudden onset suggests cerebral embolization from a cardiac (e.g., endocarditis, atrial fibrillation) or carotid artery source
  - A stuttering onset suggests in situ arterial thrombosis
- Less common etiologies include Alzheimer's dementia, postconcussion syndrome, Rasmussen's encephalitis, nonconvulsive status epilepticus, dissociative state, subdural hematoma, trauma, severe hypoglycemia, sedative-hypnotic drug intoxication, sensorineural hearing loss, herpes encephalitis, and tertiary syphilis

Types of aphasias
- Receptive (Wernicke's) aphasia
  - Inability to name objects, follow written or spoken commands, and repeat
  - Verbal (semantic, neologistic) errors are abundant; however, speech is fluent
  - Localized to the dominant posterior superior temporal lobe
- Expressive (Broca's) aphasia
  - Stuttering, nonfluent speech with literal (phonemic) errors; however, comprehension is preserved
  - Repetition is poor, but naming is preserved
  - Associated with hemiparesis
  - Localized to the inferior lateral dominant frontal lobe
- Anomic aphasia
  - Isolated inability to name a seen object
  - Localized to the angular gyrus
- Conduction aphasia
  - Isolated inability to repeat
  - Localized to the arcuate fasiculus (white matter band connecting Wernicke to Broca areas)
- Transcortical sensory aphasia
  - Similar to Wernicke's aphasia, except for preserved repetition
  - Localized to the superior posterior temporal lobe
- Transcortical motor aphasia
  - Similar to Broca's aphasia, but with preserved repetition, including urinary incontinence, echolalia (aimlessly repeating other's spoken words)
  - Localized to medial dominant frontal lobe

Workup and Diagnosis

- History and physical examination
  - History should include a complete past medical history, family history, psychiatric history, and medication history
  - Exam should include a comprehensive neurologic exam, cardiovascular exam, and head and neck exam
  - Fever and headache with aphasia suggests embolization from endocarditis or herpes simplex encephalitis
  - Gradual onset with other signs of intellectual decline suggests dementia
- The cornerstone of diagnosis is cerebral imaging (MRI has the highest sensitivity and specificity)
- Initial laboratory tests should include CBC, electrolytes, BUN/creatinine, calcium, glucose, RPR, and vitamin B_{12} level
- Consider toxicology screen
- Echocardiography (transesophageal echocardiogram is best) and blood cultures may be indicated to diagnose endocarditis
- CSF analysis and EEG to diagnose viral encephalitis versus status epilepticus
- Psychometric testing necessary for dementia
- Normal brain imaging with or without associated psychiatric signs may suggest status epilepticus, hypoglycemia, or a dissociative state

Treatment

- Embolic stroke: Anticoagulation; however, if secondary to endocarditis, do not initiate anticoagulation, because of increased risk of hemorrhage; instead, treat with antibiotics
- Thrombotic stroke: Antiplatelet therapy (e.g., aspirin or clopidogrel) and risk factor reduction (e.g., lipid and hypertension therapy)
- Viral encephalitis: IV acyclovir for 10–14 days
- Dementia: Acetylcholinesterase inhibitors are of variable effectiveness in Alzheimer's disease
- Status epilepticus: IV lorazepam and anticonvulsants
- Hypoglycemia and other electrolyte abnormalities: Correction of underlying metabolic problem
- Dissociative state: Oral or IV benzodiazepines may "break the spell" of psychiatric separation of attention from the environment; ECT may be necessary
- Speech therapy is useful to help maintain motivation to improve language function and avoid depression from communication impairment

18. Ataxia

Disorders of gait may arise from problems virtually anywhere in the nervous or musculoskeletal systems. Observation of gait is an important element of the neurologic examination. Gait abnormalities are described as slapping, stepping, or mixed. A slapping gait presents with a tendency to slap the feet firmly against the ground to improve proprioceptive input, whereas a steppage gait, as seen in patients with foot drop, involves carefully lifting the foot to prevent it from catching and tripping the patient.

Differential Diagnosis

- Orthopedic issues affecting the foot, ankle, leg, knee, or hip
- Peripheral neuropathy (sensory and/or motor)
  - Slapping gait: Sensory neuropathies may result in a tendency to slap the feet firmly against the ground to improve proprioceptive input
  - Steppage gait: Seen in patients with foot drop
  - The classic tabetic gait combines both stepping and slapping gaits
- Mononeuropathy/radiculopathy affecting the lower extremities may result in gait abnormalities (e.g., either a peroneal neuropathy or L5 radiculopathy can cause a unilateral steppage gait)
- Myelopathy
  - Patients with bilateral lower extremity weakness and hypertonicity secondary to a spinal cord lesion may exhibit a spastic gait with stiffness of both legs and a tendency toward scissoring of the legs with walking
- Brainstem or cortical lesions (e.g., multiple sclerosis, CVA)
  - Most commonly result in a hemiparetic gait with circumduction of the weak leg
- Cerebellar lesions
  - Result in an ataxic gait, which tends to be wide-based, irregular, and staggering
- Intoxications
- Parkinsonism
  - Patients exhibit stooped posture, decreased arm swing, and shuffling (take many small steps)
- Myopathies
  - Tend to produce a waddling gait because of weakness of the trunk, hip, and proximal lower extremity muscles
- Spinocerebellar ataxia
- Hereditary spastic paraparesis
- Hysterical gaits
- Inherited neuropathies (e.g., Charcot-Marie-Tooth disease)
- GALOP syndrome (gait disorder, autoantibodies, late age onset, polyneuropathy)
- Normal pressure hydrocephalus
- Infection (e.g., neurosyphillis, meningitis)
- Vitamin B_{12} or thiamine deficiency

Workup and Diagnosis

- History and physical examination
  - Note history of injury, intoxication, and the events leading to onset of gait problems
  - Careful attention should be given not only to the type of gait disturbance, but also to associated findings on neurologic exam (e.g., symmetric distal sensory loss and hyporeflexia suggest a peripheral neuropathy; circumducting gait with hemiparesis, hemisensory loss, and ipsilateral hyperreflexia suggest a cerebral lesion)
- Orthopedic imaging and consult may be indicated, especially if localized lower extremity pain is prominent
- Neuroimaging (CT/MRI) may be indicated
- EMG/nerve conduction studies may help diagnose neuropathy or myopathy
- Labs may include CBC, chemistries, RPR, vitamin B_{12} and folate levels, ESR, and other lab evaluation for neuropathy, if appropriate
- Drug screen or alcohol levels if intoxication suggested
- Anticonvulsant levels (especially phenytoin)
- Genetic testing: DNA testing is available for inherited neuropathies (e.g., CMT 1A, many of the SCAs)
- If the etiology of a gait abnormality is uncertain, a full gait analysis by a specially trained physical therapist, podiatrist, orthopedic surgeon, or neurologist is often indicated

Treatment

- Specific symptomatic measures to improve gait stability and efficiency may improve functional abilities
  - Assistive devices (e.g., canes, walkers, wheelchairs)
  - Orthotics (e.g., ankle-foot orthoses for foot drop)
  - Physical therapy
- Removing intoxicating substances if present
- Orthopedic pathologies may be resolved by rest, casting or orthotics, NSAIDs, or surgical therapy
- Peripheral neuropathy/mononeuropathy: Treat the underlying cause to improve gait or prevent worsening
- Radiculopathy: Physical therapy, medications (e.g., NSAIDs, muscle relaxants), local injection therapies (e.g., epidural injections), and/or surgical intervention
- Myelopathy: Treating the underlying cause may improve or prevent worsening of gait; spasticity may be treated with antispasticity agents (e.g., baclofen)
- Structural lesions of the brainstem, cerebellum, or cerebrum should be identified and treated if possible (e.g., multiple sclerosis)

19. Aura

A subjective sensory phenomenon that may involve any of the five senses, such as visual auras (often described as flashing lights), sensory auras (paresthesias), or auditory auras. Other auras may be described as dreamlike or déjà vu sensations, or odd odors. The type of symptom may be related to the brain area involved (e.g., visual aura suggests occipital lobe pathology).

Differential Diagnosis

- Epilepsy
  - Recurrent seizures
  - Strong family history
- Migraine with aura
  - Usually visual aura (e.g., scotoma, flashing lights) lasting less than 60 minutes
  - Usually fully reversible with rare migrainous infarction (like CVA)
  - Migraine headache follows aura within 60 minutes and lasts 4–72 hours; however, aura may occur without headache
- Partial seizure
  - 60% of patients with focal seizures have an accompanying aura
  - Aura symptoms are associated with the brain area where they originate (e.g., occipital lobe seizure results in seeing lights)
  - Simple partial seizures result in focal tonic-clonic motor activity without loss of consciousness
  - Complex partial seizures progress to decreased consciousness and unresponsiveness
- Tonic-clonic (grand mal seizure) seizures result in an abrupt loss of consciousness followed by stiffness (tonic); the patient then starts jerking (clonic) for an additional 2–3 minutes; rare aura
- Pituitary adenoma or other underlying pathology that predisposes to migraines, seizures, or altered sensations (taste, smell)
- Hallucinations (not actually an aura)
- Physiologic nonepileptic seizures
  - Usually due to an underlying physiologic cause (e.g., fever, hypoglycemia, hypo- or hyperthyroidism, renal failure, cerebral anoxia)
- Absence seizures (petit mal seizure) only rarely have an aura

Workup and Diagnosis

- History is very important
  - Type of aura (any of five senses)
  - Loss of consciousness
  - Associated activities and triggers (e.g., stress, medications, exertion, trauma, foods)
  - Postaura symptoms (e.g., headache, loss of consciousness, seizure)
  - History or family history of seizures or migraines
  - Review past medical history for head injury, stroke, dementia, intracranial infection, and alcohol or drug abuse
  - Full head, neck, and neurologic exam (look for one-sided features that suggest pathology on opposite side of brain)
  - Examine for trauma following loss of consciousness
- Initial tests may include glucose, electrolytes, calcium, magnesium, CBC, BUN/creatinine, and toxicology screen
- EEG may be indicated if seizure activity is suspected (provocative EEG with triggers gives higher yield)
  - Normal EEG does not rule out epilepsy
  - May be abnormal in migraines
- MRI to rule out cerebral pathology
- CT if physiologic seizure or trauma is involved (not indicated in patients with migraine and normal neurologic exam unless pattern of migraine has changed)

Treatment

- Migraine
  - Avoid triggers (e.g., alcohol, stress, fatigue)
  - NSAIDs and/or acetaminophen
  - 5-HT$_1$ agonists (e.g., sumatriptan) are useful during the headache phase and ergotamines (e.g., dihydroergotamine) are effective for status migraines; however, neither are effective to relieve aura
- Epilepsy
  - Status epilepticus: Stabilize patient and administer IV benzodiazepines and fosphenytoin
  - Antiepileptics if risk for recurrent seizures: Phenytoin, carbamazepine, or valproate for generalized or partial seizures; ethosuximide or valproate for absence seizures; lamotrigine or valproate for mixed seizures

20. Babinski's Sign

Babinski's sign is elicited by gently stroking the lateral sole of the foot with a slightly blunted object (e.g., cue tip) and drawing the stimulus slightly medially across the metatarsal area. A positive response has two components: Dorsiflexion of the great toe and slight abduction (fanning) of the remaining toes. A positive sign represents disinhibition of the normal spinal reflex due to damage to descending inhibitory pathways from the brain or spinal cord. It is normal in neonates due to immaturity in myelination of these pathways.

Differential Diagnosis

- Stroke is the most common cause
  - Ischemic infarction: Usually occurs in the cerebral gray matter, but may also occur in the subcortical white matter or brainstem corticospinal tracts
  - Cerebral hemorrhage: Secondary to cerebral infarction, primary hypertensive bleeding (usually in the putamen, internal capsule, or brainstem), or coagulopathy (e.g., excessive anticoagulation, trauma, surgery, tumor)
- False positive (e.g., toe withdrawal, prior podiatric surgery resulting in the appearance of chronic upgoing toe)
- Spinal cord infarction
  - Occurs in the thoracic region due to poor collateral circulation, cardiogenic embolism, or ischemia from surgical clamping during aneurysm surgery
- Spinal cord hemorrhage
  - Due to trauma, tumor, AVM, anticoagulant use
- Postictal state
- Brain abscess
- Viral encephalitis
- Embolism from bacterial endocarditis
- Meningitis or cerebritis
- Cerebral palsy
- Multiple sclerosis
- Cerebral aneurysm
- Venous sinus thrombosis
- Arteriovenous malformation
- Cavernous malformation
- Severe metabolic disturbance (e.g., hepatic, renal, or hypoxemic processes)
- Sedative-hypnotic drug intoxication
- Post cardiac-arrest state
- Degenerative brain and spinal cord disease (e.g., Alzheimer's disease, Parkinson's disease, Friedreich's ataxia)
- Neuronal storage diseases (e.g., ceroid lipofuscinosis, gangliosidoses, sialidoses)

Workup and Diagnosis

- A variety of conditions that affect the spinal cord and brain result in a positive Babinski's sign; differential diagnosis depends on localization
- Brain and spinal cord imaging are the most sensitive and specific indicators of the pathology resulting in Babinski's sign
- In patients with increased reflexes in the arms with an exaggerated finger flexor response, the likely lesion localization is in the cervical cord or brain
- In cases of unilateral positive Babinski's sign, the lesion may be in any portion of the brain or cord
- Bilateral Babinski's signs suggest a spinal cord lesion in awake patients or a brain lesion in patients with persisting delirium
- Patients with suspected stroke may undergo carotid doppler, MRA of cerebral and carotid arteries, echocardiography, and lipid and coagulability profile
- Potential tumors may require PET scanning for diagnosis
- EEG if suspect seizure activity
- Lumbar puncture and blood and CSF cultures for suspected encephalitis or cerebritis

Treatment

- Cerebral infarction: Antiplatelet or warfarin therapy, risk factor reduction (treat hypertension, hyperlipidemia, and diabetes), carotid surgery if significant stenosis, treatment of atrial fibrillation
- Cerebral hemorrhage: Surgery to relieve subdural or epidural hematoma; observation to counteract increased ICP with hyperventilation and osmotic diuresis
- Spinal cord infarction: Conservative treatment, physical therapy
- Spinal cord hemorrhage: Surgical decompression if not emanating from inside the cord
- Brain abscess: Antibiotics and drainage
- Meningitis, cerebritis, and encephalitis: Antibiotics and/or antivirals
- AVM, cavernous malformations: Radiosurgery, intra-arterial embolization
- Cerebral aneurysm: Surgical clipping, embolization
- Postictal state: Observation and anticonvulsant drugs

21. Bleeding (Excessive)

Everyone bleeds; however, most episodes of minor bleeding promptly cease with activation of the normal clotting cascade. Bleeding is considered abnormal when it occurs spontaneously without injury or if it does not stop promptly with direct pressure. Causes of abnormal bleeding are divided into vascular disorders (structural abnormalities of the blood vessels), platelet disorders (decreased number of platelets or dysfunctional platelets), and coagulation factor disorders.

Differential Diagnosis

- Drugs (e.g., aspirin, heparin, warfarin, alcohol, chemotherapy)
- Senile purpura
- Uremia
- Liver disease
- HIV
  - Platelets decrease in number due to infection of megakaryocytes
- Severe vitamin K deficiency
- DIC
- HSP
- Von Willebrand's disease
- Hemophilia
- ITP
- Heparin-induced thrombocytopenia
- Myelodysplasia
- TTP-HUS
- Leukemia
- Hereditary hemorrhagic telangiectasia
- Ehlers-Danlos syndrome
- Bernard-Soulier syndrome
- Arteriovenous malformation
- Pancytopenia
- Isolated factor deficiency

Workup and Diagnosis

- History and physical exam
  - Personal or family history of bleeding, including bleeding with minor trauma, medications, postsurgical bleeding, menorrhagia, tooth extractions
  - Rectal exam and stool guaiac testing for occult GI bleeding
  - Joint exam for hemarthrosis
- Initial laboratory tests include CBC with peripheral smear, platelet count, PT/INR (evaluates extrinsic pathway—factors X, VII, V, II, I), PTT (evaluates intrinsic pathway—XII, XI, IX, VIII, V, II, I), thrombin time (measures ability of thrombin to transform fibrinogen in fibrin), bleeding time (evaluates platelet function and capillary integrity), and urinalysis (for hematuria)
- Additional tests may be indicated
  - Fibrinogen assay
  - Urea clot lysis test (evaluates factor XIII deficiency)
  - Mixing studies (determines the presence of an anticoagulant in the blood)
  - Specific factor assays
  - Platelet adhesion and aggregation tests (to evaluate platelet function)
  - Bone marrow aspirate (to evaluate platelet production and rule out leukemia)
- Hematology consultation is often indicated

Treatment

- Initial, emergent intervention with supplemental O_2, rapid IV hydration, hemostasis (usually with direct pressure), and transfusion is necessary with brisk bleeding and/or hemodynamic compromise
- Remove offending medications (e.g., heparin)
- Uremia: DDAVP, cryoprecipitate, and treatment of renal disease
- Vitamin K deficiency: Administer parenteral vitamin K
- DIC: Treat underlying cause, administer fresh frozen plasma and cryoprecipitate
- HSP: Corticosteroids for severe cases
- von Willebrand's disease and hemophilia A: DDAVP for mild bleeding, factor VIII concentrate, cryoprecipitate
- ITP: Corticosteroids, splenectomy, IVIG in emergency
- HIT: Stop heparin
- Liver disease: Fresh frozen plasma, tranexamic acid to control epistaxis or gum bleeding, treat liver disease if possible

22. Blurred Vision

Blurred vision is one of the most common ophthalmic symptoms. It may be caused by any alteration of the optical surfaces (e.g., cataract) or the media through which the visual axis traverses (e.g., vitreous hemorrhage). History and physical examination will usually lead to a reasonable differential diagnosis. Treatment aims to restore the ideal refractive and transparent media and surfaces of the eye. Most commonly, blurred vision is due to a refractive error that can be corrected with glasses, but more serious pathology must not be missed.

Differential Diagnosis

- Refractive error
- Presbyopia (blurred near vision, starts around age 40)
- Conjunctivitis (e.g., heavy discharge)
- Macular disease
  - Age-related macular degeneration
  - Macular edema; diabetic retinopathy
  - Central serous chorioretinopathy
- Ocular media opacity
  - Corneal edema (decreased deturgescent capacity or increased intraocular pressure)
  - Uveitis (anterior or posterior)
  - Hyphema
  - Cataract
  - Vitreous hemorrhage
- Corneal irregularity or abrasion
- Dry eye; poor tear film
- Retinal detachment
- Migraine (transient blurred/absent vision)
- CNS abnormality; head trauma
- Hyperglycemia (blurring may vary from day-to-day or throughout the day)
  - Poorly controlled diabetes mellitus
  - Medication effects
  - Other (see "Hyperglycemia" entry)
- Medication or drug side effects
  - Anticholinergics
  - Antihypertensives
  - Psychotropic medications
  - Amphetamine abuse
- Vasculopathy
  - Retinal artery or vein occlusion
- Hyperviscosity; hypercoagulation
- Seizure disorders
- Extraocular muscle paralysis
  - Diplopia may be misinterpreted as blurred vision by the patient; however, this will clear with covering either eye
- Temporal arteritis
  - Blurring is variable and may be associated with superior or inferior field defects
- Acute angle-closure glaucoma
  - Associated pain and redness are common
- Myasthenia gravis
  - Ptosis, diplopia, and/or blurred vision
- Botulism
- CO_2 narcosis
- See also "Vision Loss" entry

Workup and Diagnosis

- History
  - Review the progression (sudden, gradual) and duration (minutes, days, or months) of symptoms, binocular or uniocular, near or far vision, transient or permanent
  - Past medical history (e.g., diabetes, eye or head trauma, cataracts)
  - History of associated symptoms (e.g., migraine headache, seizure activity or change in level of consciousness, stroke-like symptoms)
- Complete ophthalmologic exam
  - Best corrected visual acuity (Snellen chart or near card)
  - Improvement of vision with pinhole indicates a refractive error
  - Slit lamp exam
  - Dilated fundus exam
  - Irritated or dry eyes
- Neurologic and head and neck examination should be considered
- EEG if seizure disorder is suspected
- Initial laboratory tests may include fasting (or random) blood glucose (with a repeat glucose and Hgb_{A1C} if glucose is initially elevated), CBC, PT, and PTT

Treatment

- Glasses or contact lenses for refractive errors
- Treat underlying pathology if possible (e.g., correct hyperglycemia, cataract surgery)
- Lubrication for dry eyes
- Ocular media opacity requires medical or surgical correction
- Retinal detachment requires surgical repair
- Hyperviscosity should be treated appropriately (e.g., aspirin, discontinue cigarettes)
- Antiseizure prophylaxis for seizure disorders

23. Bowel Sounds - Decreased

Decreased bowel sounds can be as innocent as a hungry patient anticipating a next meal or as ominous as an impending abdominal catastrophe necessitating emergent laparotomy. However, the sensitivity and specificity of the auscultation of bowel sounds are quite low, differ subjectively by clinician, and will vary from one moment to the next. Before declaring an absence of bowel sounds, one should auscultate for a minimum of 5 minutes ("if you didn't hear them, you didn't listen long enough").

Differential Diagnosis

- Benign etiologies
  - Normal variant: 5–30 bowel sounds per minute is typical; however, several minutes may elapse without any sounds
  - Failure to auscultate long enough
  - Hunger
  - Auscultation immediately following abdominal palpation or percussion (examiner should always listen for bowel sounds before palpating the abdomen)
- *Complete* bowel obstruction
  - Note: Partial bowel obstructions often have *increased* bowel sounds
- Intestinal ischemia
- Adynamic ileus
  - Abdominal surgery
  - Electrolyte abnormalities (hypokalemia, hyponatremia, hypomagnesemia, uremia)
  - Drugs (e.g., narcotics, α- and β-blockers, anticholinergics, psychotropic agents)
  - Lower lobe pneumonia
  - Sepsis
  - Retroperitoneal hemorrhage
  - Vertebral compression fracture
- Peritonitis
  - Acute appendicitis (or ruptured appendix)
  - Perforated gastric ulcer
  - Perforated diverticulum or diverticulitis
  - Ruptured ectopic pregnancy
  - Ruptured abdominal aortic aneurysm
  - Pancreatitis
  - Pelvic inflammatory disease
  - Infected peritonitis
  - Solid organ injury (i.e., following trauma)
- Less common etiologies include diabetic coma, hypoparathyroidism, rib fractures, myocardial infarction, spinal injury, perforated gall-bladder, and black widow spider bite

Workup and Diagnosis

- A careful history and physical exam are crucial, including rectal exam
  - Characterization of the pain
  - Patients with peritonitis will appear very ill and have abdominal tenderness, rebound, and guarding
  - Auscultate *before* palpation
  - Auscultation of each quadrant is *not* crucial—bowel sounds radiate throughout the abdomen
- Initial labs should include CBC, electrolytes, glucose, BUN/creatinine, calcium, liver function tests, amylase, lipase, and urinalysis
- Imaging studies may include X-rays, CT scan, and ultrasound
  - Flat and upright X-rays may reveal rupture (free air) or obstruction (dilated proximal loops of bowel with air-fluid levels); thoracic and/or lumbar X-rays may reveal spinal fractures
  - Abdominal CT scan gives more anatomic detail and may better differentiate ileus from obstruction
  - Ultrasound is useful for gynecologic concerns
- Differentiate postoperative ileus from obstruction
  - Some degree of ileus is expected following laparotomy (3–5 days); prolonged ileus should be investigated
  - Both can cause nausea/vomiting, constipation or obstipation, distension, tenderness, and tympany
  - A transition point or lack of gas in the rectum may suggest an obstruction

Treatment

- Although treatment decisions should rarely (if ever) be based on bowel sounds alone, serial assessment may be a useful sign of a patient's clinical evolution
- Ileus is treated conservatively by bowel rest (NPO), IV hydration, and nasogastric decompression (for nausea and vomiting)
  - Correct electrolyte abnormalities as necessary
  - Discontinue constipating drugs (especially narcotics)
  - Prokinetic drugs (e.g., metoclopramide, erythromycin) have mixed results but are often used
  - Ambulation is encouraged
  - Decreased nasogastric output, "normal" bowel sounds, passage of flatus, improved X-rays, or patient hunger may indicate readiness to begin oral intake
- Peritonitis generally requires emergent surgical intervention; treatment is directed at the specific underlying diagnosis

24. Bowel Sounds - Increased

Despite extensive efforts to evaluate and classify the sounds of the bowel using advanced technology, correlation of sounds to physiology using manometry and/or auscultation, *meaningful interpretation of bowel sounds remains clinically futile.* The overused phrase "bowel sounds normal" has little to contribute to the clinical decision-making process in the practice of medicine today.

Differential Diagnosis

- Benign etiologies
    - Variation of normal (5–30 sounds per minute)
    - Recent meal
    - Borborygmi ("stomach growling"): Loud, rumbling and gushing sounds due to movement of large amounts of fluid and air
    - Air swallowing
- Mechanical bowel obstruction: May present with distension, hiccups, nausea/vomiting, crampy abdominal pain or spasms, constipation, or watery diarrhea
    - Adhesions from prior surgery (cause 60% of cases)
    - Neoplasms (20%): May be extra- or intraluminal
    - Hernias (10%): May be external (inguinal, femoral, ventral) or internal (diaphragmatic, congenital, mesenteric defects)
    - Crohn's disease (5%)
    - Abscess
    - Volvulus
    - Intussusception (rare in adults)
    - Colonic pseudo-obstruction (Ogilvie's syndrome)
- Diarrhea
    - Acute gastroenteritis
    - Malabsorption syndrome
    - Lactase deficiency
    - Infection
- Succussion splash: Large collection of stagnant air and fluid in the distal stomach secondary to a gastric outlet obstruction, gastroparesis, or recent large meal may be auscultated while vigorously shaking the patient
- Gallstone ileus
- Peutz-Jeghers syndrome: Polypoid hamartoma of the bowel resulting in intussusception
- Foreign body
- Carcinoid syndrome
- Hiatal hernia

Workup and Diagnosis

- A careful history and physical exam are crucial, including rectal exam
    - Vital sign assessment for fever and dehydration
    - Bowel sounds should be auscultated *before* palpation
    - Hyperactive, high-pitched "tinkles" or "rushes" ("cathedral" sounds) often occur with obstruction
    - Abdominal examination should include all hernia orifices and evaluate for signs of incarceration and strangulation
- Initial labs should include CBC, electrolytes, BUN/creatinine, glucose, calcium, liver function tests, amylase, lipase, and urinalysis
- Flat and upright (or decubitus) abdominal X-rays are helpful to diagnose obstructions
- Abdominal CT scan is the most useful test and may demonstrate the etiology
- Enteroclysis is helpful to determine the level and degree of obstruction

Treatment

- Aggressive replacement of fluids and electrolytes is crucial
- Complete bowel obstruction with signs of strangulation (e.g., fever, leukocytosis, peritonitis) requires emergent operative intervention
    - Highly selected patients with complete obstruction and no peritonitis may be managed conservatively for a short period of time, but risk development of strangulation
- Partial small bowel obstructions can usually be managed conservatively by nasogastric decompression, no oral intake, and IV fluids
    - Serial evaluations are required to detect progression to complete obstruction

25. Bradycardia

Bradycardia is defined as heart rate of less than 60 beats per minute. It is a common finding that often does not require treatment in the absence of symptoms.

Differential Diagnosis

- Sinus bradycardia
  - Heart rate <60 bpm with normal-appearing P waves before each QRS wave (narrow complex)
  - Most often due to increased vagal tone or medications (e.g., β-blockers)
  - Normally seen in healthy young adults and well-trained athletes
  - May occur with hypothermia, advanced liver disease, hypothyroidism, sinoatrial node disease, anorexia nervosa, sleep disorders, and increased intracranial pressure
- Medications (e.g., β-blockers)
- Sinus node dysfunction
  - May occur as result of sinus node fibrosis (e.g., aging) or infiltrative diseases (e.g., amyloidosis)
  - SSS: Symptomatic bradycardia with sinus node dysfunction
  - Tachycardia-bradycardia syndrome: SSS manifested by tachyarrhthymias alternating with bradyarrhthymias
- Heart block
  - First-degree AV block: Fixed prolongation of PR interval (PR ≥200 msec); results from slowed conduction through AV node
  - Second-degree AV block, Mobitz I (Wenckebach): Results from delayed conduction through AV node; progressive prolongation of PR interval occurs until a QRS is dropped (typically benign)
  - Second-degree AV block, Mobitz II: Results from disease in the bundle of His; PR is constant, but sporadic P waves are not conducted (may be life threatening because of risk of complete heart block or ventricular asystole)
  - Complete heart block: Atrial impulses are not conducted to the ventricles; thus, atrial activity occurs independent of ventricular activity (AV dissociation, with atrial rate faster than ventricular rate)
- Congenital heart block
- Aortic stenosis
- Myocardial infarction
  - More common with inferior wall MI
- Atrial fibrillation/flutter with high-degree block
- Infections (e.g., Lyme disease)

Workup and Diagnosis

- History and physical exam
  - Associated symptoms may include lightheadedness, palpitations, dyspnea, chest pain, and syncope
  - Medication history
  - Thorough review of symptoms to identify precipitants of increased vagal tone (e.g., nausea, pain, headache)
  - Assess for hemodynamic instability (blood pressure, level of consciousness), jugular venous pressure (cannon A waves are highly suggestive of AV dissociation), and soft S1 (suggests PR prolongation)
- ECG is diagnostic
- Further diagnostic tests may include echocardiogram, electrophysiologic testing, and cardiac catheterization

Treatment

- Airway, breathing, and circulation
- Sinus bradycardia: Treatment is not usually necessary
  - Treat reversible causes (e.g., withdraw medications, thyroid hormone supplementation for hypothyroidism)
  - If symptomatic or hemodynamic instability is present, administer IV atropine or epinephrine
  - Electrical pacing is indicated only in severe cases
- Remove offending medications if possible
- Sinus node dysfunction: Treat reversible causes; often requires pacemaker placement
- Wenckebach: Treatment not usually necessary
- Mobitz II: More serious than Mobitz I, because sudden cardiac death may occur
  - Pacemaker placement is indicated for symptomatic bradycardia, documented asystole >3 seconds, coexistent neuromuscular disease, or concomitant high-grade conduction disease
  - Electrophysiologic testing to determine need for pacemaker
- Complete heart block requires pacemaker

26. Breast Masses

The occurrence of a new palpable breast mass or a breast lesion on mammography is a common problem in clinical practice. Although breast lumps are a serious concern because of the risk of cancer, most breast lumps and other complaints are of benign origin. Multiple methods are available to differentiate benign from malignant breast lesions, including clinical examination, mammography, ultrasound, fine needle aspiration, and needle core or open breast biopsy. Remember that breast cancers, although rare, can occur in males.

Differential Diagnosis

- Fibroadenoma
  - Most common cause of a unilateral discrete breast mass in young women
  - May be bilateral and/or multiple
  - Common in women with "fibrocystic changes" of the breast
- Intraductal papilloma
- Fibrocystic changes
- Gynecomastia
- Breast cancer
  - Most common cause of discrete mass in women older than 50
  - Types include infiltrating ductal (most common), infiltrating lobular, and medullary carcinoma
  - Increased incidence with obesity, infertility, late first pregnancy (age >30), uterine cancer, history of breast cancer in first degree relatives (3–10-fold increase), and postirradiation
  - Usually presents with nontender breast mass, nipple discharge, or occasionally nipple bleeding
- Galactocele
  - Presents during or shortly after breast-feeding
- Cystosarcoma phylloides
- Mammary duct ectasia
- Breast abscess
- Fat necrosis
- Cyst
- Cystic mastitis
- Lymphoma
- Lipoma
- Trauma

Workup and Diagnosis

- History and physical exam should include breast examination with careful attention to area(s) of mass, supraclavicular and axillary lymphadenopathy, skin changes (e.g., dimpling, edema, erythema, ulceration, or crusting), and nipple discharge
- Bilateral diagnostic mammogram should be the initial test, but may not be helpful if below age 35 because of high breast density
  - Suggestive of malignancy: Increased density, irregular margins, spiculation, irregular microcalcifications
- Ultrasound is used as an adjunct to mammography to delineate masses that cannot be seen on mammogram, to determine whether a lesion is solid or cystic, and if age <35
- MRI may be considered for indeterminate mammogram or ultrasound
- Biopsy of masses, nonpalpable lesions, or suspicious calcifications on mammogram may be indicated
  - Fine needle aspiration extracts cells for cytologic examination to distinguish benign versus malignant
  - Core needle biopsy of solid lesions or complex cysts extracts tissue and provides a definitive diagnosis
  - Excisional biopsy is definitive and may be curative if the full lesion is removed
- Perform cytologic assessment of any nipple discharge

Treatment

- Fibroadenoma
  - Requires surgical excision for diagnosis and treatment
  - Routine follow up after excision (no increased risk of malignancy)
- Fibrocystic changes
  - Caffeine avoidance is often effective
  - Aspirate large or painful cysts
  - Vitamin E is used to reduce fibrocystic changes
  - Medical therapies (e.g., danazol, oral contraceptives) for pain relief
  - Routine follow up is sufficient unless cytologic atypia is present
- Breast cancer
  - Consultation with medical and radiation oncologist
  - Surgery, radiation, chemotherapy, and/or hormonal therapy as indicated by stage
- Galactocele
  - Needle aspiration is usually curative

27. Breast Pain & Discharge

Breast pain (or mastalgia) is a common complaint that can often be diagnosed by a careful history and physical examination. Pain and tenderness may be normal during early pregnancy and before menses. Breast discharge, however, is rarely normal except in pregnant or lactating women, and it generally requires a full workup.

Differential Diagnosis

Breast pain
- Fibrocystic change
  - Most common benign breast condition
  - Clinically present in 50% and histologically in 90% of women
- Mastitis
  - Associated with lactation
- Extramammary causes of pain (e.g., cervical radiculitis, costochondritis, herpes zoster, angina)
- Breast cancer
  - Occurs in 1/9 women (lifetime risk)
- Cyst
- Breast abscess
- Unilateral or bilateral gynecomastia
- Phylloides tumor
- Intraductal papilloma
- Fat necrosis
- Trauma
- Fibroadenoma
- Lipoma
- Pregnancy

Breast discharge
- Duct ectasia
- Galactorrhea
- Mondor's disease
- Chronic nipple stimulation
- Pregnancy
- Hypothyroidism
- Sarcoidosis
- Systemic lupus erythematosus
- Cirrhosis or other hepatic disease
- Breast cancer
  - Occurs in 1/9 women (lifetime risk)
- Intraductal papilloma
- Fibrocystic change
- Medications (e.g., phenothiazines, metoclopramide, tricyclic antidepressants, reserpine, opiates, cimetidine, androgens)
- Hypothalamic and pituitary abnormalities (e.g., prolactinoma, acromegaly, empty sella syndrome)
- Pseudocyesis

Workup and Diagnosis

- History includes past medical history, duration and pattern of pain and/or discharge, family history of breast or gynecologic cancer, and menstrual/pregnancy history
- Breast exam 7–9 days after menstrual flow
  - Fibrocystic areas: Slightly irregular, mobile, bilateral, upper outer quadrant; compression causes tenderness
  - Breast cancer: Solitary, irregular, or stellate; hard, nontender, fixed; not clearly delineated from surrounding tissue, ± lymphadenopathy
  - Mastitis: Inflamed, edematous, erythematous, indurated, tender areas, axillary lymphadenopathy
  - Nipple discharge: Bloody or serosanguinous discharge is suspicious for cancer; oral contraceptives, estrogens, or elevated prolactin levels may result in clear, serous, or milky discharge
- Diagnostic mammogram is indicated in patients >30 years old who present with solitary or dominant mass or asymmetric thickening
  - Compare with prior mammograms if possible
- Ultrasound is used to distinguish solid versus cystic
- Fine-needle aspiration, breast biopsy, cytologic exam of discharge, ductogram and/or galactogram may be indicated
- Endocrine evaluation may include prolactin levels, TSH, FSH, and LH

Treatment

- Fibrocystic changes
  - Caffeine avoidance is often effective in decreasing pain
  - Aspirate cysts or medical therapies (e.g., danazol, oral contraceptives, tamoxifen, bromocriptine, evening primrose oil, GnRH agonists, vitamin E) for pain relief
  - Routine follow up is sufficient unless cytologic atypia is present
- Breast cancer: Surgery, radiation, chemotherapy, and/or hormonal therapy as indicated by stage
- Mastitis: Warm compress, antibiotics to cover *Staphylococcus aureus* and streptococci (e.g., cephalexin); consider inflammatory breast cancer if no response after 5 days in a nonlactating female
- Abscess: Incision and drainage, antibiotics
- Cyst: Aspiration; cytology of aspirated fluid if bloody or recurrent

28. Breast Swelling

Gynecomastia, or breast swelling, refers to a noninflammatory enlargement of the male breast. It is defined histologically as a benign proliferation of the glandular tissue of the male breast and clinically by the presence of a mass extending concentrically from the nipple. Gynecomastia is common in infancy, adolescence, and in middle-aged or older adult males. Differentiate from lipomastia, which is swelling of the breast due to fatty tissue proliferation.

Differential Diagnosis

- Physiologic gynecomastia of puberty
- Persistent postpubertal/elderly gynecomastia
- Idiopathic
- Medications (e.g., estrogens, antiandrogens, spironolactone, nifedipine, digitalis, isoniazid, phenytoin, griseofulvin, cimetidine) or drugs (especially marijuana)
- Liver disease
  - Cirrhosis
  - Hepatitis
  - Hemochromatosis
- Chronic renal insufficiency
  - 50% of men on dialysis have gynecomastia
- Hypogonadism (e.g., Klinefelter's syndrome, enzymatic defects, testicular trauma or infection)
- Thyroid disease
- Pituitary disease
  - Acromegaly
  - Chromophobe adenoma
- Neoplasms
  - Breast cancer
  - Testicular cancer
  - Adrenal cancer
  - Hepatocellular carcinoma
  - Lung cancer
  - Carcinoid
- Re-feeding after starvation
- Local irradiation

Workup and Diagnosis

- History and physical exam
  - Past medical history, family history, developmental and growth history, and medication history are important
  - If patient is an adolescent with normal physical examination, the diagnosis is likely pubertal gynecomastia; gradual improvement with age supports this diagnosis
  - Signs of breast cancer may include rubbery or firm mass, concentric or asymmetric, skin dimpling, nipple retraction, discharge, and axillary lymphadenopathy
- If gynecomastia is of recent onset, painful, or tender, initial laboratory evaluation may include β-hCG, LH, testosterone, TSH, estradiol, liver function tests, BUN/creatinine, prolactin, and DHEA-S
- Mammogram may be indicated to evaluate for cancer
- Ultrasound may distinguish normal glandular tissue from worrisome solid lesions
- Karyotype to diagnose Klinefelter's syndrome (XXY)

Treatment

- Many cases regress spontaneously without treatment
- Discontinue offending medications if possible
- Three types of medical therapies are available for elderly patients with severe pain, tenderness, or embarrassment
  - Androgens (e.g., testosterone, dihydrotestosterone, danazol)
  - Antiestrogens (e.g., clomiphene, tamoxifen)
  - Aromatase inhibitors (e.g., testolactone)
- Surgical therapy may be indicated if no response to medical therapy
  - Liposuction
  - Direct surgical excision
- Treat underlying medical conditions when possible

29. Breath Sounds (Decreased)

Decreased breath sounds represent either decreased flow of air through the airway or decreased transmission of sound across the chest wall. Lung pathology is a common etiology; however, physical causes such as obesity can be a less obvious etiology. A careful history and thorough physical examination can differentiate potentially life-threatening processes that require emergent intervention from chronic and/or benign processes. Determining whether the decrease in breath sounds is an acute or chronic process, and identifying accompanying symptoms and signs, will narrow the differential significantly.

Differential Diagnosis

Decreased airflow through respiratory tree
• Airway obstruction
  –Aspirated foreign body
  –Asthma
  –Bronchitis
  –Bronchiolitis
  –Croup
  –Epiglottitis
  –Neoplasm
  –Goiter
• Alveolar or interstitial processes
  –Pulmonary edema
  –Pneumonia
  –Pleurisy
  –Sarcoidosis
• Decreased lung expansion
  –Atelectasis
  –COPD or emphysema
  –Bronchiectasis
  –Kyphosis or scoliosis
  –Increased abdominal girth (e.g., ascites, obesity, pregnancy)
  –Pulmonary fibrosis
  –Diaphragmatic paralysis
  –Abdominal, chest wall, or pleuritic pain

Obstructed transmission of sound
• Obesity
• Pleural effusion
• Pneumothorax, hemothorax, or chylothorax
• Pleural thickening
• Large pulmonary embolus
• Less common etiologies ("zebras") include cystic fibrosis, alveolar hemorrhage, BOOP, now called COP, pneumonectomy (postsurgical), systemic lupus erythematosus, vocal cord paralysis, vocal cord dyskinesia, and psychogenic

Workup and Diagnosis

• History and physical examination
  –History should include associated symptoms (e.g., fever, dyspnea, wheezing, chest pain) and a detailed past medical, surgical, and exposure history
  –Physical examination should include vital signs; examination of oral cavity and neck for evidence of mass, foreign body, or tracheal deviation; inspection and palpation of the chest wall to assess for symmetric movement; percussion and auscultation of all chest fields for related abnormalities (e.g., rhonchi, wheezes, rales, rubs, egophony)
• Initial labs may include CBC, pulse oximetry, arterial blood gas, and TSH
• Chest X-ray is the initial imaging test
  –Associate the area of decreased breath sounds to hyperlucency or increased opacity on chest X-ray
  –Tracheal shift to a side with a density and decreased breath sounds likely signifies atelectasis or endobronchial obstruction
  –Tracheal shift away from a side with hyperlucency and decreased breath sounds may indicate tension pneumothorax
• Lateral neck X-ray may be indicated to rule out epiglottitis ("thumb sign")
• If there is evidence of external airway compression, chest and neck CT scans may be needed for further evaluation
• Pulmonary function testing

Treatment

• Closely monitor airway, breathing, and circulation
• Administer supplemental O_2 as needed
• Treat underlying etiology (e.g., removal of foreign body, bronchodilators, steroids)
• Emergent interventions may be necessary (e.g., chest tube insertion)

30. Cardiomegaly

Cardiomegaly is defined as enlargement of the heart above the normal size. When looking at a chest X-ray, one must be sure that an anterior-posterior view is being used, because the heart may appear falsely enlarged on a posterior-anterior view. When true cardiomegaly is present, further evaluation by echocardiography or other definitive testing is indicated to identify the cause of the enlargement.

Differential Diagnosis

- Congestive heart failure
- Ischemic heart disease
- Hypertension (with left ventricular hypertrophy)
- Valvular disease (primarily MR, AS, AR)
- Hypertrophic cardiomyopathy
- Congenital heart disorders (e.g., ASD, VSD, PDA, coarctation of the aorta, Ebstein's anomaly, tetralogy of Fallot)
- Idiopathic cardiomyopathy
- Alcoholic cardiomyopathy
- Lung disease (leading to right-sided enlargement)
    - Pulmonary embolus
    - COPD
    - Cor pulmonale
    - Primary pulmonary hypertension
- Subacute bacterial endocarditis
- Myocarditis
- Renal failure (risk of pericardial effusion)
- Anemia
- Scleroderma
- Systemic lupus erythematosus
- Sickle cell disease
- Marfan's syndrome
- Pregnancy
- Drugs (numerous drugs are cardiotoxic)
- Postradiation
- Normal, "athletic" heart
- Mediastinal mass
- Kyphoscoliosis
- Rheumatoid arthritis
- Less common etiologies include infiltrative diseases (e.g., amyloidosis, hemochromatosis, atrial myxoma, endocardial fibroelastosis, Fabry's disease, Hurler's syndrome, Pompe's disease), epicardial fat pad, carcinoid, acromegaly, hyper- or hypoparathyroidism, and severe cases of hypocalcemia, hypomagnesemia, and/or hypophosphatemia

Workup and Diagnosis

- Complete history and physical exam
    - Associated symptoms may include fatigue, dyspnea at rest and/or on exertion, palpitations, dizziness, or syncope
    - Note use of alcohol or recreational drugs
    - Family history of heart disease or sudden death
- Chest X-ray and ECG
- Echocardiogram is indicated in all patients to evaluate for valvular disease, chamber size, wall motion abnormalities, and ventricular function
- Stress testing if coronary artery disease is suspected
- Cardiac catheterization may be indicated to evaluate for coronary artery disease and valvular disease
- Laboratory studies may include CBC, ESR, electrolytes, BUN/creatinine, glucose, TSH, calcium, magnesium, and phosphorus
- Blood cultures are indicated in some cases
- Consider ANA, rheumatoid factor, and screening for pheochromocytoma (i.e., urinary metanephrines and VMA) and hemochromatosis (i.e., iron studies) in selected patients

Treatment

- Stabilize airway, breathing, and circulation
- Treat underlying cause
- Discontinue offending drugs
- Administer antiarrhythmics, digoxin, diuretics, and/or afterload and preload reducers as clinically indicated
- Periodic follow-up is based on severity of condition
- Transplant may be necessary in end-stage symptomatic heart failure that is refractory to medical treatment
    - Implantable ventricular assist devices may be indicated for severe heart failure patients to serve as a temporizing measure until heart transplantation occurs

31. Carotid Bruits

A carotid bruit is a blowing sound or murmur over the carotid artery, heard best with the bell of the stethoscope. It is usually associated with carotid stenosis secondary to atherosclerosis and may imply an increased risk of stroke, depending on the degree of stenosis and history of TIA or short-lived, stroke-like symptoms.

Differential Diagnosis

- Internal carotid artery stenosis
- External carotid artery stenosis
- Normal (nonstenotic), yet tortuous, carotid arteries
- Heart murmur with radiation to the neck (e.g., aortic stenosis)
- Excessive compression of the stethoscope over the neck vessels, resulting in deformity of vessel wall and turbulence
- Hyperthyroidism
  –Results in hyperdynamic circulation, tachycardia, and hypertension
- Takayasu's arteritis
  –Decreased pulses and bruits may occur over the abdominal aorta, carotid arteries, brachial arteries, and subclavian arteries
- Fisher's contralateral systolic bruit
  –Heard over the carotid bifurcation, eyeball, and/or skull on the "normal side" due to increased flow, as the "silent" side is completely occluded

Workup and Diagnosis

- Complete history and physical exam, with special attention to cardiac risk factors, TIA symptoms, cardiovascular exam, and neurologic exam
  –Bruit pitch increases as stenosis worsens, but may become silent when full occlusion occurs
  –Amaurosis fugax: Described as a "shade coming down over the eye" contralateral to the stenosis
- Laboratory evaluation includes lipid panel, CBC, glucose, electrolytes, homocysteine level (an independent risk factor for stroke), vitamin B_{12} and folate levels, TSH, and ESR
- Carotid duplex ultrasound will evaluate the degree of stenosis
- MRA, CTA, or arteriography is indicated to better evaluate symptomatic stenosis that may require surgery

Treatment

- Patients with symptomatic stenosis (i.e., presence of TIA symptoms in the appropriate distribution) and >70% carotid stenosis confirmed on duplex ultrasound should strongly consider carotid endarterectomy
- Symptomatic patients with 50–69% stenosis have greater benefit from surgery than from medical approach
- Asymptomatic patients and those that cannot tolerate surgery should begin aspirin (60–325 mg/day) and/or antiplatelet therapy (e.g., ticlopidine, clopidogrel)
- Smoking and alcohol cessation
- Treat hypertension, diabetes, and hyperlipidemia
- Carotid angioplasty is currently under study
- Patients with underlying disease processes require appropriate treatment

32. Chest Pain

Although most cases of chest pain are due to benign etiologies, such as gastroesophageal reflux or a muscle strain, life-threatening etiologies must be assessed and treated immediately if present. There are five primary etiologies of acute, life threatening chest pain: Aortic dissection, myocardial infarction, esophageal rupture, tension pneumothorax, and pulmonary embolism. Note that clinical improvement following use of antacids does not rule out the possibility of a cardiac etiology.

Differential Diagnosis

- Cardiovascular etiologies
  - Myocardial infarction
  - Angina
  - Acute coronary syndrome
  - Pulmonary embolus
  - Pericarditis
  - Arrhythmias
  - Mitral valve prolapse
  - Aortic stenosis
  - Aortic dissection
  - Cardiac tamponade
- Pulmonary etiologies
  - Pneumonia
  - COPD
  - Asthma
  - Pneumothorax
  - Tension pneumothorax
  - Hemothorax
  - Empyema
  - Pneumomediastinum
  - Lung cancer
- Gastrointestinal etiologies
  - Esophagitis/GERD
  - Gastritis
  - Peptic ulcer disease
  - Perforated ulcer
  - Esophageal spasm
  - Pancreatitis
  - Esophageal rupture
  - Pneumoperitoneum
- Musculoskeletal etiologies
  - Muscle strain or spasm
  - Intercostal muscle spasm
  - Costochondritis
  - Trauma (e.g., rib fracture)
- Zoster
- Cancer (e.g., lymphoma)
- Panic disorder
- Less common etiologies include Tietze's syndrome, Pott's disease (tuberculosis of the spine), xyphodenia, cholecystitis, peritonitis, liver cancer, and hepatitis

Workup and Diagnosis

- History and physical examination
  - Assess onset, duration, location, radiation, type of pain, and exacerbating and alleviating factors
  - Cardiovascular evaluation includes assessment of heart sounds, murmurs, gallops or rubs, and carotid bruit
  - All patients require a rectal exam (e.g., to assess for occult bleeding due to GI etiologies, to assess for occult bleeding before initiating anticoagulation)
  - Risk factors for coronary artery disease include smoking, hyperlipidemia, diabetes, and a personal or family history of coronary artery disease
- Initial evaluation may include pulse oximetry, CBC, electrolytes, BUN/creatinine, calcium, glucose, PT/INR/PTT, ECG, chest X-ray, and cardiac enzymes
- Patients with suspected coronary artery disease may require stress testing, echocardiogram, and/or cardiac catheterization
- Further studies to consider include arterial blood gas, liver function tests, amylase and lipase, CT of chest and abdomen, VQ scan, peak flow testing and pulmonary function tests, arteriogram, bronchoscopy, EGD, and/or esophagram
- Transesophageal echocardiogram and/or CT scan or MRI of the chest may be required to rule out aortic dissection (if widened mediastinum is present on X-ray)

Treatment

- Attention to airway, breathing, and circulation
- All patients with suspected coronary artery disease should initially be treated with supplemental O_2, aspirin, and nitroglycerin; morphine may be added if pain does not subside
- If an acute myocardial infarction is suspected, β-blockers, ACE inhibitors, heparin (usually low molecular weight heparin, enoxaparin), thrombolytic therapy or primary angioplasty (PTCA), and/or glycoprotein IIb/IIIa inhibitors (e.g., eptifibatide, abciximab, or tirofiban) may be indicated
- Treat other etiologies as appropriate (e.g., antiarrhythmics and/or cardioversion for arrhythmias, pericardiocentesis for cardiac tamponade, H2 blockers or PPIs for GERD and peptic ulcer disease, antibiotics for pneumonia, bronchodilators and steroids for asthma)
- Emergent surgery for aortic dissections that involve the aortic arch proximal to left subclavian artery (type A); strict blood pressure control for type B dissections that only involve the aorta distal to left subclavian artery

33. Chorea

Chorea (Greek for "dance") refers to continuous, rapid, and abrupt jerking movements, which are involuntary and often possess a writhing quality. These movements often interfere with the ability to complete daily activities. A characteristic feature is an inability to maintain voluntary sustained contractions. When chorea is proximal and of large amplitude, it is called ballismus.

Differential Diagnosis

- Huntington's disease (chronic progressive hereditary chorea)
  - Autosomal dominant transmission
  - Associated with psychiatric symptoms and progressive dementia
  - Caudate atrophy on neuroimaging studies
  - Marker on chromosome 4
- Sydenham's chorea
  - Symptoms follow febrile illness (20–30% of cases are associated with group A strep)
  - Seen in rheumatic fever
  - Peak ages: 5–13 years
  - More common in females
- Systemic lupus erythematosus
- AIDS
- Hyperthyroidism
- Chorea gravidarum
  - Develops in the first 4–5 months of pregnancy
  - Resolves following delivery
- Drug-induced (e.g., levodopa, stimulants, anticonvulsants, antidepressants, neuroleptics, oral contraceptives)
- Stroke
- Neoplasm
- Wilson's disease
  - Autosomal recessive disorder
  - Deficiency in copper metabolism
  - Associated with hepatic dysfunction, dystonia, dysarthria
- Benign hereditary chorea
  - Autosomal dominant
  - Onset before age 5
  - Symptoms are nonprogressive
- Neuroacanthocytosis
  - Etiology unknown
  - Characterized by chorea and deformed erythrocytes
- DRPLA
  - Most common in Japan
  - Characterized by chorea, ataxia, epilepsy, and dementia

Workup and Diagnosis

- History and physical examination
  - Clinical diagnosis is sufficient for Sydenham's chorea
  - Huntington's disease may present with psychiatric symptoms (e.g., depression) before other manifestations; onset of symptoms typically occurs in the fourth and fifth decades of life
  - The appearance of Kayser-Fleischer rings in the cornea on slit-lamp exam is diagnostic for Wilson's disease
- Neuroimaging (CT, MRI) to rule out mass lesions and Huntington's disease (cerebral/basal ganglion atrophy)
- Genetic testing for Huntington's disease
- Echocardiography to diagnose carditis
- Throat culture or serology (ASO) for streptococcal infection
- Low level of serum ceruloplasmin and elevated 24-hour urine copper in Wilson's disease
- Thyroid function tests to rule out hyperthyroidism
- ANA to rule out lupus
- Neuroacanthocytosis: Acanthocytes appear on peripheral smear with clinical symptoms of chorea, dystonia, and tics
- DRPLA: Imaging studies may reveal cerebral and cerebellar atrophy

Treatment

- Huntington's disease: Antidepressants may reduce depressive symptoms; neuroleptics (e.g., haloperidol, clozapine) may suppress choreic movements; disease is progressive and fatal; genetic counseling is suggested
- Sydenham's chorea is usually self-limited with symptom resolution within 15 weeks
- Acute rheumatic fever: Corticosteroids may shorten course of chorea; antibiotic therapy with penicillin for at least 10 days
- Drug-induced chorea: Discontinue or reduce dosage of implicated medications; atypical neuroleptics are associated with decreased risk of involuntary movements
- Chorea gravidarum may require delivery
- Wilson's disease: Copper-chelating agents
- Neuroacanthocytosis: Usually fatal within 9 years of symptom onset
- Specific therapy for lupus, hyperthyroidism, AIDS

34. Chronic Pain

Chronic pain is historically undertreated and underdiagnosed. It is defined as pain that persists beyond the recognized time for the body to heal (usually 4–6 weeks). Although acute pain serves a physiologic purpose, chronic pain without a physiologic role becomes a disease state in and of itself. It is usually categorized as diffuse or regional depending on the symptom distribution. Be aware of the high rate of psychiatric co-morbidities that exist with these conditions.

Differential Diagnosis

- Headache
  - Migraine headache
  - Cluster headache
  - Tension headache
  - Cervical radiculopathy
  - Temporomandibular joint syndrome
- Low back pain
  - Myofascial pain
  - Lumbar radiculopathy
  - Spinal stenosis
  - Facet syndrome
- Musculoskeletal
  - Soft tissue injury
  - Repetitive strain syndromes
  - Myofascial pain syndrome
  - Fibromyalgia
  - Arthritis
- Neuropathic
  - Diabetic neuropathy
  - Post-herpetic neuralgia
  - Cervical radiculopathy
  - Reflex sympathetic dystrophy (chronic regional pain syndrome)
  - Phantom limb
  - Postoperative thoracotomy
- Cancer pain syndromes
  - Bony pain secondary to metastasis
  - Visceral pain secondary to mass effects
  - Postradiation neuritis or mucositis
- Pelvic/abdominal
  - Endometriosis
  - Fibroids
  - Irritable bowel syndrome
  - Interstitial cystitis
- Psychiatric
  - Depression
  - Anxiety
  - Somatization
  - Physical, sexual, and/or emotional abuse
  - Malingering

Workup and Diagnosis

- History of symptoms should include onset, location, character, intensity, duration, radiation, aggravating and alleviating factors, and associated symptoms, as well as detailed past medical and surgical histories, how the symptoms affect the patient's life, and any previous evaluations and treatments
- Physical examination should include a comprehensive evaluation of each region where symptoms are described, including all affected joints and soft-tissue regions; complete mental status examination including affect, mood, ideation, and insight; and comprehensive evaluations of individual systems consistent with the patient's description of presentation
- Labs may be indicated depending on the distribution of symptoms and associated organ systems, possibly including CBC, BUN/creatinine, electrolytes, glucose, and calcium
  - ESR or CRP to evaluate for inflammatory conditions
  - CPK to evaluate for myopathies
- Imaging may be helpful, but should be targeted to specific conditions (e.g., plain films or CT scan for bony abnormalities or radiculopathy, MRI for soft-tissue mass or neural lesions, bone scan for reflex sympathetic dystrophy)
- Consider EMG

Treatment

- NSAIDs are often used, especially for inflammation
- Narcotics are usually reserved as adjuvant therapy after more conservative measures have failed; concern about addiction is a common barrier to use
- Tricyclic antidepressants and anticonvulsants are useful for neuropathic pain
- SSRIs are effective for fibromyalgia
- Spinal delivery of pain medication may be useful for radicular pain and reflex sympathetic dystrophy
- Tramadol is often used as a bridge between NSAIDs and narcotics
- Physical/occupational therapy is often very useful in a variety of conditions, especially reflex sympathetic dystrophy, low back pain, and fibromyalgia
- Alternative therapies may be useful as primary treatment or adjuvant therapy for chronic pain syndromes
- Psychiatric evaluation may be indicated for potential primary psychiatric conditions and co-morbidities
- Consider referral to a pain specialist

35. Constipation

Constipation is a common complaint that must be accurately defined by the patient before initiating an extensive evaluation. Constipation may include fewer than three bowel movements (BMs) in a week, excessive straining during BMs, a feeling of incomplete evacuation after BM, or passage of hard or pellet-like stools. The time of onset of constipation, amount of fluid and fiber in the diet, history of back trauma, neurologic problems, malignancy, medication history, and previous pattern of BMs may be helpful in reaching the correct diagnosis.

Differential Diagnosis

- Medications
  - Narcotic analgesics
  - Antihypertensives (e.g., calcium channel blockers)
  - Tricyclic antidepressants
  - Aluminum hydroxide in antacids
  - Iron supplements
- Inadequate dietary fiber or liquid intake
- Neurological dysfunction
  - Diabetes mellitus
  - Multiple sclerosis
  - Hirschsprung's disease
- Mechanical difficulties
  - Colorectal cancer
  - Hernia
  - Diverticulitis
  - Inflammatory bowel syndrome
  - Adhesion
  - Stricture
  - Torsion
  - Volvulus
- Metabolic and endocrine
  - Hypothyroidism
  - Hypercalcemia
  - Hypokalemia
- Chronic laxative abuse

Workup and Diagnosis

- History and physical examination
  - Specific attention to medication history, diet, and thyroid examination
  - Abdominal examination: Note any surgical scars, palpate for masses (stool) and hepatosplenomegaly, check for hernias; however, note that examination results are often normal
  - Rectal examination: Determine presence of stool, masses, hemorrhoids, fistulas, abscesses, or fissures; resting and squeezing sphincter tone; when patient bears down, relaxation of anal tone and perineal descents should be palpable (the absence of relaxation or inadequate perineal descents raises the suspicion of obstructive defecation)
- Initial laboratory testing may include CBC, electrolytes, BUN/creatinine, glucose, calcium, phosphate, thyroid function tests, and fecal occult blood test
- Consider a stool examination for ova and parasites, and flexible sigmoidoscopy or colonoscopy (colonoscopy if age greater than 50, new onset of constipation without cause, or blood in stool)

Treatment

- If history, physical, and evaluation are all negative, a series of lifestyle modifications and conservative treatments are indicated
  - Increase fiber and fluid intake
  - Exercise
  - Avoid causative medications
  - Saline cathartics: Magnesium-containing compounds and phosphate enemas work by osmotic effect; avoid in renal insufficiency; for acute cases only
  - Hyperosmotic nonabsorbing sugars (e.g., lactulose) may be used for long-term management and are less toxic
  - Lavage solutions may be used for refractory constipation and impactions
  - Enemas: Low volume tap water or sodium phosphate (FLEET) may be used for severe constipation
  - A combination of suppositories (glycerin or bisaccodyl) and enemas (phosphate) will soften impactions; however, digital disimpaction may be necessary

36. Cough - Nonproductive

Initial history of cough should include an assessment of the production of sputum. Additionally, associated history and physical findings, with particular attention to the quantity, quality, and circumstances surrounding coughing episodes and social details (such as history of smoking, farm work, or allergen exposure), are also important in identifying the etiology. A persistent, nonproductive cough caused by ACE inhibitor usage must not be overlooked, as it is both concerning and annoying to the patient and can be remediated by adjusting the medication regimen.

Differential Diagnosis

- Smoker's cough
- Postnasal drip (e.g., chronic sinusitis, allergic rhinitis)
    - Most common cause of chronic cough in nonsmokers
- GERD
    - Second most common cause of chronic cough in nonsmokers
- Asthma/reactive airway disease
    - Classic triad of chronic cough, dyspnea, and wheezing
- ACE inhibitor use
- Acute bronchitis
    - Most commonly caused by viruses (e.g., influenza, adenovirus, rhinovirus, RSV)
    - Postviral bronchitis may last beyond 6 weeks
- Pneumonia
    - "Typical" pneumonia (e.g., *Streptococcus pneumoniae, Haemophilus influenzae,* or influenza/parainfluenza viruses) is characterized by acute or subacute onset of fever, dyspnea, fatigue, pleuritic chest pain, and cough
    - "Atypical" pneumonia (e.g., *Mycoplasma, Legionella, Chlamydia*) is characterized by more gradual onset, dry cough, headache, fatigue, and minimal lung signs
- Aspirated foreign body
    - Abrupt onset of unilateral wheezing or stridor, cough, decreased breath sounds
    - Leading cause of home accidental death in children younger than 6 (boys > girls)
- Lung cancer
    - 90% of cases due to smoking (other risk factors include radon, asbestos, pollutants)
- COPD (emphysematous variant)
- Sarcoidosis
- Cryptogenic organizing pneumonia
    - Most commonly occurs following viral infection or exposure
- Congestive heart failure
- Filarial disease
- Aspiration

Workup and Diagnosis

- Complete history and physical examination
    - Note acute (<3 weeks) versus chronic or recurrent
- Initial tests may include CBC, pulse oximetry, ESR, peak flow measurements, PPD, and eosinophil count
- Chest X-ray and/or CT if patient has concerning symptoms (e.g., weight loss, hemoptysis, fever)
- Consider blood and sputum cultures
- Initial empiric treatment of postnasal drip (antihistamine, decongestant, nasal steroids), asthma (trial of bronchodilators or a methacholine challenge test), and/or GERD (proton pump inhibitor) may be advisable
- If imaging is normal and empiric treatment for GERD does not resolve symptoms, proceed with upper GI endoscopy or esophageal pH monitoring
- Consider CT of sinuses or nasolaryngoscopy to evaluate for sinusitis
- Consider bronchoscopy to identify subtle pulmonary causes
- Consider cardiac workup if pulmonary and GI evaluations are negative

Treatment

- Cessation of cigarette smoking and/or ACE inhibitors
- Postnasal drip: Treat underlying etiology (e.g., antibiotics for sinusitis, antihistamines and/or nasal steroids for allergies)
- GERD: Lifestyle modifications (e.g., weight loss, dietary changes to eliminate predisposing agents, avoid alcohol and tobacco, avoid food within 4 hours of bedtime, sleep with head of bed elevated), anti-ulcer/antacid medications (H2 blockers, proton pump inhibitors), anti-reflux surgery (fundoplication)
- Asthma: Avoid triggers; use inhaled β_2 agonists (e.g., albuterol) and anticholinergics (e.g., ipratropium), inhaled or oral steroids (delayed onset 2–6 hours), children may benefit from magnesium or cromolyn
- Acute bronchitis: Inhaled β_2 agonists (e.g., albuterol); since most cases are of viral origin, antibiotics are usually not indicated; increased fluid intake; antitussive
- Pneumonia: Appropriate oral or IV antibiotics

37. Cough - Productive

Initial history of cough should include an assessment of the production of sputum, and the quantity, quality, and circumstances of the sputum production and coughing episodes. Additionally, associated history and physical findings, with particular attention to inciting factors such as history of smoking, farm work, allergen exposure, etc., are important in identifying the etiology as well. Culture and Gram stain of the sputum is necessary in all but the most obvious cases of productive cough such as upper respiratory infection.

Differential Diagnosis

- Postnasal drip (e.g., chronic sinusitis, allergic rhinitis)
  - Most common cause of chronic cough in nonsmokers
- Acute bronchitis
  - Most commonly caused by viruses (e.g., influenza, adenovirus, rhinovirus, RSV)
  - Bacteria are much less common (e.g., *Streptococcus pneumoniae, Mycoplasma, Haemophilus influenzae*)
- Pneumonia
  - May be community-acquired, hospital-acquired, or due to aspiration
  - "Typical" pneumonia (e.g., *S. pneumoniae, H. influenzae,* influenza virus) has acute or subacute onset of fever, dyspnea, fatigue, pleuritic chest pain, and productive cough
  - "Atypical" pneumonia (e.g., *Mycoplasma, Legionella, Chlamydia, Pneumocystis carinii*) has more gradual onset, dry cough, headache, fatigue
- Smoker's cough
- Lung cancer
  - 90% of cases due to smoking (other risk factors include radon, asbestos, pollutants)
- Asthma with secondary infection
- COPD (chronic bronchitis component)
- Congestive heart failure
  - Associated with "frothy" sputum
- Tuberculosis

Workup and Diagnosis

- Complete history and physical examination
  - Note acute (<3 weeks) versus chronic or recurrent
- Initial tests may include CBC, pulse oximetry, ESR, peak flow measurements, PPD, chest X-ray, blood cultures, sputum Gram stain and culture, and acid-fast stain for tuberculosis
- Pulmonary function tests with or without methacholine challenge
- Chest CT and/or sputum cytology if patient has concerning symptoms (e.g., weight loss, hemoptysis, fever)
- Initial empiric treatment for postnasal drip (antihistamine, decongestant, nasal steroids)
- Consider CT of sinuses or nasolaryngoscopy to evaluate for sinusitis
- Consider bronchoscopy with possible bronchoalveolar lavage and/or biopsy

Treatment

- Cessation of cigarette smoking
- Administer supplemental O_2 if necessary
- Postnasal drip: Treat underlying etiology (e.g., antibiotics for sinusitis, antihistamines and/or inhaled steroids for allergies)
- Acute bronchitis: Inhaled β_2 agonists (e.g., albuterol); since most cases are of viral origin, antibiotics are usually not indicated; increased fluid intake; antitussive
- Pneumonia: Oral (e.g., macrolide, doxycycline, quinolone) or IV antibiotics (third-generation cephalosporin and a macrolide; or a second-generation quinolone)
- COPD: Inhaled bronchodilator therapy with β_2 agonists (e.g., albuterol) and anticholinergics (e.g., ipratropium); systemic corticosteroids; antibiotics (e.g., azithromycin, doxycycline) should be administered in severe exacerbations or secondary infections; noninvasive mechanical ventilation by CPAP or BiPAP may be necessary

38. Crackles/Rales

Rales, also known as crackles, are caused by the opening of collapsed airways. They are discontinuous, nonmusical breath sounds that may be fine (soft, 5–10 milliseconds in duration, high-pitched) or coarse (slightly louder, 20–30 milliseconds in duration, lower in pitch). Distinguish from rhonchi, which are caused by air flowing through airway secretions and are continuous (250+ milliseconds) musical sounds of low pitch (versus wheezes).

Differential Diagnosis

- Pneumonia
  - May be community-acquired, hospital-acquired (i.e., due to residence in any health care facility or nursing home in the preceding 10–14 days), or due to aspiration
  - "Typical" pneumonia (e.g., *Streptococcus pneumoniae, Haemophilus influenzae*) is characterized by acute or subacute onset of fever, dyspnea, fatigue, pleuritic chest pain, and productive cough
  - "Atypical" pneumonia (e.g., *Mycoplasma, Legionella, Chlamydia,* influenza/parainfluenza viruses) is characterized by more gradual onset, dry cough, headache, fatigue, and minimal lung signs
- Pulmonary edema
  - Leakage of fluid into the interstitium and alveoli due to elevated capillary pressure (cardiogenic) or abnormal capillary permeability (noncardiogenic)
  - Cardiogenic pulmonary edema: LV failure (e.g., MI, cardiomyopathy), valve disease, high output states (e.g., thyrotoxicosis), volume overload, hypertensive emergency
  - Noncardiac pulmonary edema: Sepsis, inhalation injury, drugs (e.g., narcotics), renal failure, high altitude, aspiration, pancreatitis, seizure, trauma, emboli (fat, air, amniotic fluid), CNS injury, airway obstruction (e.g., croup, foreign body)
- Atelectasis
  - May be acute (e.g., postoperative) or chronic (due to airlessness, infection, bronchiectasis, lung destruction and fibrosis)
- Interstitial lung disease
  - A group of disorders characterized by inflammation and fibrosis of alveolar walls and the interstitium (e.g., sarcoidosis, asbestosis, scleroderma)
- Bronchiolitis
- Bronchiectasis
- Bronchospasm (e.g., asthma)
- Congenital heart disease
- Bronchoalveolar carcinoma
- Cryptogenic organizing pneumonia

Workup and Diagnosis

- History and physical examination
  - Percussion may reveal dullness
  - "E" to "A" changes (egophony) may be present in lobar pneumonia, atelectasis, and postinfectious bronchiolitis
- Initial laboratory studies may include CBC, pulse oximetry, electrolytes, BUN/creatinine, glucose, and calcium
- Chest X-ray is generally the initial test
  - CHF: Interstitial and alveolar edema, especially in dependent regions; cephalization; Kerley B lines (if chronic); cardiomegaly; may see pleural effusion
  - Interstitial disease: Reticulonodular or interstitial pattern (diffuse lines and/or small nodules)
  - Atelectasis: Decreased lung volume (retracted ribs, deviation of heart and trachea to the affected side, overinflation of contralateral lung); triangular shadow with apex pointing to hilum; opacification
  - Bronchiolitis: Patchy infiltrate, pleural fluid
  - Bronchiectasis: Bronchial dilation, thickened walls
- Arterial blood gas will evaluate for barriers to oxygen diffusion (increased A-a gradient), hypoxemia, and hypercapnia
- High-resolution chest CT scan can detect early disease and small lesions unidentifiable on chest X-ray, can distinguish inflammation from fibrosis, and will confirm bronchiectasis ("signet ring" sign)
- Biopsy and bronchoalveolar lavage may be necessary to diagnose interstitial lung disease

Treatment

- Attention to airway, breathing, and circulation
- Administer supplemental O_2
- Cardiogenic pulmonary edema: Vasodilators (e.g., IV nitroglycerin, ACE inhibitors), loop diuretics (e.g., IV furosemide), morphine, and inotropes
- Noncardiogenic edema generally requires only supportive care; treat underlying etiology (e.g., surgical correction of valvular lesions)
- Interstitial lung disease: Remove offending agent and/or stop smoking; treat the underlying etiology; systemic steroids are beneficial in some patients; other immuno-suppresives may be indicated (e.g., methotrexate, cyclosporine, azathioprine); lung transplant may be considered in end-stage patients
- Atelectasis: Aggressive respiratory therapy, including incentive spirometry, mobilization, and/or positioning of patient to drain the affected lung; encourage coughing, suctioning, or vigorous respiratory/physical therapy; PEEP or CPAP; antibiotics for infection

39. Cyanosis

Cyanosis is a bluish discoloration of the skin or mucous membranes that is caused by significantly decreased oxygenation of the blood. It may be generalized or confined to the periphery.

Differential Diagnosis

Central cyanosis (cyanosis of lips and mucous membranes)
- Pulmonary disease
  - Severe pneumonia
  - Pulmonary edema
  - Pulmonary arteriovenous fistulas
  - Tension pneumothorax
  - Severe COPD or asthma
  - Adult respiratory distress syndrome
  - Lung cancer
  - Obstruction (e.g., tracheal foreign body or stenosis)
  - High altitude exposure
  - Decreased respiration with oversedation
  - Sleep apnea
- Congenital heart disease with shunting
  - Tetralogy of Fallot
  - Transposition of the great vessels (most common cause of cyanosis in the immediate newborn period)
  - Tricuspid atresia
  - Truncus arteriosus
- Cardiovascular disease
  - Cardiogenic shock (e.g., massive MI)
  - Severe valvular heart disease
  - Cor pulmonale
  - Massive pulmonary embolus
- Abnormal hemoglobin
  - Methemoglobinemia: Usually caused by drugs or chemicals (e.g., sulfa, nitrites, benzene derivatives) or genetic defects
  - Hemoglobin Kansas
  - Sickle cell disease
- Toxins/poisons (e.g., carbon monoxide, nitroprusside, cyanide)

Peripheral cyanosis (cyanosis of phalanges, earlobes, and nose)
- Increased resistance to blood flow
  - Raynaud's phenomenon
  - Acrocyanosis
  - Superior vena cava obstruction
  - Venous hypertension
  - Arterial embolism
  - Exposure to cold air or water
- Decreased cardiac output
  - Shock
  - Congestive heart failure
  - Mitral stenosis
- Increased blood viscosity
  - Polycythemia vera

Workup and Diagnosis

- History and physical examination
  - Clubbing of the fingers or toes may indicate congenital heart disease or chronic pulmonary disease
  - Blood pressure, capillary refill, and heart and lung exam are always indicated
  - Pulses and neurologic function in all involved extremities must be evaluated in peripheral cyanosis
- Initial labs include pulse oximetry, CBC, electrolytes, BUN/creatinine, glucose, arterial blood gas (to assess oxygenation, CO level, and presence of methemoglobin), and ECG
- Chest X-ray and/or CT scan to evaluate for lung pathology and heart size
- Echocardiogram will assess ventricular function and valves, and rule out structural abnormalities
- Pulmonary function tests
- Cardiac enzymes may be indicated to rule out MI
- Hemoglobin electrophoresis may be indicated to evaluate hemoglobin structure
- For peripheral cyanosis isolated to one limb, arterial Doppler studies or angiogram may be indicated to rule out embolus
- Pulmonary angiogram may be indicated to rule out an arteriovenous fistula or massive pulmonary embolism

Treatment

- Administer supplemental oxygen to all patients
  - Cyanosis and hypoxemia due to (most) lung disease and carbon monoxide poisoning will quickly improve upon oxygen administration
- Respiratory support with intubation and mechanical ventilation may be necessary
- Treat shock as necessary with IV fluids, vasopressors, and correction of underlying cause
- Treat underlying etiologies as appropriate

40. Delirium

An acute confusional state caused by a disturbance in global cortical function. Features include disturbance of consciousness, change in cognition, fluctuations of symptoms, and evidence that the condition is secondary to an underlying medical condition. Frequently, multiple etiologies are present simultaneously. Delirium occurs in 30% of older medical patients during hospitalization. Patients with delirium experience prolonged hospitalization, functional decline, and are at high risk for institutionalization.

Differential Diagnosis

- Dementia
- Medical etiologies
  - Infections (e.g., UTI, pneumonia, encephalitis, meningitis)
  - Drug toxicity, including alcohol
  - Drug withdrawal (especially benzodiazepines)
  - Fluid, electrolyte, and metabolic disorders (e.g., hyponatremia, hypoglycemia, hypercalcemia, uremia, hypercarbia)
  - CHF
  - Hypoxia (multiple causes, including CHF)
  - Medications (e.g., antiarrhythmics, antidepressants, neuroleptics, analgesics, GI medications)
  - Stroke
  - Cerebral ischemia (multiple causes)
  - Complex partial seizure disorder is associated with an alteration of awareness
- Psychiatric etiologies
  - Depression
  - Psychotic illness
  - "Sundowning": Behavioral deterioration occurs during evening hours (typically occurs in demented institutionalized patients)

Workup and Diagnosis

- History should include evaluation of memory difficulties, disorientation, incoherent speech, and level of attention, and a discussion with patients' family caregivers
  - Risk factors include advanced age, cognitive impairment (including dementia), psychiatric conditions, and severe chronic medical illness
  - Mini-mental status examination
- Physical examination should include vitals, state of hydration, infectious foci, and neurologic exam, with complete investigation into possible medical etiologies
- Initial labs may include serum electrolytes, BUN/creatinine, glucose, calcium, magnesium, CBC, and urinalysis
- Pulse oximetry and/or arterial blood gas may be indicated to screen for hypoxia and/or hypercarbia
- Thyroid function tests and vitamin B_{12}/folate levels
- Imaging studies (e.g., head CT, chest X-ray), blood and urine cultures, and/or lumbar puncture may be indicated
- EEG is indicated if suspect seizure disorder
  - Slowing of α rhythms and unusual slow-wave activity are common in delirium

Treatment

- Delirium is usually reversible with correction of the underlying cause
  - Discontinue possible contributing medications
  - Treat infection if present
  - Correct metabolic or electrolyte abnormalities
- Pharmacologic therapy
  - Antipsychotics (e.g., haloperidol) for hallucinations, delusions, or illusions
  - Benzodiazepines (e.g., lorazepam) for anxiety, agitation, insomnia, or alcohol withdrawal
- Environmental supports (e.g., calendars, direction signs) to help with orientation
- Psychosocial support
- Physical restraints paradoxically increase patient agitation; thus, other alternatives (e.g., safe environment, door alarms) should be used initially

41. Delusions

Delusions are firmly held, stable, but false beliefs that are not consistent with educational or cultural background and are not given up even in the face of contrary evidence. They are an essential feature of psychosis. Delusions take many forms, such as persecutory or grandiose ideas, thoughts of being controlled or of a partner's infidelity, ideas of reference (believing neutral external events have specific personal meaning), or religious.

Differential Diagnosis

- Schizophrenia
  - Delusions are the key symptom
  - Complex, disorganized, persecutory thoughts; ideas of reference; thoughts of being controlled
  - Hallucinations (usually auditory)
  - Thought disorders
  - Catatonic or disorganized behavior
  - Disorganized speech
  - Minimum 6 month duration
  - Social/occupational dysfunction
- Mania or hypomania
  - Delusions are usually grandiose
  - Associated with frantic, ill-considered activity (e.g., hypersexuality, gambling, overspending), irritability, reduced sleep, and reduced appetite
  - Bipolar with depression
- Psychotic depression
  - Delusions of guilt, worthlessness in context of depressed mood, loss of interest/pleasure (anhedonia), suicidal ideas/plans, and sleep/appetite disturbance
- Delirium
  - Disorganized thought, fluctuating awareness, misperceptions, paranoid fears
  - Temporary
  - "Delusions" not fixed
- Dementia
  - Delusions often seen in context of global cognitive decline
- Chronic psychostimulant and alcohol abuse
  - Psychosis with delusions can develop
- Schizoaffective disorder
- Delusional disorder
  - Rare condition
  - Well-formed, specific, fixed delusions (e.g., of being loved, persecuted, having specific somatic abnormality)
  - Persistent, but does not interfere with other areas of functioning
  - No other psychiatric symptoms
- Illicit drugs (e.g., LSD, mescaline, phencyclidine, mushrooms, amphetamines)
- Alzheimer's disease (usually paranoid type)
- Hyperparathyroidism

Workup and Diagnosis

- Careful history is necessary to distinguish between psychiatric syndromes
  - Mental status examination is required, including suicidal ideation/plan
  - Past, family, and social history may shed light on diagnosis
  - Consider interviewing family and/or friends
  - Drug and alcohol history and appropriate workup if present
  - Dementia assessment, including mini-mental status examination and appropriate workup if present
- Consider CBC, electrolytes, calcium, glucose, BUN/creatinine, pulse oximetry, and TSH

Treatment

- Antipsychotic medications are effective more for behavioral control, associated symptoms (e.g., hallucinations), and distress than for complete elimination of delusions
  - Newer antipsychotics (e.g., risperidone, olanzapine, quetiapine) cause fewer dystonic side effects; however, may cause weight gain and diabetes
  - Administer IM haloperidol if patient is unable or unwilling to take oral medications in the acute setting
  - In acute disorders in young patients, higher end of dose range used; in older patients, low doses are preferred
- Mood stabilizers (e.g., lithium, valproic acid) for manic patients and antidepressants (e.g., SSRIs) for depression
- Psychotherapy may provide structure and support but usually does not eliminate delusions
- Environmental support and safety management is necessary in impaired patients, severe chronic schizophrenia, and dementia

42. Dementia

Dementia is a syndrome of premature neuronal death in focal brain regions. More than 50 illnesses may cause dementia. It affects 1% of the population by age 60, and this prevalence doubles every 5 years to reach 30–50% by age 85. Common findings include aphasia (language disorder of speech, comprehension, naming, reading, and writing), apraxia (inability to perform previously learned tasks such as combing hair or "saluting the flag"), and agnosia (impaired recognition or comprehension of specific auditory, visual, and tactile stimuli).

Differential Diagnosis

- Alzheimer's disease is the most common cause of dementia
- Lewy body dementia
- Multi-infarct dementia
- Parkinson's disease
- Alcohol/drugs
- Vitamin deficiency (B_{12}, thiamine)
- CNS infections
  - HIV encephalitis
  - Meningitis
  - Herpes encephalitis
  - Creutzfeldt-Jacob disease
  - Cerebral abscess
  - Neurosyphilis
- Depression (pseudodementia)
- Head trauma
- Pick's disease
- Chronic subdural hematoma
- Huntington's disease
- Chronic hydrocephalus
- Paraneoplastic encephalitis
- Hypothyroidism
- Cerebral vasculitis
- Systemic lupus erythematosus (lupus cerebritis)
- Wilson's disease
- Chronic hypoglycemia or hypocalcemia
- Uremic encephalopathy
- Dialysis dementia
- Multiple sclerosis
- Hydrocephalus
- Postanoxic dementia

Workup and Diagnosis

- Important to distinguish dementia from delirium (acute metabolically induced state of fluctuating consciousness) and depression
- A complete history and physical are essential to rule out underlying medical, neurologic, or psychiatric illnesses that may mimic symptoms of dementia
  - Mini-mental status exam
  - Medication history should be elicited to identify drugs that may contribute to cognitive changes (e.g., analgesics, sedatives, anticholinergics, antihypertensives)
- Labs may include CBC, electrolytes, calcium, BUN/creatinine, liver function tests, glucose, thyroid function tests, vitamin B_{12} and folate, screening for inflammatory/infectious causes, and toxicology screen
- CT without contrast to rule out structural lesions (e.g., infarct, malignancy, hydrocephalus, extracerebral fluid collection)
- EEG is not routinely used; however, it may identify toxic/metabolic disorders or Creutzfeldt-Jakob disease
- Genetic testing may be indicated if family history suggests Alzheimer's disease (especially early-onset)
  - Mutations of chromosomes 1, 14, 21
  - Increased frequency of apolipoprotein $\epsilon4$ allele
- CSF analysis may be useful in some cases
- HIV and syphilis (RPR) testing if known risk factors

Treatment

- Treat reversible causes (e.g., hypothyroidism, vitamin deficiency, cerebral vasculitis, neurosyphilis, HIV)
- Manage nonreversible etiologies, including genetic risks, health care planning, and help groups (e.g., Alzheimer's Association)
- Alzheimer's disease: Anticholinesterases (e.g., tacrine, donepezil) may improve cognitive function; selegiline and α-tocopherol may delay progression
- Vascular dementia: Treat risk factors (e.g., discontinue tobacco use, lower blood pressure and lipids)
  - Note that lost cognitive function will not return despite treatment
- Parkinson's disease: Dopamine and dopamine agonists; anticholinergics improve function but do not affect progression of disease; selegiline may slow disease progression

43. Diarrhea - Acute

Diarrhea is defined as an increase in the volume of bowel movements. Acute diarrhea is designated as being of less than 4 weeks' duration. Many patients describe increased frequency or decreased consistency of bowel movements as diarrhea, so the clinician should be certain to identify whether the patient indeed suffers from diarrhea.

Differential Diagnosis

- Infectious etiologies
  - Acute (viral) gastroenteritis
  - "Traveler's diarrhea": *Shigella, Salmonella,* enterotoxigenic *E. coli, Campylobacter*
  - Rotavirus
  - Norwalk virus
  - *Yersinia enterocolitica*
  - *Clostridium difficile* (pseudomembranous enterocolitis): Follows antibiotic use
  - Giardiasis: Foul-smelling, explosive diarrhea
  - Enterovirus
- Lactose intolerance
- IBS: Alternating diarrhea and constipation
- Ischemic colitis: Associated with history of atherosclerotic disease (CAD, PVD, AAA)
- Inflammatory bowel disease (ulcerative colitis, Crohn's disease)
- Medications (e.g., laxatives, antibiotics, anticholinergics, chemotherapy, metformin)
- Malabsorption syndromes
- Vasculitis
- Neoplasia
- Appendicitis
- Adrenal insufficiency
- Hyperthyroidism
- HIV
- Less common etiologies include *E. coli* O157:H7 (commonly associated with raw meat; invasive, bloody diarrhea), *Cryptosporidium, Cyclospora, Isospora belli,* typhoid fever

Workup and Diagnosis

- History and physical examination
  - Proper history should include travel history, woodland exposure (*Giardia*), immune status, and sick contacts
  - Blood pressure and pulses, including orthostatics
  - Full abdominal examination
  - Back, genital, and rectal examinations
  - Skin examination (e.g., jaundice, turgor)
  - Signs of dehydration (e.g., loss of jugular pulsations, dry mucous membranes, skin tenting, orthostasis)
- Stool examination and culture are usually indicated
  - Fecal leukocytes suggest for infectious causes
  - Fecal lactoferrin suggests laxative abuse
  - Ova and parasites (for *Giardia* and *Cryptosporidium*) should be considered in at-risk patients with persistent diarrhea
  - Stool cultures may identify *Salmonella, Shigella, Campylobacter, Yersinia,* or *E. Coli*
  - Test stool for *C. difficile* toxin, if suspected
  - Stool osmolar gap is elevated in osmotic and malabsorptive diarrhea and decreased in infectious/secretory diarrhea
- Initial laboratory studies may include CBC, electrolytes, BUN/creatinine, glucose, urinalysis, liver function tests, and hepatitis serologies
- Therapeutic trial of a lactose-free diet or lactose intolerance testing may be useful
- Barium enema, colonoscopy, and/or flexible sigmoidoscopy may be indicated
- Consider HIV testing

Treatment

- Treatment is generally supportive
- Fluid resuscitation (oral, if possible, or IV)
- Antimotility agents: Opiates (e.g., loperamide) and parasympathetic inhibitors (e.g., diphenoxylate plus atropine); former concerns that these agents may slow the clearance of pathogens have been disproved
- Antibiotic therapy is reserved for severe disease
  - Most authorities recommend empiric treatment with a fluoroquinolone or trimethoprin-sulfamethoxasole in patients with severe or bloody diarrhea, fever, or fecal leukocytes
  - If *Giardia, C. difficile,* or *E. histolytica* is suspected, treat empirically with metronidazole
  - Antibiotic therapy increases the risk of hemolytic-uremic syndrome in children with *E. coli* O157:H7
  - There is no good evidence that antibiotics prolong the carrier state in *Salmonella* infections
- Advise patient to hydrate with glucose-containing, caffeine-free beverages, and to avoid lactose, sorbitol-containing gum, and raw fruit until symptoms subside

44. Diarrhea - Chronic

Chronic diarrhea is defined as increased volume bowel movements persisting for more than 4 weeks. Mechanisms of diarrhea are categorized as increased secretion, decreased absorption, osmotic diarrhea, or abnormal intestinal motility. Many patients mistakenly identify increased frequency or decreased consistency of bowel movements as diarrhea, so the clinician should be certain to identify whether the patient indeed suffers from diarrhea.

Differential Diagnosis

- Diarrhea due to deranged motility presents with alternating diarrhea and constipation, bloating, mucus or blood in the stool, relief of abdominal pain upon defecation, worsening diarrhea with stress
  - IBS: Usually presents in the morning, seldom at night; more common in women; rectal urgency
  - Diabetic neuropathy: Uncontrolled, explosive, postprandial diarrhea; usually seen in patients with neurologic dysfunction and uncontrolled blood sugar
  - Hyperthyroidism
  - Postileal resection
  - Scleroderma
  - Carcinoid syndrome: Diaphoresis and diarrhea
- Secretory diarrhea will persist even after a 48–72 hour fast; stool osmotic gap <50
  - Bacterial gastroenteritis
  - Bile acid malabsorption
  - Colitis
  - Hyperthyroidism
  - Collagen vascular diseases (SLE, MCTD, scleroderma)
  - Neuroendocrine tumors (e.g., VIPoma, gastrinoma, carcinoid)
- Osmotic diarrhea will cease upon fasting; stool osmotic gap >100 mOsm/kg
  - Malabsorption (celiac sprue, nontropical sprue, Whipple's disease)
  - Nonabsorbable substances (e.g., laxatives, lactose, magnesium)
- Inflammatory diarrhea presents with blood and mucus in the stools, urgency, fevers
  - Inflammatory bowel disease
  - Behçet syndrome
  - Invasive bacterial disease (*Campylobacter jejuni*)
  - Intestinal neoplasm

Workup and Diagnosis

- History should include appearance of bowel movements (e.g., bloody, mucusy, greasy, color, consistency), recent travel history, associated symptoms (e.g., abdominal pain), and timing
- Physical examination
  - Blood pressure and pulses, including orthostatics
  - Abdominal, back, genital, and rectal examinations
  - Skin examination (e.g., jaundice, turgor)
  - Signs of dehydration (e.g., loss of jugular pulsations, dry mucous membranes, tenting, orthostatics)
- Stool examination
  - Blood suggests an inflammatory process
  - WBCs suggest an inflammatory or infectious process
  - 72-hour stool collection for fecal fat with Sudan stain will diagnose malabsorption or oil-containing laxatives
  - Stool electrolytes should be measured to calculate stool osmolality $[2(K^+ + Na^+)]$ and osmotic gap [calculated stool osmolality $- 300 \times$ (normal stool osmolality)]
  - Stool culture (including culture for parasites) is indicated if infectious causes are suspected
  - Stool pH
- Initial lab tests may include CBC, electrolytes, LFTs, BUN/creatinine, calcium, glucose, urinalysis, and TSH
- Endoscopy (flexible sigmoidoscopy, colonoscopy with biopsy, or EGD for small bowel biopsy)
- Breath hydrogen test for lactose intolerance
- Abdominal CT, small bowel series, and/or barium enema may be indicated

Treatment

- Fluid resuscitation: Oral, if possible, or IV (e.g., normal saline or lactated Ringer's)
- Nonspecific antidiarrheal agents (e.g., loperamide, codeine, tincture of opium) and fiber supplementation may be attempted initially
- Diabetic neuropathy: Control blood sugar, metoclopramide may be used
- Irritable bowel syndrome: High-fiber diet, anticholinergics
- Inflammatory bowel disease is treated with steroids for acute exacerbations and daily prophylactic therapy with 5-aminosalicylic agents
  - Bowel resection may be necessary
- Lactose intolerance: Lactose-free diet
- Diseases of malabsorption: Gluten-free diet, long-term antibiotics
- Intestinal neoplasm: Consultation with gastroenterology, oncology, and/or surgery

45. Diplopia

Diplopia, or double vision, is a common ophthalmologic complaint. Diplopia may be horizontal, vertical, or diagonal. It occurs secondary to paralysis, paresis, and/or restriction of the extraocular muscles. Most cases are binocular, due to misalignment of the two eyes. Monocular diplopia is rarely a "true" diplopia; rather, it is a "ghosting" or superposition of images. True monocular diplopia is caused by very rare CNS lesions. Note that diplopia may be the presenting symptom for life-threatening conditions (e.g., aneurysm, CVA). As a rule of thumb, a pupillary abnormality suggests more severe pathology.

Differential Diagnosis

Binocular diplopia
- Decompensated phoria (ocular deviation)
- Third nerve palsy (vertical and horizontal diplopia)
  - Compressive lesions (especially if pupil is involved), including aneurysm, cavernous sinus or orbit tumor, pituitary apoplexy, and uncal herniation
  - Ischemic microvascular disease (e.g., diabetes mellitus, hypertension)
  - Midbrain infarct
  - Giant cell arteritis
  - Herpes zoster
  - Leukemia
  - Meningitis
  - Subarachnoid hemorrhage
  - Ophthalmoplegic migraine
  - Trauma
- Fourth nerve palsy (vertical diplopia): Etiologies include trauma, ischemic microvascular disease, congenital, multiple sclerosis, and other causes as above
- Sixth nerve palsy (horizontal diplopia): Etiologies include ischemic microvascular disease, trauma, increased ICP (bilateral palsy), tumor, multiple sclerosis, post-LP, sarcoidosis/vasculitis, pontine infarct, and other causes as above
- Myasthenia gravis
- Orbital disease (e.g., Graves' orbitopathy, orbital inflammation, tumor)
- Cavernous sinus or superior orbital fissure syndrome (multiple CN involvement)
- Postocular surgery
- Trauma
- Brown's syndrome (restriction of superior oblique tendon)
- Internuclear ophthalmoplegia (MS, CVA)
- Vertebrobasilar insufficiency (vertigo)
- Botulism

Monocular diplopia
- Refractive error (high astigmatism)
- Corneal opacity or irregularity
- Cataract
- Dislocated lens or lens implant
- Extrapupillary openings
- Macular disease
- Retinal detachment
- Nonphysiologic

Workup and Diagnosis

- History, neurologic, and ocular examinations
  - Note onset, duration, associated symptoms (e.g., eye or orbit pain, headache, erythema), trauma, and past history (e.g., diabetes, HTN, CVA, infection, thyroid disease)
  - Complete neurological exam: Note focal neurological deficits, cranial nerve involvement, cerebellar signs, and symptoms of demyelination (e.g., abnormal Romberg)
  - Ocular exam: Vision, pupil size and reaction, eye motility ductions and versions, ptosis, fundus exam (optic nerve edema or pallor), visual field defect, proptosis, and ice test (myasthenia gravis)
- Consider ophthalmology consultation
- If suspect CNS lesion, MRI is usually the test of choice
- If suspect orbital etiology (e.g., trauma, thyroid), CT is usually superior
- MRI/MRA (and/or angiography) is indicated immediately in cases of pupil-involving third nerve palsy, if age <50 (to rule out demyelinating disease), if no improvement over 3 months, aberrant regeneration, multiple cranial nerve or systemic neurologic involvement exists
- Further testing may include Tensilon test and acetyl-cholinesterase receptor antibodies to rule out myasthenia gravis, fasting blood glucose and HgbA1C to rule out diabetes, ESR or CRP to rule out giant cell arteritis (urgent temporal artery biopsy is indicated if arteritis is strongly suspected), thyroid function tests and orbital ultrasound or CT for Graves' orbitopathy
- Lumbar puncture may be necessary (after head CT is done, to rule out increased intracranial pressure)

Treatment

- Treat the underlying etiology
- Patch one eye (usually the involved eye) as necessary
  - In children <10 years old, avoid patching and monitor for development of amblyopia
- Document magnitude of ocular deviation and/or diplopia to determine improvement or stability between exams (measured with prisms by ophthalmologist)
- Prisms in glasses for small stable deviations
- Strabismus surgery for symptomatic diplopia in primary and reading positions if deviation is stable for more than 6 months, for manifest head tilt, or for improving appearance

46. Displaced PMI

The normal point of maximal impulse, or PMI, should be routinely palpated in all patients during a cardiac examination. The normal PMI lies in the left midclavicular line between the fourth and fifth ribs, and normally is no more than 2–3 centimeters in diameter. In the normal heart, the PMI represents the apical impulse of the left ventricle. Displacement of the PMI gives clues to the presence of abnormalities of the heart and, when coupled with inspection and auscultation, assists in correct diagnosis.

Differential Diagnosis

- Left ventricular hypertrophy
  - PMI is enlarged
- Left ventricular enlargement
  - Inferolateral displacement of PMI
  - Seen in aortic regurgitation, mitral regurgitation, and dilated cardiomyopathy
- Right ventricular dilation
  - Lateral displacement of PMI
  - Seen in CHF
- Right-sided tension pneumothorax
  - Lateral displacement of PMI
- Massive pleural effusion
  - Lateral displacement of PMI
- Left ventricular aneurysm
  - Inferolateral displacement of PMI
- Aortic aneurysm
  - Pulsation of right second intercostal space
- Right ventricular hypertrophy
  - Epigastric, subxyphoid pulsations
  - Right ventricular heave
- Dilated pulmonary artery
  - Pulsation over left second and third intercostal space

Workup and Diagnosis

- History and physical examination
  - Dyspnea suggests CHF, pleural effusion, pulmonary hypertension, or pneumothorax
  - Orthopnea and lower extremity edema suggest CHF
  - Chest pain (coronary artery disease, pulmonary embolism, aortic dissection)
  - Decreased exercise tolerance (CHF, pulmonary hypertension, right heart failure)
  - Elevated JVP (CHF, right heart failure)
  - Rales (CHF)
  - Decreased BS, dullness to percussion (pleural effusion)
  - Hyperresonance (pneumothorax)
- Chest X-ray is helpful in diagnosis of CHF, pleural effusion, pneumothorax
- Echocardiogram to assess chamber size, wall thickness, ventricular function, presence/absence of apical aneurysm, and indirect measurement of PA pressure
- CT, MRI, and/or transesophageal echocardiogram for aortic aneurysm/dissection

Treatment

- Left ventricular hypertrophy: Mainstay of therapy is blood pressure control
- Tension pneumothorax: Needle decompression, chest tube
- Pleural effusion: Thoracentesis or observation and diuretics
- Right heart failure: Treat underlying etiology (e.g., hypoxia, pulmonary hypertension); diuretics only for symptomatic relief of lower extremity edema
- Aortic aneurysm: Surgical correction if symptomatic, abdominal aneurysm >5 cm, thoracic aneurysm >6 cm (>5.5 cm in Marfan's syndrome), rapidly expanding (>0.5 cm/year), or thrombotic/embolic complications

47. Dizziness/Lightheadedness & Vertigo

Dizziness/lightheadedness, a sensation of nearly losing consciousness, must be distinguished from vertigo, a sense of impulsion (spinning), either of the environment or of the patient. Dizziness/lightheadedness usually results from a decrease in cerebral blood flow, resulting in momentary attention deficit (lasting milliseconds); vertigo usually occurs due to inner ear pathology. However, both dizziness/lightheadedness and vertigo may occur secondary to primary CNS pathology.

Differential Diagnosis

Dizziness/lightheadedness
- Transiently decreased cerebral blood flow
    - Hyperventilation
    - Vasovagal response
    - Congestive heart failure
    - Aortic stenosis
    - Hypertrophic cardiomyopathy
    - Hemorrhage
    - Dehydration or hypotension
    - Carotid sinus pressure
    - Cerebral artery thrombosis or embolism
    - Cardiac arrhythmia
    - Autonomic dysfunction (e.g., Shy-Drager syndrome)
    - TIA
    - Hypoxemia
    - Anemia
- Primary CNS dysfunction not associated with decreased blood flow
    - Migraine
    - Seizure
    - Severe electrolyte disturbance
    - Elevated intracranial pressure
- Panic attack
- Hyperventilation and/or anxiety
- Ictal aura
- Basilar migraine
- Drug intoxication (e.g., alcohol, sedatives, centrally-acting α-blockers)
- Allergic reactions
- Postconcussion syndrome
- Carbon monoxide poisoning

Vertigo
- Peripheral vertigo (inner ear pathology)
    - Benign positional vertigo (>20% of cases)
    - Ménière's disease
    - Labyrinthine trauma
    - Labyrinthitis (viral)
    - Nonspecific or recurrent vestibulopathy
    - Bilateral vestibular loss
    - Acoustic neuroma
    - Autoimmune inner ear disease
- Central vertigo (CNS pathology)
    - Multiple sclerosis
    - Brainstem tumors
    - Labyrinthine trauma
    - Epileptic vertigo
    - Vertebrobasilar insufficiency
    - Tabes dorsalis
    - Friedreich's ataxia

Workup and Diagnosis

- A complete history and physical exam should include signs of dehydration, questions about excessive pressure on the neck, headaches, palpitations, history of heart disease, hearing loss, cardiac auscultation, orthostatic blood pressures, and complete ENT (including Weber's and Rinne's tests) and neurologic exams (gait)
- Laboratory evaluation may include CBC, electrolytes, calcium, glucose, BUN/creatinine, BNP, ESR, carbon monoxide level, pulse oximetry and/or arterial blood gas, eosinophil count, and stool occult blood testing
- Further testing may include ECG, 24-hour ECG monitoring, echocardiography, electronystagmography, hearing evaluation, head CT, EEG, MRI (head and/or labyrinth) and/or MRA (head or vertebrobasilar circulation)
- Vertigo may be evaluated with several specific maneuvers
    - Dix-Hallpike maneuver: Patient is sitting; rapidly move to supine position with head over back of table; observe for nystagmus (type and duration); repeat with head facing to the left and right (nystagmus that does not fatigue or is vertical is unlikely to be BPV)
    - Barany maneuver (Nylan-Barany maneuver) is similar to the Dix-Hallpike maneuver, but less sensitive

Treatment

- Treat the underlying disorder of lightheadedness
    - Rehydrate patient as necessary
    - Compensate for heart failure with inotropic agents, diuretics, and ACE inhibitors
    - Surgical intervention for valvular incompetence
    - Treat prodromal stroke (TIA) with aspirin or warfarin
    - Carotid endarterectomy for significant carotid stenosis
    - Acute migraine treatment with NSAIDs or triptans (e.g., sumatriptan); prophylaxis with valproate or tricyclic antidepressants;
    - Phenytoin or carbamazepine for seizures and auras
- Vertigo
    - Meclizine and/or reassurance and time are usually sufficient for benign positional vertigo
    - Modified Epley and/or particle repositioning maneuvers for positional symptoms
    - Diuretics and/or surgery for Ménière's disease
    - Central causes require disease-specific therapy

48. Dry Skin (Xerosis)

Xerosis, or dry skin, is extraordinarily common. Simple measures, such as daily emollient use, can make a big difference in patients' lives. More than 99% of cases are benign.

Differential Diagnosis

- Dry skin is a very common problem
  - Low humidity and cold temperatures make winter xerosis and "winter itch" common complaints
  - Mild xerosis can cause impaired skin barrier function and allow irritants and allergens to more easily affect the skin
  - Most common on the legs, but often affecting the entire skin surface
  - Can present with severe pruritus without much evidence of a rash
- Severe xerosis is common in the elderly, and can cause eczema craquelé
  - Patient's legs often have scale that resembles cracked porcelain
  - Secondary erythema and excoriations occur because of the persistent itch
- Ichthyoses vulgaris
  - Very common cause of dry skin
  - A genetic defect in skin barrier function, leading to a higher risk of atopic dermatitis
  - Patients often have hyperlinearity of their palmar skin and xerotic fish scale on their legs
- Many genetic conditions, such as the large family of ichthyoses (including X-linked ichthyoses, Netherton's disease), lead to severely dry skin in association with other systemic manifestations
- Hypothyroidism and hyperthyroidism can also cause marked xerosis and/or itch
- Anemia
- There is an uncommon association between lymphoma and marked xerosis
- HIV
- Sarcoidosis
- Liver and biliary disease, and renal insufficiency, are commonly associated with xerosis and marked pruritus
- Diabetes mellitus
- Medications (e.g., niacinamide)
- Atopic dermatitis

Workup and Diagnosis

- A complete history should be taken that includes social, family, environmental, and exposure history; past medical history; a focused physical examination should also be performed, including thyroid, entire skin surface, and other exam
- Most cases of xerosis are secondary to environmental factors; If the xerosis is very severe or of acute onset, or is associated with intractable pruritus or other systemic symptoms, consider checking a CBC, thyroid function tests, BUN/creatine, and liver function tests
- Young, at-risk patients with severe xerosis, especially of recent onset, may be considered for HIV testing
- If the patient fails to respond to conservative therapy, age-appropriate malignancy screening should be considered

Treatment

- Emollients and humectants should be incorporated into the patient's daily routine; Avoid harsh antibacterial soaps, and avoid long, hot baths or showers; Apply rich creams (e.g. Keri lotion[R], Eucerin[R]) that are fragrance-free and hypoallergenic immediately after bathing and twice daily
- Hydroxyzine and even phototherapy can be helpful to these patients. Bile acid-sequestering medications can help liver patients with xerosis and pruritus
- Topical steroid ointments are sometimes necessary to control the pruritus until the skin barrier function is restored
- Compliance is a problem in xerosis patients who don't want to put greasy or heavy creams on their skin
- Systemic retinoids are sometimes used as adjuvant therapy for patients with certain genetic ichthyoses
- For the rare patient that has an associated malignancy, the xerosis should improve once the malignancy is eradicated

49. Dysarthria

Dysarthria implies poor speech articulation, as opposed to aphasia or impoverished intelligence due to mental retardation or dementia. Pain is not a feature of dysarthria, nor is poor education. Speech and reading comprehension are completely unaffected in pure dysarthria. Speech therapy is an essential part of treatment to prevent aspiration and optimize communication.

Differential Diagnosis

- Neurological causes
  - Lesions of upper motor neurons: Stroke, tumor, abscess, degeneration (e.g., Parkinson's disease); voluntary motor pathways to cranial nerve nuclei 9, 10, and 12 are affected
  - Lesions of lower motor neuron: Brainstem stroke, amyotrophic lateral sclerosis, hypothyroidism, diabetic nerve infarction
  - Lesions of the neuromuscular junction: Myasthenia gravis, prolonged effects of anesthesia, botulism, nerve gas/organophosphate poisoning; all cause oropharyngeal or glossal weakness
  - Lesions of muscle: Polymyositis, dermato-myositis, inherited muscle diseases such as myotonic muscular dystrophy, mitochondrial diseases
- Structural causes
  - Tumors of the lips, tongue, squamous cell epithelium of the vocal cords and oropharynx
  - Polyps or salivary gland dysfunction resulting in xerostomia (dry mouth)
  - Hypoglossal nerve damage due to surgical traction from carotid endarterectomy
- Less common etiologies include glossitis (amyloidosis, hypothyroidism, anaerobic infection), acute dystonic reaction, unrecognized foreign accent, mild cerebral palsy, sedative/anticonvulsant intoxication, poor dentition or ill-fitting dentures, cleft palate

Workup and Diagnosis

- History and physical examination, with focus on past medical history and a comprehensive ENT and neurologic exam
- Upper motor neuron lesions: Cerebral imaging (especially MRI) is indicated to distinguish ischemic from hemorrhagic infarction, and an abscess from a tumor
- Lower motor neuron lesions: MRI is vastly superior to CT; labs may include TSH, glucose tolerance testing, and toxicology screen in patients with suspected metabolic causes or sedative drug intoxication
- EMG with nerve conduction tests is indicated in suspected cases of ALS
- Neuromuscular junction lesions often present with fluctuations of dysarthria; myasthenia gravis antibody testing may be indicated; ECG and telemetry are indicated in various poisonings
- Muscle lesions: Genetic testing for heritable causes; creatine phosphokinase level and EMG testing for acquired causes
- Structural causes: Proper ENT examination with indirect laryngoscopy and MRI of the oropharynx if masses are suspected or palpated

Treatment

- Speech therapy is often necessary to relearn oral movements and communication skills, prevent aspiration, and motivate the patient
- Treat underlying etiologies as necessary
  - ALS does not improve
  - Dysarthria may improve with treatment of diabetes and/or hypothyroidism
  - Myasthenia gravis improves with pyridostigmine and immunosuppression
  - Pralidoxime and atropine for nerve gas poisoning
  - Antitoxin and close ICU observation for botulism
  - Steroids for polymyositis and dermatomyositis
- Surgical intervention may be necessary for structural causes

50. Dysmenorrhea

Dysmenorrhea, or painful menstruation, is one of the most common gynecologic complaints. It is divided into two broad categories: Primary dysmenorrhea refers to severe uterine cramping during ovulatory menses and in the absence of demonstrable pelvic disease; secondary dysmenorrhea is painful menstruation in the presence of underlying pelvic disease (e.g., endometriosis).

Differential Diagnosis

- Primary dysmenorrhea
  - Symptoms develop before age 25
  - Pain occurs with onset of bleeding, then gradually diminishes
- Secondary dysmenorrhea
  - Endometriosis (uterosacral ligament nodules, severe dysmenorrhea)
  - Adenomyosis (enlarged uterus, menorrhagia, age 40–50, parous)
  - Acute PID (acute adnexal and cervical motion tenderness, fever, discharge, and/or new-onset dysmenorrhea)
  - Chronic PID (due to scarring)
  - Uterine leiomyoma/fibroids (enlarged, mobile uterus, menorrhagia)
  - Ovarian cysts (new dysmenorrhea, unilateral fullness)
- Mental health issues
  - Somatization
  - Substance abuse
  - Depression
  - Sexual abuse
- Extrapelvic disorders
  - Irritable bowel syndrome
  - Appendicitis
  - Urinary tract infection
  - Inflammatory bowel disease
  - Diverticulitis
  - Cholecystitis
- Fibromyalgia
- Malformations of the müllerian ducts
- Interstitial cystitis
- Intestinal or uteropelvic junction obstruction
- Malignancy (e.g., uterine, ovarian)
- Ectopic pregnancy

Workup and Diagnosis

- History, physical, pelvic, and rectal examination will often identify the diagnosis
- Patients unresponsive to an initial trial of NSAIDs and oral contraceptives may have pelvic pathology (secondary dysmenorrhea)
- Initial labs include CBC, urinalysis, β-hCG, wet mount, KOH prep, and gonorrhea and *Chlamydia* cultures, which may uncover pathology associated with secondary dysmenorrhea
- Abdominal and/or vaginal (with vaginal probe) ultrasound may be used to detect pelvic masses (e.g., ovarian cysts, uterine leiomyoma)
- Hysterosonogram if intrauterine pathology is suspected
- Hysteroscopy should follow abnormal hysterosonogram
- Abdominal and/or pelvic CT scan will evaluate gynecologic and abdominal pathology
- Laparoscopy may be both diagnostic and therapeutic
- Culdocentesis may be indicated if ruptured ectopic pregnancy is suspected; however, rarely used today, because of the advent of ultrasound

Treatment

- Primary dysmenorrhea is initially treated with NSAIDs
  - High-dose ibuprofen may be administered beginning the day before the onset of menses
  - Oral contraceptives with or without NSAIDs may be effective when NSAIDs alone are inadequate
  - Low-fat vegetarian diet, a fish oil supplement, and vitamin E may reduce pain severity
- Patients unresponsive to NSAIDs and oral contraceptives should be evaluated for pelvic pathology (secondary dysmenorrhea)
  - Endometriosis: GnRH analogs, danazol; laparoscopy in severe cases; treat infertility if necessary
  - Adenomyosis: Hysterectomy is treatment of choice
  - Leiomyoma: Removal, embolization, hysterectomy
  - Pelvic inflammatory disease: Antibiotics, oral contraceptives (to prevent ectopic pregnancy), treat infertility if necessary
  - Treat depression and/or anxiety as necessary

51. Dyspareunia

Dyspareunia is defined as painful and/or difficult sexual intercourse. There is a large differential requiring detailed history and physical exam. Distinguish primary dyspareunia (dyspareunia occurs from the outset of sexual experience) from secondary dyspareunia (dyspareunia was preceded by painless intercourse).

Differential Diagnosis

- Definitions
  - Sexual pain disorder: Persistent or recurrent genital pain of nonorganic cause associated with sexual stimulation, thus causing personal stress; subcategories include dyspareunia and vaginismus
  - Superficial dyspareunia: Pain or dysfunction felt upon initial penetration
  - Deep dyspareunia: Pain or dysfunction felt deep within the pelvis during intercourse
  - Vaginismus: Painful involuntary spasm of the vagina, preventing intercourse
  - Vulvar vestibulitis: A chronic and persistent clinical syndrome characterized by severe pain with vestibular touch or attempted vaginal entry, tenderness in response to pressure within the vulvar vestibule, and physical findings confined to various degrees of vestibular erythema
  - Vulvodynia: Chronic vulvar discomfort (e.g. burning, stinging, irritation, rawness)
- Neurologic etiologies: Nerve damage or infection, dysesthetic (essential) vulvodynia
- Gynecologic etiologies: Gynecologic tumors (e.g., vulvar, cervical, uterine, ovarian, or rectal cancer; fibroids), Bartholin's gland inflammation
- GI: Constipation, irritable bowel syndrome, colitis, diverticulitis, GI tumors (in pelvis)
- Urinary: Interstitial cystitis, urethritis, urethral diverticulum
- Infectious: Endometritis, vaginitis, PID, salpingitis, vulvovaginitis, herpes genitalis, post-herpetic neuralgia, Bartholin's abscess
- Dermatologic etiologies: Vaginal atrophy, lichen sclerosis, Behçet syndrome, contact dermatitis
- Musculoskeletal: Pelvic floor myopathy, fibromyalgia, levator ani myalgia, dysfunctional vaginismus
- Endocrine: Estrogen deficiency, endometriosis
- Psychiatric: Female sexual dysfunction(s)
- Iatrogenic: Surgical (e.g., pelvic adhesions, episiotomy, strictures), pharmacologic (drying soaps or agents, topical medications, OCPs)
- Trauma: Vaginal lacerations or ecchymoses
- Primary pain disorder
- Severely retroverted uterus
- Imperforate hymen

Workup and Diagnosis

- History and physical examination with pelvic and rectal exams
  - Timing: Onset (e.g., upon entry, after intercourse), duration, persistence after intercourse, prior occurrence(s)
  - Associations: Symptoms may occur with all vaginal or vulvar contact, with intercourse only, with exams only, with masturbation, or with memories or recollections of prior occurrences or traumatic experiences
  - Alleviating and aggregating factors during intercourse
  - Qualifiers: Burning, sharp, dull, aching, throbbing, stabbing
  - Old medical records may be of crucial importance
  - Include complete psychiatric history and exam
- Cervical and/or vulvar cultures and microscopic evaluation of normal saline and potassium hydroxide wet mounts should be done
- Imaging studies may be indicated, including pelvic and/or abdominal ultrasound and/or CT scan
- Management of psychiatric causes is particularly challenging and requires specific and specialized therapy
- Consider gynecology and/or psychiatry consult

Treatment

- Treatment varies depending on etiology
- Infections require appropriate antimicrobials
- Steroids or topical treatment may be indicated for dermatologic causes
- Topical treatments or oral hormone replacement may be indicated for endocrine-related causes
- Psychological causes may require counseling with behavioral feedback and/or pharmacological treatment
- Symptoms refractory to initial treatment of proper duration require prompt reconsideration and further workup
- Referral may be necessary for specialized cases or cases with psychiatric components

52. Dysphagia

Dysphagia refers to difficulty in swallowing (distinguish from odynophagia, which refers to painful swallowing). Pathologies that affect voluntary skeletal muscle generally exhibit as difficulty initiating swallowing; if involuntary smooth muscle of the esophagus is affected, sensation of incomplete swallowing tends to occur.

Differential Diagnosis

- Intrinsic esophageal lesions
  - Gastric acid reflux
  - Esophageal webs and rings
  - Radiation-induced inflammation and stricture formation
  - Trauma
  - Esophageal perforation
  - Diverticula
  - Malignancy
  - Postsurgical
  - Foreign body retention
- Extrinsic lesions
  - Anterior cervical osteophyte
  - Mediastinal mass (e.g., thymoma, teratoma, lymphoma, carotid/aortic aneurysm)
  - Post-thoracic surgery or anterior cervical discectomy
  - Enlarged thyroid
  - Thyroglossal duct cyst
- Aberrant motility
  - Hypertensive lower esophageal sphincter
  - Nutcracker esophagus
  - Scleroderma
  - Achalasia
  - Diffuse esophageal spasm (DES)
- Neurological causes
  - Myopathies (e.g., polymyositis, inherited)
  - Neuromuscular junction disorders (e.g., myasthenia gravis, botulism)
  - Polyneuropathies (e.g., diabetic, Guillain-Barré syndrome, toxin-related)
  - Brainstem stroke
  - ALS
- Less common etiologies ("zebras") include globus hystericus (psychogenic dysphagia), anxiety disorders, hypothyroidism, amyloidosis, dysphagia lusoria (extrinsic esophageal compression due to aortic arch anomalies), left atrial enlargement, and Chagas' disease

Workup and Diagnosis

- History and physical examination
  - History should include onset, duration, and severity; dysphagia with liquid versus solids; past medical history, including anxiety and other psychiatric illnesses; prior dysphagia or caustic substance exposure; and other head and neck problems
  - Exam should include a thorough head, nose, mouth, neck/thyroid, and abdominal examination, and observation of the patient swallowing
- Oropharyngeal dysphagia: Difficulty initiating swallowing
  - Barium swallow will identify area of swallowing lesion (usually done by speech therapist)
  - EMG/nerve conduction tests to rule out neurologic causes (e.g., myasthenia gravis, ALS)
  - Elevated CPK level suggests muscle disease
  - Brain MRI if CVA is suspected
- Esophageal dysphagia: Sensation of food sticking seconds after initiating swallowing
  - Solids: Barium swallow is less invasive than endoscopy and is frequently sufficient for diagnosis
  - Liquids and/or solids: Esophageal manometry and barium swallow visualization (scleroderma, DES)
- In general, endoscopy and biopsy by a trained gastroenterologist (or surgeon) is necessary for suspected cancer and various therapeutic interventions

Treatment

- Acute mechanical obstructions require urgent endoscopy to relieve the obstruction and prevent potential perforation
- Dysphagia with gastroesophageal reflux disease can be minimized with promotility agents or proton pump inhibitors, weight loss, and avoiding offending foods
- Chronic mechanical obstruction from webs, rings, and strictures require endoscopic treatment or thoracic surgery; balloon dilation may be considered
- Lower esophageal spasm may improve with anticholinergic antispasmodics or the injection of botulinum toxin
- Polymyositis: Glucocorticoids.
- Myasthenia gravis: Muscarinic agents (pyridostigmine), glucocorticoids
- ALS, stroke: Speech therapy evaluation, anticholinergics to prevent saliva aspiration

53. Dyspnea

Dyspnea is defined as an abnormally uncomfortable awareness of breathing. It is one of the cardinal symptoms of cardiac and pulmonary disease, but may also result from abnormalities of the chest wall, neurologic disorders, and anxiety. A complete history and physical exam focused on the chest, abdomen, and cardiovascular and pulmonary systems are generally sufficient to narrow the differential, which can be further refined with an appropriate diagnostic and laboratory evaluation.

Differential Diagnosis

- Asthma
  - Classic triad of chronic cough, dyspnea, and wheezing
- COPD; chronic bronchitis
- Pulmonary edema (acute or chronic)
  - Cardiogenic pulmonary edema: LV failure (e.g., MI, cardiomyopathy), valve disease, high-output states (e.g., thyrotoxicosis), volume overload, hypertensive emergency
  - Noncardiac pulmonary edema: Sepsis, inhalation injury, drugs (e.g., narcotics), renal failure, high altitude, aspiration, pancreatitis, seizure, trauma, emboli (fat, air, amniotic fluid), CNS injury, airway obstruction (e.g., croup, foreign body)
- Coronary artery disease
  - May present without chest pain ("anginal equivalent")
- Pneumonia
- Pleural effusion
  - Common causes: CHF, pneumonia, cancer, pulmonary embolus, connective tissue disease (e.g., SLE, rheumatoid arthritis), pancreatitis, and renal or liver disease
- Pulmonary embolism
  - Risk factors (Virchow's triad) present in 90% of cases: Venous stasis (e.g., immobility, pedal edema), endothelial damage (e.g., recent trauma or surgery, burns, indwelling catheters, IV drug use), hypercoagulability (e.g., malignancy, obesity, pregnancy, HRT/OCP)
- Pneumothorax
- Interstitial lung disease
  - A group of disorders characterized by inflammation and fibrosis of alveolar walls and the interstitium
- Pulmonary hypertension
  - Primary pulmonary HTN: No identifiable cause
  - Secondary pulmonary HTN: Due to underlying disease (e.g., mitral stenosis, PE, COPD)
- Less common etiologies ("zebras") include pericardial disease, chest wall abnormality, tracheal obstruction, neuromuscular diseases, and psychogenic

Workup and Diagnosis

- Thorough history and physical exam
  - Note onset (sudden or chronic, progressive)
  - Timing (persistent or intermittent)
  - Associated symptoms (e.g., chest discomfort, syncope)
- Initial laboratory studies should include CBC, BUN/creatinine, calcium, electrolytes, thyroid function tests, pulse oximetry (resting, ambulatory, and nocturnal), and chest X-ray
- ABG will identify barriers to oxygen diffusion (increased A-a gradient), hypoxemia, and chronic hypercapnia
- ECG may reveal evidence of MI, right ventricular strain (e.g., due to PE, pulmonary hypertension), dysrhythmias, and/or bundle branch block
- Pulmonary function tests are indicated to identify restrictive or obstructive disease and barriers to diffusion
- BNP may be useful, if the etiology is uncertain, to distinguish CHF from other causes of dyspnea
- Echocardiogram to establish a diagnosis of structural heart disease, LV dysfunction, or elevated PA pressure
- Chest CT scan, V/Q scan, and/or lower extremity dopplers if PE is suspected
- Sputum culture and blood cultures may be necessary in cases of pneumonia

Treatment

- Attention to airway, breathing, and circulation
- Administer supplemental O_2 as needed
- Asthma: Avoid triggers; bronchodilation with inhaled β_2 agonists (e.g., albuterol) and anticholinergics (e.g., ipratropium); inhaled, oral, and/or IV steroids
- COPD: Inhaled bronchodilators (e.g., albuterol, ipratropium); systemic corticosteroids; antibiotics (e.g., azithromycin, doxycycline) in severe exacerbations; mechanical ventilation (CPAP or BiPAP)
- Cardiogenic pulmonary edema: Vasodilators (e.g., IV nitroglycerin, ACE inhibitors), loop diuretics (e.g., IV furosemide), morphine, digoxin, and/or inotropes
- Noncardiogenic edema generally requires only supportive care; treat underlying etiology (e.g., surgical correction of valvular lesions)
- Pleural effusion: Address underlying cause; diagnostic or therapeutic thoracentesis may be indicated; pleurodesis for recurrent effusions
- Pneumothorax: 100% O_2 accelerates resorption

54. Dysuria

Dysuria is a painful or burning sensation during or immediately after urination. This is a common symptom in primary care; nearly 20% of women aged 20–55 will have one episode of dysuria per year. Women have episodes of acute dysuria much more frequently than men. The most common cause of dysuria in adult women is lower urinary tract infection.

Differential Diagnosis

- Lower urinary tract etiologies (male)
  - Infectious cystitis: *E. coli* (#1 cause), *Staphylococcus saprophyticus, Proteus, Klebsiella, Enterococcus*
  - Acute prostatitis
  - Benign prostatic hypertrophy
  - Epididymitis/urethritis: *Chlamydia,* gonorrhea, *E. coli, staphylococcus aureus*
  - External infections (e.g., herpes)
  - Allergic reaction to contraceptives, soaps, lotions
  - Malignancy (urethral or bladder cancer)
  - Urethral strictures
- Lower urinary tract etiologies (female)
  - Infectious cystitis: *E. coli* (#1 cause), *Staphylococcus saprophyticus, Proteus, Klebsiella, Enterococcus*
  - Acute urethritis: *Chlamydia,* gonorrhea
  - Vaginitis: *Candida,* herpes
  - Atrophic vaginitis
  - Allergic reaction to contraceptives, soaps, lotions
  - Malignancy: Urethral cancer, bladder cancer
  - Urethral strictures
  - Vaginitis (*Trichomonas,* bacterial vaginosis)
- Upper urinary tract etiologies
  - Pyelonephritis: Fever, chills, nausea, vomiting, and CVA tenderness
  - Urolithiasis: Acute onset of dysuria with associated flank pain, with or without hematuria
- Reiter's syndrome
  - Genital ulcers, conjunctivitis, and arthritis
- Noninfectious cystitis (e.g., drugs, radiation, granulomatous, allergic)
- Behçet syndrome
  - Oral and genital ulcers, arthritis, and uveitis
- Trauma
- Rectal fissure
- Psychogenic (e.g., conversion disorder)

Workup and Diagnosis

- History and physical examination
- Male genital exam with gonorrhea/chlamydia test, culture, Gram stain
  - Tender, boggy, swollen prostate suggests prostatitis (avoid prostatic massage, because of risk of bacteremia)
  - Tender epididymitis and testicles suggest infection
  - Generally enlarged prostate associated with nocturia and increasing frequency suggests BPH
- Female genital exam with KOH prep, wet mount, Gram stain, and DNA tests/culture as indicated
  - Thin, papery vaginal tissue suggests atrophic vaginitis
  - *Candida* discharge is thick, cheesy, and white; pruritic
  - *Chlamydia* discharge is scant, watery and gradual onset
  - Gonorrhea discharge is profuse, yellow-green with abrupt onset, intracellular gram-negative diplococci
  - Bacterial vaginosis discharge is pruritic, with clue cells on wet mount and a fishy odor with KOH (whiff test)
  - *Trichomonas* discharge is frothy, grey-green, with pruritis and mobile organisms on wet mount
- Urinalysis should be done in all patients
  - Hematuria suggests urolithiasis, pyelonephritis, or cystitis; painless hematuria suggests bladder cancer
  - Positive nitrites, leukocyte esterase, or WBCs with suprapubic tenderness suggests uncomplicated cystitis
- Urine culture is indicated if positive urinalysis and in pregnant women, diabetic or immunocompromised patients, or males with urethral discharge

Treatment

- Cystitis/prostatitis: Appropriate antibiotics
  - Begin with empiric therapy and adjust to sensitivities
  - Noninfectious cystitis: Remove offending medications or allergens if possible
- Pyelonephritis: Outpatient antibiotic treatment in patients who tolerate liquids and have no significant co-morbidities; otherwise, admit for IV hydration and antibiotics
- Urolithiasis: Hydration, pain control while attempting to pass stones; urology referral if stones will not pass
- Atrophic vaginitis: Consider estrogen creams or systemic replacement if other symptoms
- BPH: Symptomatic relief with α-blockers, 5α-reductase inhibitors, or saw palmetto extract
- Sexually transmitted diseases
  - Treat specific etiology and screen for coexistent STDs (e.g., HIV, hepatitis B)

55. Ear Pain

Ear pain is an extremely common presenting complaint in both primary care and otolaryngology practices. The description of the onset, character, and location of pain, along with a careful physical examination, identify most common causes of ear pain. Otitis media (infection/inflammation of the inner ear) and otitis externa (infection/inflammation of the ear canal) cause most ear pain. The vast majority of otitis media cases are caused by viruses; thus, deciding when to use antibiotics is a common medical issue.

Differential Diagnosis

- Otitis media
  - Most cases are of viral origin
  - Red tympanic membrane with decreased mobility
  - Male > female; peak incidence 6–18 months
  - Risk factors include day care, supine bottle feeding, smoking in household, siblings with otitis media, anatomic abnormalities (e.g., Down's syndrome)
- Eustachian tube dysfunction
  - Common in young children
- Otitis externa
  - Pain upon movement of tragus
- Malignant (necrotizing) otitis externa
  - Usually due to *Pseudomonas*
  - Mostly seen in diabetics
- Referred pain
  - TMJ: May result in ear pain, jaw pain, neck pain, and/or headache
  - Dental infection, trauma, or orthodontic intervention (e.g., tightening of braces)
  - Pharyngitis or tonsillitis
  - Post-tonsillectomy/adenoidectomy
  - Retropharyngeal abscess and other ENT deep-space infections
  - Cervical adenitis
  - Sinusitis/rhinitis
  - Laryngitis
  - Trigeminal neuralgia
  - Esophagitis
  - Cervical spine arthritis
  - Parotiditis/sialoadenitis (including mumps)
  - Angina/acute coronary syndrome
- Foreign body in ear canal (including impacted cerumen)
- Reaction to topical agents
- Trauma: Laceration, abrasion, barotrauma (e.g., deep sea diving, airplane)
- Cellulitis
- Tympanostomy tube obstruction
- Myringitis bullosa
- Furunculosis (localized abscess)
- Varicella or herpes simplex/zoster infection in the ear canal
- Mastoiditis
  - Ear protrudes anteriorly
- Tumor
- Eczema/psoriasis
- Mumps

Workup and Diagnosis

- History and physical examination, including otoscopic exam with pneumatic otoscopy and complete head and neck examination
  - Pain upon traction of pinna suggests otitis externa (hyperemic external canal)
  - Bulging, red, immobile tympanic membrane is consistent with acute otitis media (with or without otorrhea secondary to perforation)
  - Retracted, immobile tympanic membrane may be seen in serous otitis media
  - Mass lesion behind tympanic membrane suggests cholesteotoma or tumor
  - Tonsillar asymmetry or uvular deviation suggests peritonsillar abscess or mass
- Tympanometry may reveal otitis media with effusion, eustachian tube dysfunction, or tympanostomy tube obstruction
- Audiometry to evaluate for hearing loss
- Consider culture of otorrhea if perforation (not canal) or complicated (e.g., recurrent infection, spread of infection such as meningitis or mastoiditis)
- Lateral neck X-ray will diagnose retropharyngeal mass or abscess
- Head CT is indicated if intracranial lesion or basilar skull fracture is suspected
- Consider CBC and ESR if suspect malignant necrotizing otitis media
- Check glucose in recurrent severe otitis externa

Treatment

- If patient is in distress, immediately stabilize airway, breathing, and circulation
- Pain control with acetaminophen, NSAIDs, warm compress, and topical benzocaine solution
- Otitis media: Most patients with risk factors (e.g., persistent fever, immunocompromise) should be treated with appropriate antibiotics
  - Serous otitis media that persists for >3 months may require a course of corticosteroids or myringotomy
- Otitis externa: 8% aluminum acetate ± 2% acetic acid (especially eczematous otitis externa), antibiotics, steroid drops
- Malignant otitis externa: IV antipseudomonal or antistaphylococcal antibiotics
- Cerumen and foreign bodies: Remove with a curette
- Pharyngitis/tonsillitis: Appropriate antibiotics
- Barotrauma: Pinch nose, then exhale with mouth closed to equalize pressure; decongestants
- TMJ: NSAIDs, physical therapy, dental bite adjustment

56. Elbow Pain/Swelling

The elbow joint is formed by the radius, ulna, and distal humerus. Trauma is a common cause of injury. Injuries frequently result from falling on an outstretched hand and may be associated with nerve injuries (axillary, radial, ulnar, and/or median nerves); furthermore, the elbow is the third most commonly dislocated large joint, with posterior dislocation most common.

Differential Diagnosis

- Trauma
- Fracture
  - Radial head fracture is most common: Usually due to a fall on an outstretched arm, resulting in pain with supination
  - Olecranon fracture: Pain with extension
  - Distal humerus fractures are less common
- Dislocation
  - Nursemaid's elbow (subluxation of the radial head) occurs in young children who were pulled by an outstretched arm; children will refuse to move the arm
  - In adults, dislocations generally occur secondary to falling on an outstretched arm; 80% are associated with an olecranon fracture
- Bursitis: Due to trauma, inflammation, infection
- Epicondylitis
  - Degeneration of the tendinous insertion at the lateral or medial epicondyles
  - Lateral epicondylitis ("tennis elbow"): Due to extensor muscle overuse (results in pain with pronation and wrist dorsiflexion)
  - Medial epicondylitis ("golfer's elbow"): Due to flexor muscle overuse (results in decreased grip strength and pain with pronation or wrist flexion)
- Ulnar nerve entrapment
  - Usually in the groove of the posterior aspect of the medial epicondyle
  - Occurs acutely after direct trauma or with prolonged pressure or overuse
  - Causes acute medial aching with numbness and tingling in fourth and fifth digits
- Osteoarthritis
- Rheumatoid arthritis
- Gouty arthritis
- Infection
- Distal biceps tendon rupture
- Pronator syndrome
  - Median nerve entrapment distal to elbow from racquet or throwing sports
  - Anterior pain and distal paresthesias
  - Pain with resisted pronation
- Radial tunnel syndrome
  - Compression of the radial nerve as it crosses the head of the radius
- Loose body (e.g., bone fragment)

Workup and Diagnosis

- History and physical examination
  - Include careful exam of the hand, wrist, elbow, and shoulder of the affected side
  - Evaluate for pain, paresthesias, bony point tenderness, crepitus on palpation, swelling and ecchymosis, limited range of motion, and neurovascular compromise (e.g., coolness, pallor, loss of distal pulses)
- Standard X-rays include A/P, lateral, and oblique views
- Aspiration may be diagnostic as well as therapeutic for bursitis; send for cultures and crystals
- Occasionally, nerve conduction tests are indicated to evaluate nerve entrapment and/or carpal tunnel syndrome
- Rarely, an MRI is indicated; may be considered if the treatment is not progressing as planned

Treatment

- General principles of fracture management include immobilization, analgesia, NSAIDs, and elevation
- Immediate anatomic reduction is required in cases of neurovascular compromise
- Nondisplaced fractures should be immobilized with the elbow flexed at 90°
- Displaced or intra-articular fractures usually require open reduction with internal fixation
- Joint aspiration may relieve pain if effusion is present
- Epicondylitis is treated with rest, NSAIDs, and physical therapy
- Elbow dislocation requires reduction followed by splint immobilization
- Splinting may be beneficial
- Reduction of a subluxed radial head (nursemaid's elbow) is performed by placing the thumb over the radial head while supinating, then flexing, the forearm

57. Epistaxis

Bilateral or posterior nasal epistaxis (nosebleed) suggests a medical etiology; unilateral epistaxis suggests a physical cause or local structural abnormality. Because the nose protrudes from the face, trauma is a common etiology. Further, the thin mucosal surface often becomes dry and cracked, exposing the rich blood supply beneath. The majority of bleeds originate from irritation to the anterior aspect of the nasal septum, Kiesselbach's area (seen easily with nasal speculum, the "picking zone").

Differential Diagnosis

- Bilateral or posterior nasal epistaxis usually indicates a medical etiology
  - Bleeding disorder (e.g., leukemias, aplastic anemia, thrombocytopenia, von Willebrand's disease, hemophilia, liver failure)
  - Clotting disorders (e.g., liver failure, snake bite, infection, DIC)
  - Trauma (e.g., facial fracture)
  - Ectopic menstruation due to endometriosis
  - Hypertension (usually severe)
- Unilateral or anterior epistaxis usually indicates a physical cause or local structural abnormality
  - Irritation of the nose due to the common cold is the most common cause
  - Dryness of nasal mucosa (e.g., low humidity)
  - Allergic rhinitis
  - External trauma (e.g., fist fight)
  - Internal trauma (e.g., nose-picking)
  - Foreign body
  - Nasal polyps (often secondary to allergy, aspirin, or cystic fibrosis)
  - Status/post-sinus surgery
  - Bleeding from a sinus is an uncommon presentation of bony fracture from trauma or infection
  - Neoplasm: Most common malignancy is squamous cell carcinoma
  - Telangiectasias (can also be posterior epistaxis)
  - Arteriovenous malformation (can also be posterior epistaxis
- Infection
  - Sinusitis
  - Rhinitis
  - Scarlet fever
  - Malaria
  - Typhoid fever
- Septal deviation or perforation
  - In the presence of nasal perforation without significant trauma, cocaine use should be suspected

Workup and Diagnosis

- History and physical examination
  - History of nasal irritation or trauma, rhinorrhea, allergy symptoms, bleeding of other areas (e.g., gums, hematuria), prior epistaxis, sinus and/or tooth pain, frequency and inciting factors (e.g., dry air), and exposures (e.g., nasal sprays, cocaine)
  - Inspect for evidence of septal perforation or deviation and for the source of bleeding
  - Washing the area with normal saline or 1:1,000 epinephrine may increase visibility
  - Blood seen in the mouth without evident nasal bleeding suggests a posterior bleed
- Labs are only necessary in cases that do not respond to treatment: Include a CBC with platelet count, PT/PTT, and bleeding time
- Occasionally, leukemia or other bone marrow changes may present with epistaxis and/or bleeding from other sites (e.g., gums, urinary tract, rectal bleeding); thus, a bone marrow biopsy may be indicated if the clinical picture suggests one of these conditions
- CT scan of the sinuses and nasal area may be indicated to search for neoplasms of the nasopharynx and sinuses
- Consider biopsy of suspicious areas and/or nasolaryngoscopy, especially in smokers

Treatment

- Resuscitation with IV fluids or possibly blood transfusion may be necessary for severe blood loss
- Tilt head forward to prevent posterior blood drainage
  - Apply continuous pressure by pinching nares together for 5–10 minutes
  - Pressure applied between the upper lip and gum may help in some difficult cases
  - If no improvement, pack nose with vasoconstrictor-soaked gauze and a heavy coat of petroleum jelly for 10 minutes
- If a bleeding vessel is identified (usually on the septal surface), apply silver nitrate to it for 5 seconds
- If a posterior bleed is suspected, apply pressure with specialized nasal balloons and packing or Foley catheter
- Further treatment may be indicated based on etiology
- Vitamin K, fresh frozen plasma, clotting factor replacement, and/or platelet transfusion may be necessary for bleeding disorders
- Consider ENT consult for some cases (e.g., trauma, intractable bleeding, neoplasm)

58. Facial Paralysis & Bell's Palsy

Differentiate supranuclear facial palsy from peripheral (nuclear) facial palsy. Supranuclear palsy involves predominantly the lower part of the face. Emotional responses may be intact (e.g., the patient may not be able to show you his teeth but will smile in response to a joke). Peripheral, or nuclear facial, palsy affects all ipsilateral muscles of facial expression, resulting in paralysis of the entire ipsilateral side. The mouth is pulled at an angle to the normal side and may droop on the affected side, facial creases are effaced, and the eyelid may not close.

Differential Diagnosis

- Bell's palsy (idiopathic facial palsy of lower motor neuron type)
  - Most common cause of facial nerve paralysis
- Lyme disease
- Tumors that invade the temporal bone (e.g., cholesteatoma, carotid body tumor)
- Ramsay Hunt's syndrome
  - Association of facial palsy with herpes zoster eruption in the pharynx and external auditory canal
  - Eighth cranial nerve often affected as well
- Acoustic neuroma
  - May compress the facial nerve
- Pontine lesions
  - Secondary to infarcts, demyelinating processes, or tumors
  - Signs of brainstem involvement may be associated
- Facial diplegia or bilateral facial palsy
  - Guillain-Barré syndrome (associated with ascending areflexic motor paralysis)
  - Heerfordt's syndrome (a form of sarcoidosis; also known as uveoparotid fever)
- Diabetic neuropathy
- Leprosy
- Melkersson-Rosenthal syndrome
  - Recurrent facial palsy, labial edema, and tongue plication
- Sarcoidosis

Workup and Diagnosis

- History and physical examination, with complete ENT and neurologic exams
  - Associated neurologic deficits may occur (e.g., weakness of the arm or leg, aphasia) due to involvement of surrounding brain areas in a vascular event
  - Depending on the site of interruption, the patient may have hyperacusis, a loss of taste over the anterior 2/3 of tongue, deafness, tinnitus, dizziness, or associated brainstem signs
  - Bell's palsy is a clinical diagnosis with testing reserved for atypical presentations or slowly resolving cases; make sure there are no herpetic lesions in the pharynx or external auditory canal; also pay special attention to assessing the eighth cranial nerve, as it courses very close to the facial nerve
- Initial labs may include CBC, glucose, ESR, and Lyme titer
- Head MRI
- In cases of supranuclear palsy, a workup for CVA, demyelinating processes, and/or tumors may be indicated; include CT, MRI, and CSF studies

Treatment

- Bell's palsy
  - IV acyclovir and corticosteroids may lead to better recovery and less neuronal degeneration
  - Tape eye and use eye shade to protect the eye during sleep
  - Massage of weakened muscles
  - Electrical stimulation of paralyzed muscles in cases with delayed recovery
- In other cases, treat the inciting causes (e.g., control of blood pressure and hyperlipidemia in patients with CVA, antibiotics for patients with Lyme disease, antivirals in Ramsay Hunt's syndrome, steroids for sarcoidosis)
- Consider neurologic referral

59. Fatigue

Fatigue is a very common, although nonspecific, presenting symptom that refers to the sensation of exhaustion during or after usual activities, or a feeling of inadequate energy to begin these activities. Fatigue is a difficult clinical complaint because there are many possible explanations. This difficulty is compounded by the subjective nature of the complaint and the potential seriousness of some of the etiologies. A thorough history and physical exam are crucial in narrowing down the differential and identifying serious causes.

Differential Diagnosis

- Infectious
  - Acute viral or bacterial infection
  - Chronic infection (e.g., subacute bacterial endocarditis, osteomyelitis, tuberculosis, HIV, viral hepatitis, mononucleosis)
- Hematologic
  - Anemia
  - Thrombotic thrombocytopenic purpura
  - Polycythemia vera
- Cardiac
  - Congestive heart failure
  - Congenital heart disease
  - Valvular heart disease
  - Coronary artery disease
- Pulmonary
  - COPD
  - Obstructive sleep apnea
  - Poorly controlled asthma
- Endocrine
  - Hypothyroidism/hyperthyroidism
  - Diabetes, types I and II
  - Pregnancy
  - Perimenopause
  - Addison's disease
- Rheumatologic
  - Rheumatoid arthritis
  - Systemic lupus erythematosus
  - Sjögren's syndrome
  - Polymyalgia rheumatica
- Gastrointestinal
  - Inflammatory bowel disease
  - Portal hypertension (e.g., cirrhosis)
- Acute or chronic renal failure
- Neurologic
  - Parkinson's disease
  - Multiple sclerosis
- Psychiatric (e.g., depression, anxiety or panic disorder, anorexia nervosa or bulimia, somatization disorder)
- Malignancy
- Chronic fatigue syndrome
- Fibromyalgia
- Tension headache
- Primary obesity
- Medication side effects (e.g., β-blockers, phenytoin, digitalis, antidepressants, muscle relaxants, hypnotics)
- Drug intoxication or withdrawal (e.g., alcohol, opioids, benzodiazepines, barbiturates, cocaine)

Workup and Diagnosis

- Complete history and physical exam are essential, including screening for malignancy, chronic infection, chronic cardiopulmonary disease, and psychiatric disease
- Initial workup may include CBC, chemistries, glucose, calcium, urinalysis, liver function studies, TSH, stool guaiac, and age-appropriate cancer screening (e.g., PAP smear, mammography, flexible sigmoidoscopy, PSA)
- Further testing based on history and physical findings may include chest X-ray (for dyspnea, cough, abnormal lung exam), ECG (for chest pain, dyspnea), echocardiogram (heart murmur), appropriate cultures and/or serology if infection is suspected (e.g., PPD, HIV, hepatitis), malignancy workup, pregnancy test, ANA, ESR, RF, and Lyme titers
- Further testing based on abnormal initial labs may include anemia workup (reticulocyte count, iron studies, vitamin B_{12} and folate levels, hemoglobin electrophoresis), hepatitis workup (GGTP, viral hepatitis serologies, ultrasound of the liver), renal ultrasound, bone marrow biopsy, colonoscopy, and thyroid function tests
- Appropriate imaging studies based on initial workup may include head CT/MRI, abdominal ultrasound or CT, cardiac stress testing, bone X-rays and/or bone scan

Treatment

- Treatment is targeted at specific underlying medical problems, if determined (e.g., thyroid disease, chronic infection, malignancy)
- Stop or change offending medications
- Consider trial of antidepressant therapy and/or cognitive behavioral psychiatric therapy
- Regularly scheduled physical activity
- Improve sleep hygiene
- Referral to support groups
- Discontinue offending medications
- Chronic fatigue syndrome and fibromyalgia are often treated with supportive care, healthy diet, moderate exercise, and low-dose antidepressants
- Weight loss for obesity

60. Fever

Fever is defined as an elevation of normal body temperature (37°C, or 98.6°F). True fever occurs when the body adopts a new thermoregulatory "set point" secondary to the release of pyrogenic cytokines in response to bacteria, viruses, or other exogenous sources (e.g., malignancy). Hyperthermia, on the other hand, is an elevation of body temperature without resetting of the thermoregulatory mechanism. This occurs when heat production outstrips the body's ability to disperse excess heat.

Differential Diagnosis

- Infection is the most common cause
  - Viral (e.g., influenza, HIV, hepatitis, herpes simplex encephalitis, mononucleosis, adenovirus)
  - Bacterial (e.g., pneumonia, endocarditis, tuberculosis, meningitis, pyelonephritis, appendicitis, cholecystitis, cellulitis)
  - Lyme disease
  - Malaria
  - Syphilis
  - Tularemia
  - Intra-abdominal abscess
- Malignancy
  - Lymphoma (Hodgkin's and non-Hodgkin's)
  - Lymphoproliferative disorders
  - Renal cell carcinoma
  - Leukemia
  - Hepatocellular carcinoma
- Rheumatologic disorders
  - Temporal arteritis/giant cell arteritis
  - Adult-onset Still's disease
  - Systemic lupus erythematosus
  - Sarcoidosis
  - Rheumatoid arthritis
- Drug fever
  - Often temporally associated with the initiation of a new medicine
  - Often associated with a rash (biopsy reveals leukocytoclastic vasculitis)
  - Eosinophilia is common
- Pulmonary embolism
  - Mild fever is often present
  - Other findings of thromboembolic disease (e.g., leg swelling, dyspnea) may be present
- Osteomyelitis
- Occult abscess
- Malignant hypothermia

Workup and Diagnosis

- Complete history and physical examination
  - In most cases, the cause of fever will be suggested during the history and physical
  - Note characteristics of the fever, maximum temperature, presence of diurnal variation, and recent travel
- Initial laboratory studies may include CBC with differential, electrolytes, BUN/creatinine, glucose, calcium, urinalysis, urine cultures, liver function tests, and ESR
- Blood cultures, including thick smear of the blood to evaluate for parasites (e.g., malaria)
- Chest X-ray may reveal focus of infection (e.g., pneumonia, tuberculosis, malignancy)
- Lumbar puncture for CSF analysis may be indicated
- CT scan of chest and abdomen may reveal an occult infection, abscess, or malignancy
- Echocardiogram is indicated if suspect infective endocarditis or aortitis (syphilis)
- Tagged white cell scans may be used to localize abscess
- Bone marrow biopsy may be indicated if leukemia or a myelodysplastic syndrome is suspected

Treatment

- Initial treatment of fever includes antipyretics (e.g., acetaminophen, NSAIDs)
- Infection should be treated with appropriate antimicrobial therapy and tailored as antibiotic sensitivities are identified
  - Many cases of deep-seated infection or abscess require percutaneous or surgical drainage
- Fever due to malignancy will usually regress with surgical debulking, chemotherapy, and/or radiation directed at the primary tumor
- Rheumatologic disorders may require NSAIDs, steroids, methotrexate, hydroxychloroquine, or other cytotoxic agents
- Dantrolene for malignant hypothermia

61. Flank Pain/CVA Tenderness

Pain and/or tenderness on the side of the trunk from the ribs to the ileum is often associated with renal disease; however, nonrenal etiologies are very common. Of course, renal disease should be strongly suspected in the case of costovertebral angle tenderness and concurrent urinary complaints.

Differential Diagnosis

- Degenerative disk disease and/or disk herniation is the most frequent cause of pain
- Muscle spasm or cramping
- Trauma
- Nephrolithiasis/urolithiasis (renal or ureteral calculi or stones) is the most common urinary tract etiology
- Pyelonephritis (acute or chronic)
  - *E. coli* is the most common cause of upper and lower urinary infections, followed by *Staphylococcus saprophyticus*
  - Acute pyelonephritis is usually a complication of a lower UTI
  - Chronic pyelonephritis is usually associated with obstruction
- Perirenal (kidney) abscess
- Acute pancreatitis
- Glomerulonephritis
- Herpes zoster
- Bacterial cystitis
- Polycystic kidney disease
- Renal infarction or trauma
- Papillary necrosis
- Duodenal ulcer
- Cholecystitis or biliary colic
- Pneumonia
- Appendicitis
- Obstructive uropathy
- Ectopic pregnancy
- Cervicitis
- Renal or bladder cancer
- Leaking or ruptured abdominal aortic aneurysm

Workup and Diagnosis

- History should include onset, duration, quality, intensity, and location of pain; radiation; associated symptoms (e.g., nausea/vomiting, fever, dysuria, hematuria, rash); history of recent trauma or illness; and family history of renal disease or cancer
- Exam should include complete cardiovascular, pulmonary, abdominal, and genitourinary exam, and pelvic exam if suspect cervicitis or ectopic pregnancy
  - Turner's sign (bluish discoloration at flank) and/or Cullen's sign (bluish discoloration at the umbilicus) indicate retroperitoneal hemorrhage and may be present in cases of pancreatitis or ruptured AAA
  - Initial labs may include CBC, ESR, electrolytes, BUN/creatinine, calcium, amylase/lipase, liver function tests, pregnancy test, blood cultures, urinalysis, and urine culture
- Urine cytology, cystoscopy, and biopsy may be indicated if renal or bladder cancer is suspected
- Renal or abdominal ultrasound or abdominal CT scan
- Spiral CT scan without contrast is the gold standard to diagnose stones and urinary tract obstruction
- Intravenous pyelography has high sensitivity/specificity for stones, urinary tract obstruction, and renal cysts
- Voiding cystourethrography
- Lumbosacral X-ray may be indicated to evaluate for degenerative joint disease
- Lumbosacral MRI may be indicated to evaluate for disk disease

Treatment

- Disk disease: NSAIDs and physical therapy; surgery is rarely indicated
- Muscle spasm: Rest, physical therapy, analgesics
- Renal calculi: Increased fluid intake, analgesics, consider surgery
- Pyelonephritis, cystitis, and perirenal abscess: Antibiotics and increased fluid intake
- Pancreatitis: Analgesics, antibiotics, consider surgery
- Glomerulonephritis: Antibiotics (if poststreptococcal), loop diuretics, antihypertensive agents
- Polycystic kidney disease: Manage blood pressure
- Renal infarction: Surgery, antihypertensive, streptokinase
- Papillary necrosis: Dialysis, treat underlying cause
- Cholelithiasis: Cholecystectomy, analgesics
- Appendicitis and ectopic pregnancy: Surgery
- Renal and bladder cancer: Surgical resection, chemotherapy, and radiation

62. Gallops & Extra Heart Sounds

Cardiac auscultation should be performed in a systematic manner. Normal heart sounds (S_1, S_2) should be identified, and the precordium should be examined for gallops (S_3, S_4) and additional heart sounds.

Differential Diagnosis

- S_3 gallop
  - Low-frequency diastolic sound following S_2, best heard with bell
  - May be heard normally in healthy young adults
  - The presence of an S_3 in a patient over 40 suggests ventricular enlargement, often secondary to chronic mitral regurgitation, decreased left ventricular ejection fraction, elevated left atrial pressure, acute pulmonary edema, or high-output states (e.g., thyrotoxicosis, pregnancy)
  - Right ventricular infarct
  - Hypertrophic cardiomyopathy
- S_4 gallop
  - Low-frequency diastolic sound preceding S_1, best heard with bell
  - May be normally heard in healthy older adults
  - Occurs with hypertensive heart disease, aortic stenosis, hypertrophic cardiomyopathy, pulmonary hypertension, coronary artery disease
- Midsystolic click
  - Most commonly due to mitral valve prolapse
- Summation gallop
  - Fusion of S_3 and S_4 with tachycardia
  - Results in a loud diastolic filling sound
- Pericardial knock
  - Early diastolic sound
  - Common in constrictive pericarditis (with or without pericardial calcification)
- Opening snap
  - High-frequency, early diastolic sound
  - Most commonly due to mitral stenosis, tricuspid stenosis, ventricular septal defect, thyrotoxicosis
- Early systolic ejection sound (ejection click)
  - Associated with a bicuspid aortic valve, mitral or tricuspid prolapse, aortic stenosis, prosthetic valves
- Tumor "plop" secondary to atrial mycoma

Workup and Diagnosis

- History and physical examination
- ECG is indicated in all patients
  - Atrial fibrillation is often seen in mitral stenosis
  - Left atrial enlargement is seen in mitral stenosis or mitral regurgitation
  - Left ventricular hypertrophy is seen in patients with hypertensive heart disease, hypertrophic cardiomyopathy, or bicuspid aortic valve
- Chest X-ray may reveal valvular calcification, pulmonary edema, or left ventricular enlargement
- Echocardiogram is used to assess chamber size, wall thickness, ventricular function, valvular abnormalities, and left ventricular outflow obstruction
- Consider cardiology consult

Treatment

- Left ventricular hypertrophy: Blood pressure control
- Mitral regurgitation: Endocarditis prophylaxis, afterload reduction with ACE inhibitors, and diuretics to control volume status, if needed; valve repair (preferred) or replacement may be indicated for severe disease
- Aortic stenosis or bicuspid aortic valve: Valve replacement is often indicated for asymptomatic critical AS, symptomatic AS, and severe AS with LV dysfunction independent of symptoms
- Hypertrophic cardiomyopathy: High-dose β-blockers and calcium channel blockers are the mainstay of medical therapy; diuretics, if indicated, should be used cautiously; septal myomectomy or alcohol septal ablation for left ventricular outflow tract obstruction
- Mitral stenosis: Endocarditis prophylaxis; β-blockers, calcium channel blockers, or digitalis to slow ventricular rate and prolong diastolic filling; mitral valvulotomy or valve replacement for moderate-to-severe disease

63. Genital Skin Lesions

Skin lesions in the genital area are common, and the etiology can range from simple irritation to sexually transmitted diseases to malignancy. The appearance of the lesion, the presence of pain and/or itching, and a description of how the lesion has changed over time can help narrow the differential diagnosis. Be careful not to miss the characteristic chancre of syphilis, which will be a painless ulceration that resolves spontaneously, but may infect others and lead to the serious consequences of secondary or tertiary syphilis.

Differential Diagnosis

- Herpes simplex virus (HSV-1 and HSV-2) is the most common cause of genital lesions in the U.S.
  - Presents with prodromal tingling and genital discomfort before lesions
  - Lesions are always painful and appear as grouped vesicles on an erythematous base
- Condyloma acuminatum ("warts," HPV)
  - Etiologic agent is human papilloma virus
  - Lesions usually painless and pearly with a smooth surface but may be filiform, fungating, and lobulated
- Tinea cruris
  - Inguinal erythema with itch or tenderness
  - Always spares the scrotum
- Candida intertrigo
  - Inguinal erythema with itch or tenderness
  - Often very red with satellite lesions
  - Frequently involves the labia or scrotum
- Syphilis
  - Primary stage: Painless solitary ulcer (chancre) on labia, penis, or oral mucosa that heals in 2–3 weeks
  - Secondary stage: Condyloma lata (moist hypertrophic papules on genital and oral regions)
  - Tertiary stage: Cardiac, neurologic, and other systemic effects
- Molluscum contagiosum
  - Multiple, very small, painless, flesh-colored nodules with umbilicated centers
- Chancroid
  - Etiologic agent is *Haemophilus ducreyi*
  - Painful, solitary, and erythematous lesions
  - May present with dyspareunia and/or dysuria
- Erythrasma
- Lymphogranuloma venereum
- Granuloma inguinale
- Behçet syndrome
  - Oral and genital ulcers, retinitis, uveitis
- Lichen planus
- Scabies
- Zoon's plasma cell balanitis
- Less common etiologies ("zebras") include inverse psoriasis, seborrheic dermatitis, genital squamous cell carcinoma, extramammary Paget's disease, plaque psoriasis, and fixed drug eruptions

Workup and Diagnosis

- History and physical examination including a sexual history and a complete skin exam
  - Separate lesions into painless and painful categories; however, note that an initially painless lesion may become painful following a secondary infection
- Viral culture is gold standard for HSV detection
- Tzanck test may be used to detect HSV and will reveal multinucleated giant cells and intranuclear inclusions
- RPR or VDRL serum tests screen for syphilis, but become positive only 6–8 weeks after primary infection
  - These tests have high false-positive rates
  - Serum FTA is more specific for syphilis
  - Early diagnosis of primary disease requires dark-field microscopic evaluation of infected tissue or IgM assay
- Culture or Gram stain to detect chancroid
- Condyloma acuminata can be diagnosed by applying acetic acid to lesions, which will turn acetowhite
- Molluscum contagiosum is diagnosed by appearance
- Wood's lamp may be used to detect erythrasma
- Shave biopsy is diagnostic for psoriasis, Zoon's, and neoplasms
- Lesions in older patients that are changing in size, appearance, or texture should always be biopsied to rule out carcinoma
- All patients with a suspected STD require a full workup for HIV, syphilis, hepatitis B and C, and pregnancy

Treatment

- Herpes simplex virus: Antivirals (e.g., acyclovir) are best given within 24 hours of outbreak to reduce severity and duration of disease; acetaminophen, NSAIDs, and cool baths for symptomatic relief
- Condyloma acuminata: Destruction of lesions with podophyllin, cryotherapy, cantherone, trichloroacetic acid, or laser can ablate lesions; topical immunotherapy with imiquimod or squaric acid is also successful
- Tinea cruris: Topical (e.g., terbinafine) or oral antifungals (e.g., terbinafine, fluconazole)
- Syphilis: Antibiotics (e.g., penicillin)
- Molluscum contagiosum: Cryotherapy for mild disease; surgical removal for moderate disease
- Chancroid: Antibiotics (e.g., azithromycin)
- Low-potency topical steroids are necessary to treat psoriasis, Zoon's balanitis, and seborrheic dermatitis
- If a red or white plaque persists despite topical therapy, biopsy the lesion to rule out carcinoma

64. GI Bleeding - Hematemesis

Hematemesis refers to vomiting of clots, fresh blood, or "coffee grounds" and generally represents bleeding from the upper GI tract (i.e., proximal to the ligament of Treitz). May be associated with black, tarry stools (melena). The spectrum of upper GI bleeding varies from occult hemorrhage that presents as anemia to acute, life-threatening hemorrhage resulting in hypotension and shock. Sources of life-threatening upper GI bleeding include peptic ulcer disease, esophageal varices, and Mallory-Weiss tears.

Differential Diagnosis

- Peptic ulcer disease is the most common etiology of upper GI bleeding
  - Increased risk with NSAID, steroid, or alcohol use; smoking, stress (e.g., ICU and trauma patients), or infections (*Helicobacter pylori,* CMV, herpes simplex virus)
- Nasopharyngeal or oropharyngeal sources of bleeding
- Esophageal etiologies
  - Esophageal varices (common in alcoholics and cirrhotic patients)
  - Erosive esophagitis: Infectious (e.g., *Candida,* HSV, CMV), corrosive ingestion, or pill-induced
  - Esophageal or gastric carcinoma
  - Esophageal or gastric polyps
- Gastric etiologies
  - Gastric ulcer
  - Gastritis
  - Arteriovenous malformations: Osler-Weber-Rendu syndrome (cutaneous telangectasias, recurrent nosebleeds), idiopathic angiomas, radiation-induced telangiectasias, blue rubber bleb nevus syndrome
  - Mallory-Weiss tear secondary to repetitive vomiting
  - Dieulafoy's lesion: Erosion of the mucosa overlying an artery in the stomach causes necrosis of the arterial wall and resultant hemorrhage
  - Gastric varices: Secondary to splenic vein thrombosis
  - Benign or malignant tumors
- Duodenal etiologies
  - Duodenal ulcer
  - Erosion of a pancreatic tumor into the duodenum
  - Aortoenteric fistula: Must be suspected in any patient with a known aortic graft (e.g., prior AAA repair or occlusive aortic disease)
- Systemic etiologies
  - Coagulopathies (e.g., hemophilia)
  - Thrombocytopenia
  - Anticoagulation therapy (e.g., warfarin)
  - Hereditary hemorrhagic telangiectasia
  - Leukemia
  - Connective tissue disease

Workup and Diagnosis

- Evaluate the severity of bleeding (e.g., signs of shock, orthostatic hypotension, decreased hematocrit) and begin immediate resuscitation if necessary
- Identify the source of bleeding
  - Nasogastric tube insertion to verify upper GI bleeding
  - Upper GI endoscopy (EGD) is diagnostic in most cases (identifies the source of bleeding in 90% of patients) and may be therapeutic
  - Angiography (radionuclide or conventional) is indicated for severe bleeds, if endoscopy is not available, or if endoscopy is inconclusive
  - If patient has a known aortic graft (prior aneurysm repair or aortic occlusive disease), a high index of suspicion for an aortoenteric fistula
- Initial labs should include CBC, coagulation workup (PT/PTT/INR, bleeding time, platelet count), glucose, electrolytes, BUN/creatinine, calcium, liver function tests, and toxicology screen (e.g., for alcohol)
  - Elevated BUN/creatinine ratio suggests upper GI bleed
  - Abnormal prothrombin time suggests coagulopathy
  - Serial hemoglobin/hematocrit measurements are necessary as they may be initially high until volume is replaced; then may decrease
- ECG may be indicated to rule out cardiac ischemia secondary to severe anemia, especially in patients with known diabetes and/or coronary heart disease

Treatment

- Ensure adequate airway, breathing, and circulation
- Stabilize and resuscitate patients as necessary
  - Insert two large-bore IV lines
  - Administer IV fluids (Ringer's lactate or normal saline)
  - Type and cross match two units of packed RBCs
  - Correct coagulopathies if present (e.g., fresh frozen plasma, vitamin K, platelets)
  - Consider blood transfusion
- Identify and treat the source of bleeding
  - IV octreotide (vasoconstrictor) infusion
  - Vasopressin for significant variceal bleeding (contraindicated in CAD or CVA patients)
  - Endoscopy with injection of vasoconstrictors (e.g., epinephrine), sclerosing agents, or electrocautery
  - Angiography with visualization of bleeding vessel and subsequent embolization
  - Surgical control of bleeding if all else fails
- H2 blockers or proton pump inhibitors may be started for suspected peptic ulcer disease or gastritis

65. GI Bleeding - Melena & Hematochezia

Lower GI tract bleeding occurs distal to the ligament of Treitz (which separates the duodenum from the jejunum) and refers to the passage of either bright red blood per rectum (hematochezia), maroon stools, or black, tarry stools (melena). Hematochezia suggests either bleeding from the lower intestinal tract or very brisk bleeding from higher in the intestinal tract. Melena suggests that the blood has had time to be processed by the intestinal tract, implying slower bleeding that originates higher in the intestinal tract.

Differential Diagnosis

- Anatomic lesions
  - Diverticular bleeding causes 30–50% of all cases of massive rectal bleeding; associated with mild, crampy pain, but can be painless; *not* associated with diverticulitis
  - Meckel's diverticulum
- Vascular lesions
  - Angiodysplasia (arteriovenous malformation): Most frequent cause in older patients; bleeding tends to be episodic and self-limited; painless; increased risk with increased age
- Neoplastic lesions
  - Colon cancer or polyps: Causes 10% of cases of lower GI bleeding in patients >50 years; generally low-grade, recurrent bleeding
  - Rectal cancer
  - Small bowel tumors
- Inflammatory lesions
  - Colitis/ulcers (e.g., inflammatory bowel disease, infectious colitis, ischemic colitis, radiation colitis)
  - Ischemic colitis generally presents with abdominal pain
  - Ulcerative colitis more associated with gross rectal bleeding
  - Crohn's disease more commonly associated with diffuse crampy abdominal pain, whereas ulcerative colitis is more localized to left lower quadrant
- Anorectal lesions
  - Hemorrhoids are the most common cause of rectal bleeding in patients younger than 50 years old; usually painless bleeding
  - Fissures
  - Polyps
  - Idiopathic rectal ulcers
- Aortoenteric fistula: Must be suspected in any patient with a known aortic graft (e.g., prior aortic aneurysm repair or occlusive aortic disease)
- Idiopathic in up to 15% of cases
- Upper GI bleeding
- Systemic bleeding disorders (e.g., hemophilia, excessive anticoagulation, thrombocytopenia)

Workup and Diagnosis

- Evaluate the severity of bleeding (e.g., signs of shock, orthostatic hypotension, decreased hematocrit)—if impending shock or exsanguination, emergent resuscitation (see below) and surgical intervention are indicated
- Determine the source of bleeding
  - Rectal examination
  - Rule out upper GI bleeding by nasogastric tube aspiration or upper GI endoscopy
  - Abdominal X-ray to rule out perforation or obstruction (before initiating colonoscopy)
  - Colonoscopy is usually diagnostic for the bleeding source
  - Angiography is used for active, heavy bleeding and/or if colonoscopy is inconclusive
  - Tagged RBC scan is helpful for Meckel's diverticula
- Initial labs should include CBC, coagulation workup (PT/PTT/INR, bleeding time, platelet count), glucose, electrolytes, BUN/creatinine, LFTs, albumin, toxicology screen (e.g., for alcohol), and stool ova/parasites culture
- ECG may be indicated to rule out cardiac ischemia secondary to severe anemia, especially in patients with known diabetes and/or CAD

Treatment

- Ensure adequate airway, breathing, and circulation
- Stabilize and resuscitate patients as necessary
  - Insert two large-bore IV lines
  - Administer IV fluids
  - Type and cross match two units of packed RBCs
  - Administer blood transfusion if necessary
  - Correct coagulopathies if present (e.g., fresh frozen plasma, vitamin K, platelets)
- Several options are available to treat persistent bleeding: Endoscopic sclerotherapy, electrocautery, or laser coagulation; angiographic embolization; or resection
- Diverticular hemorrhage: Resection may be indicated
- Angiodysplasia: Endoscopy or resection
- Colorectal cancer and/or polyps: Excision or resection
- Infectious colitis: Appropriate antibiotic regimens
- Inflammatory bowel disease: Steroids and aminosalicylates; resection for severe disease
- Aortoenteric fistula requires repair of bowel, graft excision, and extra-anatomic bypass graft

66. Halitosis

Halitosis, or bad breath, may be acute or chronic, depending on the underlying cause. It may indicate the need for improved dental hygiene or may be a symptom of an underlying infection or chronic disease. Oral causes constitute about 90% of the etiologies of halitosis, whereas nasal causes constitute nearly 10%; thus, other etiologies are relatively uncommon.

Differential Diagnosis

- Head and neck etiologies
  - Foods (e.g., onion, garlic)
  - Dental conditions (periodontal disease, gingivitis, denture odor, dental abscesses, food particles not cleaned from teeth)
  - Postnasal drip
  - Dry mouth (xerostomia): Mouth breathing, side effect of medications, salivary gland disease, dehydration
  - Nasal foreign body
  - Gastroesophageal reflux disease
  - Chronic sinusitis
  - Allergic rhinitis
  - Tonsillar disease (e.g., streptococcal pharyngitis)
  - Zenker's (pharyngoesophageal) diverticulum: Presents as dysphagia, regurgitation, cough, and extreme halitosis
  - Tobacco or alcohol use
- Systemic etiologies
  - Diabetes mellitus, especially with ketoacidosis
  - Uremia
  - Pulmonary disorders (e.g., bronchiectasis, pneumonia, neoplasms, tuberculosis)
  - Trimethylaminuria (fishy breath odor)
  - Liver failure (fetor hepaticus)
  - Menstruation may exacerbate halitosis

Workup and Diagnosis

- Careful dental and medical history, including dental hygiene habits and dietary history
  - Note associated symptoms that suggest systemic etiology (e.g., cough, nasal congestion)
  - Odor after sleeping, dieting, or exercising suggests xerostomia
  - Odor upon talking suggests postnasal drip
  - Bleeding gums suggests periodontal disease
- Dental examination to rule out treatable dental causes (e.g., periodontal disease)
- Physical examination should include careful oral, nasal, sinus, neck, pulmonary, and abdominal examinations
  - Assess odor from mouth and nose separately
  - Small malodorous whitish stones on tongue suggest tonsilloliths
  - Place dentures into plastic bag for several minutes and then smell to evaluate for denture odor
  - Spoon test involves scooping mucous/saliva from back of tongue and evaluating for malodor; if present, suggests postnasal drip
  - Nasolaryngoscopy if nasal cause is suspected but specific cause cannot be identified
- Zenker's diverticulum is diagnosed by contrast barium swallow

Treatment

- Maintain good oral hygiene (e.g., brush teeth at least twice per day, floss daily, treat underlying periodontal disease)
- Avoid exacerbating medications or foods
- Tongue cleaning with toothbrush
- Gargle with chlorhexidine mouthwash twice a day for a week to assess improvement
- Treat postnasal drip (e.g., antihistamines, nasal steroids, polyp removal)
- Treat sinusitis with appropriate antibiotics
- Decrease or eliminate alcohol and tobacco use
- Zenker's diverticulum may require surgical resection if symptomatic
- Treat other underlying medical diseases (e.g., diabetic ketoacidosis, uremia, GERD)

67. Hallucinations

Hallucinations are psychotic symptoms in which patients perceive stimuli that do not exist. Any of the five senses (auditory, visual, tactile, gustatory, or olfactory) may be involved, with auditory hallucinations being the most common. Patients may believe the hallucinations to be true or they may identify them as false. Distinguish all hallucinations from illusions, the misinterpretation of real but ambiguous stimuli. The patient's medical and psychiatric condition, as well as the type and duration of hallucinations, are important in reaching the correct diagnosis.

Differential Diagnosis

- Delirium
  - Develops over hours to days
  - Fluctuates throughout the day
  - Causes include dehydration, drug-induced, electrolyte imbalance, UTI, URI, hypoglycemia, and alcohol or drug withdrawal
  - Occurs in 10–30% of hospital patients
  - Drug-induced delirium (e.g., cocaine, β-blockers, alcohol, corticosteroids, pseudoephedrine, dopaminergic drugs)
- Alcohol withdrawal (delirium tremens)
  - Often presents in hospitalized patients about 3 days after admission
  - Commonly presents with tactile hallucinations (e.g., formication—the sense of insects crawling over body)
  - May be accompanied by seizure activity
- Hallucinogenic syndromes (e.g., LSD, marijuana, mescaline, phencyclidine, mushrooms, amphetamines)
- Schizophrenia
  - Auditory hallucinations are most frequent; visual hallucinations occur in about 50% of patients, tactile in 20%, olfactory in 6%
  - Progresses to positive psychotic symptoms (e.g., hallucinations, delusions, thought disorder) and/or negative symptoms (e.g., anhedonia, poor concentration, flattened affect, poor social/personal function)
  - 1% incidence in the general population, males > females
- Schizophreniform disorder
- Schizoaffective disorder
- Post-traumatic stress disorder
- Dementia
- Systemic lupus erythematosus
  - Auditory hallucinations caused by corticosteroids; visual and tactile by lupus psychosis
- Bipolar disorder
- Psychotic depression
- Postpartum major depression
- Mass lesions
- CNS infections/encephalitis
- Seizures
- Occipital lobe injury
- Heavy metal ingestion
- Lewy body dementia

Workup and Diagnosis

- History and physical examination
  - In caring for patients with major psychiatric illness, follow three important principles: Know the patient's drug regimen, work with psychiatrist if changes are needed, and remember that chronic psychiatric patients have difficulty communicating medical history and needs
  - Diagnosis of schizophrenia requires two positive or negative symptoms present for 1 month and signs continuing for at least 6 months (DSM-IV criteria)
  - Assess for suicidal/homicidal ideations
  - Note timing of hallucinations (e.g., following alcohol or drug use, at random, under stress)
- Initial labs may include electrolytes, glucose, calcium, BUN/creatinine, albumin, liver function tests, alkaline phosphatase, magnesium, phosphate, CBC, ECG, pulse oximetry, urinalysis, toxicology screen, and drug levels
- Chest X-ray may be indicated for infectious etiologies of delirium; lumbar puncture may be indicated
- Further tests, if delirium is suspected, include vitamin B_{12} and folate levels, ANA, ammonia, and heavy metal screen
- EEG may reveal slowing activity in delirium, low-voltage fast activity in alcohol withdrawal
- Psychiatric consult after medical causes of psychosis are ruled out

Treatment

- Treat hallucinations symptomatically with antipsychotic drugs (e.g., haloperidol, risperidone, olanzapine)
- Delirium: Treat underlying cause (e.g., hydration, proper nutrition, oxygen, thiamine, and glucose)
- Alcohol/sedative withdrawal: Monitor and treat for seizures with benzodiazepines
- Schizophrenia: Traditional antipsychotics (e.g., haloperidol, chlorpromazine)
  - Extrapyramidal side effects (parkinsonism, akathisia, dystonia) are common
  - Neuroleptic malignant syndrome (hyperthermia, rigidity, hypertension, tachycardia) may rarely occur in first week of treatment and can be fatal
  - Clozapine carries a 1% risk of fatal agranulocytosis

68. Hand and Foot Rashes

Hand and foot rashes do not all look alike: Look for the subtle clues discussed below and obtain a detailed exposure and health history to narrow the differential. Be sure to evaluate the full extent of the skin rash before finalizing your differential diagnosis. Dyshidrotic and irritant eczema are by far the most common etiologies of hand and foot rashes.

Differential Diagnosis

- Dyshidrotic eczema (pompholyx)
  - Very common idiopathic skin disease
  - Affects one or both hands and/or feet in the thenar eminence, palms and/or soles, and sides of fingers and toes
  - Causes itching, scaling, and erythema, and minute vesicles and painful fissures
  - Usually chronic and intermittent, and often exquisitely pruritic
- Irritant or allergic hand eczema
  - Very common
  - Difficult to distinguish from dyshidrosis because both are vesicular and very itchy
  - Flares occur during work/hobbies, with improvement on vacation when away from the irritant or allergen
- Tinea manus (hand) and tinea pedis (foot)
  - Presents as itchy, diffuse, light scale, and/or maceration; prominent on palmar, plantar (moccasin distribution), and interdigital surfaces
  - Erythema is rarely present
  - Often "two hands and one foot" or "two feet and one hand" are affected
- Scabies
  - Presents as short (a few millimeters), linear burrows and vesicles on the hands and feet (web spaces), belt region, and/or intertriginous spaces
  - Intensely pruritic, especially at night
  - Often many members of the household unit affected
  - Definitive diagnosis made by visualizing the scabies mite in a skin scraping
- Psoriasis
  - Often affects the hands and/or feet
  - Well-demarcated, erythematous plaques with adherent scale, or can present as a focal or diffuse pustular eruption
  - Look for associated nail dystrophy or other skin involvement
- Reiter's disease
  - Uveitis, urethritis, and arthritis
- Pityriasis rubra pilaris
  - Well-demarcated bright salmon or red plaques on the palms or soles
- Keratoderma
  - Focal or diffuse thickening of the skin of the palms or soles
- Erythema multiforme
- Infection (secondary syphilis, varicella meningococcemia)

Workup and Diagnosis

- History and physical examination
  - Note chronic exposure to chemicals or potential irritants at work or in hobbies
  - Any family history of psoriasis or allergy/atopy
  - Look closely for the presence of small, clear "water blisters" under the skin that may indicate pompholyx
  - Examine nails for evidence of coexisting onychomycosis (very common in cases of tinea pedis and manus, and a nidus for frequent reinfection), "oil spots," or nail pitting (may suggest psoriasis)
  - Examine joints for arthritis (psoriasis/Reiter's), eyes (Reiter's), and genitalia (psoriasis/Reiter's)
- KOH preparation from scale scraped from the palms, soles, or between the toes to determine presence of branching hyphae of tinea or scabies mites
- Culture any intact pustules
- Consider performing a patch test to rule out allergic contact dermatitis
- A punch biopsy may be helpful to distinguish psoriasis or PRP from the other common eczematous diseases of the hands and feet
- Fungal culture of nail clipping if onycholysis (nail thickening) present
- Dermatology referral is often indicated in resistant cases

Treatment

- Pompholyx, psoriasis, and most noninfectious hand eczemas are treated with topical high potency steroid ointments (e.g., temovate, diprolene) for short periods
- Irritant eczema: Bland heavy emollients (e.g., petroleum jelly, mineral oil, various cream formulations with a dimethicone base) will rehydrate the skin to prevent recurrence of irritant or other types of dermatitis; avoid wet-work, irritants, and harsh soaps
- Tinea manum and pedis
  - Topical antifungal preparations or a short course of oral fluconazole or terbinafine (2 weeks)
  - If onychomycosis is present (confirmed by nail clipping and PAS stain or culture), treat with oral antifungals for 6–12 weeks to prevent recurrence
- Topical or systemic phototherapy with PUVA can significantly improve palmoplantar eczemas that are refractory to topical monotherapy
- Systemic methotrexate and cyclosporine are also used to treat severe dyshidrotic disease or psoriasis

69. Headache

Headache is one of the most common primary care complaints. It may be an isolated or recurrent event; it may be idiopathic or secondary to an underlying structural lesion; or it may simply require an analgesic for pain relief or a complete and detailed workup for its source. One must distinguish benign causes of headache from malignant and life-threatening causes and treat appropriately.

Differential Diagnosis

- Tension-type headache
  - Most common cause of headache
  - Diffuse, bilateral, band-like pain
  - Lasts for hours to days
  - May occur on a fairly regular basis
- Migraine headache
  - Throbbing unilateral or bilateral pain
  - May last for days
  - May have preceding aura (flashing light)
  - Triggers include foods, drugs, or stress
- Meningitis
  - May present with fever, photophobia, neck stiffness, nausea/vomiting, papilledema
  - Brudzinski's sign: Neck pain upon passive flexion of neck
  - Kernig's sign: Neck pain and involuntary flexion upon passive extension of knee with hips flexed
- Head trauma
- Medications
- Carbon monoxide exposure
- Sinusitis
- Temporomandibular joint syndrome or dental pain
- Withdrawal from alcohol, barbiturates, caffeine, or other substance
- Temporal arteritis
  - Pain/tenderness over temporal area/jaw
  - Occurs uniquely in patients over 50
  - Blindness may occur
- Mass lesions (e.g., tumor, hematoma)
  - Daily, progressive headache
  - May awaken from sleep
  - Focal neurologic signs
- Subarachnoid hemorrhage
  - Sudden onset of "worst headache of my life"
  - Neck stiffness
  - Loss of consciousness
- Cluster headache
  - Severe, unilateral pain
  - Lasts minutes to hours
  - Occurs daily for months, then remits for months or even years
- Glaucoma
  - Retro-orbital pain
- Chronic daily headache or rebound headache (e.g., secondary to chronic analgesic use)
- Benign intracranial hypertension

Workup and Diagnosis

- History and physical exam often make the diagnosis
  - History should focus on onset, duration, frequency, possible triggers, severity, quality (e.g., throbbing, band-like), accompanying symptoms (e.g., aura, photophobia, visual changes, nausea/vomiting, lacrimation, nasal congestion), constitutional symptoms (e.g., weight loss, fever), medications, and dietary history
  - Is this first and/or worst headache of life?
  - Exam should include a complete neurologic exam, visual/retinal exam, head/neck, and gait exam
- Possible serious etiologies and need for further workup are suggested by the following red flags: Constitutional symptoms, new headache in a patient over 50, sudden onset, awakening from sleep, mental status changes, focal neurologic signs, visual/motor/balance disturbance, papilledema
- CT will identify hemorrhage and mass lesions and rule out increased intracranial pressure
- MRI will identify posterior fossa tumors
- Lumbar puncture is indicated if CT is normal but still suspect hemorrhage, infection, or tumor
- Serologies for bacterial, viral, and other causes of meningitis or encephalitis
- Elevated ESR suggests temporal arteritis or infection
- Carboxyhemoglobin measurement if history suggests carbon monoxide poisoning

Treatment

- Tension-type headache: Regular exercise, stress management, tricyclic antidepressants, analgesics
- Migraine headache: Avoid triggers; serotonin agonists (e.g., sumatriptan), NSAIDs, ergotomines
- Temporal arteritis: High-dose corticosteroids
- Meningitis: Search for and treat the primary source (e.g., pneumonia, sinusitis, neoplasm)
  - Urgent antimicrobial administration for infections
  - Treat inflammatory causes with steroids
- Subarachnoid hemorrhage requires attention to airway, breathing, and circulation, and management of increased intracranial pressure (maintain normal blood pressure; hypertension may cause the aneurysm to rebleed, hypotension may cause cerebral ischemia); administer nimodipine to prevent cerebral vasospasm, seizure prophylaxis with IV phenytoin, surgery
- Cluster headache: Oxygen inhalation for 5–10 minutes; serotonin agonists, ergotamines, and/or methysergide

70. Hearing Loss

Hearing loss affects about 10% of the U.S. population. Two broad categories of hearing loss exist, conductive and sensorineural. Conductive hearing loss results from any process that prevents sound from reaching the inner ear. Sensorineural hearing loss refers to nerve-type hearing loss in either the inner ear or the auditory nerve. Early diagnosis allows early intervention, which has important implications in speech and language development in children.

Differential Diagnosis

- Conductive hearing loss: Results from any process preventing sound from reaching the inner ear
  - Obstruction of the ear canal, usually due to cerumen impaction or foreign body
  - Otitis media with middle ear effusion (most common in children but also occurs in adults)
  - Chronic otitis media: Permanent change in the ear (e.g., tympanic membrane perforation, ossicular chain discontinuity and fixation, cholesteatoma) secondary to otitis media
  - Congenital atresia of the external auditory canal
- Sensorineural hearing loss: Nerve type hearing loss, either in the inner ear or the auditory nerve
  - Presbycusis is the most common form
  - Noise-induced hearing (occupational or nonoccupational)
  - Hereditary sensorineural hearing loss, usually autosomal recessive heritance
  - Medications (e.g., aminoglycosides, chemotherapeutics, diuretics)
  - Ménière's disease: Hearing loss, tinnitus, vertigo, and aural fullness
  - Acoustic neuroma: Results in unilateral hearing loss and tinnitus as the initial symptoms in 90% of patients
  - Alport's syndrome: Hereditary nephritis, sensorineural deafness, ocular abnormalities)
- Mixed hearing loss (both conductive and sensorineural hearing loss)
  - Wardenberg's syndrome
  - Prolonged QT syndrome variant
  - Other causes of congenital deafness
  - Meningitis
  - Vascular (e.g., embolism, thrombosis, hemorrhage)
  - Viral (e.g., mumps, measles, influenza, varicella, adenovirus, EBV)

Workup and Diagnosis

- Otologic history should include duration of hearing loss, laterality, otorrhea, tinnitus, associated dizziness, family history, and a focused medical history (e.g., exposure to gentamicin, history of infections)
- Weber's and Rinne's tuning fork testing may be used to determine conductive hearing loss versus sensorineural; however, audiogram is the definitive test
- Otoacoustic emission and auditory brainstem response are objective tests of nerve function; these are increasingly being used to screen for hearing loss in newborns
- CT scan of the temporal bones may be helpful in evaluating conductive hearing loss
- MRI with gadolinium is indicated for all patients with unilateral sensorineural hearing loss or tinnitus to evaluate for acoustic neuroma

Treatment

- In many cases, the physical exam is therapeutic, because it involves cleaning the ear canal
- For middle ear effusions, a course of antibiotics and observation is usually sufficient; if symptoms persist, myringotomy and tube placement may be indicated
- Hearing aids are helpful for most cases of conductive or sensorineural hearing loss
- Middle ear implantable devices for moderate to severe sensorineural hearing loss
- Cochlear implants may be indicated for severe to profound sensorineural hearing loss if hearing aids are of minimal or no benefit
- Reconstructive middle ear surgery may be necessary, and includes tympanoplasty and stapedectomy
- Prevention of additional hearing loss by ear protection

71. Heartburn

Heartburn is a term commonly used by patients and must be carefully evaluated to ensure accurate understanding of the symptoms. Typically, the term "heartburn" describes a substernal and/or epigastric burning pain associated with a "sour stomach" sensation and/or a sour, acidic taste in the back of the mouth or throat. Though esophageal pathologies are most common, clinicians must immediately assess the patient for life-threatening conditions, such as myocardial ischemia/infarction, ruptured aortic aneurysm, and perforating peptic ulcer disease.

Differential Diagnosis

- Distinguish between esophageal pain (reflux) and cardiac pain (angina)
- Coronary artery disease
  - Angina/ischemia
  - Myocardial infarction
  - Pericardial disease
- Esophageal pathology
  - Gastroesophageal reflux disease
  - Hiatal hernia
  - Motility disorders with decreased peristaltic clearance (e.g., achalasia)
  - Peptic ulcer disease
  - Gastritis
  - Infectious esophagitis (e.g., *Candida,* HIV, CMV, HSV): Common in immunosuppressed patients
  - Barrett's esophagus
  - Esophageal carcinoma (commonly squamous cell)
  - Strictures, webs, or rings
  - Esophageal diverticulum
  - Scleroderma
  - Esophageal varices
  - Mallory-Weiss tear
  - Esophageal atresia or fistula
- Caustic agent ingestion with resultant mucosal injury
- Myasthenia gravis
- Chagas' disease
- Pulmonary embolism
- Muscle strain
- Asthma
- Pregnancy

Workup and Diagnosis

- Distinguish between esophageal pain (reflux) and cardiac pain (angina)
- History and physical exam often make the diagnosis
- Be sure to appropriately rule out coronary artery disease in unexplained cases of chest pain
  - ECG
  - Cardiac enzymes
  - Stress testing
- Initial diagnostic test for esophageal etiologies may be a therapeutic challenge with H2 blockers or proton pump inhibitors; further evaluation is indicated only for patients who fail initial therapy or may have serious pathology
- Endoscopy (with biopsy and *Helicobacter pylori* testing) will verify reflux esophagitis and other pathology (e.g., stricture) and rule out Barrett's esophagus and esophageal carcinoma
- Ambulatory esophageal pH monitoring may be used to evaluate patients with atypical reflux symptoms and normal endoscopy
- Double contrast barium swallow may identify early stages of reflux esophagitis, ulcers, strictures, and folds
- Esophageal manometry will diagnose motility disorders, decreased peristalsis, and esophageal spasm
- Biopsy is diagnostic for Barrett's esophagus, carcinoma, sclerosis, and infection

Treatment

- Lifestyle modification is the initial therapy for most cases of esophageal pathology
  - Elevate head of bed (for nocturnal symptoms)
  - Avoid reflux-inducing foods (e.g., fat, chocolate, caffeine, alcohol, acidic foods)
  - Decrease total caloric intake, smoking, and stress
  - Promote salivation with chewing gum or lozenges
  - Avoid tight-fitting garments
- Acid suppressive medications are indicated for significant reflux and/or failed lifestyle modifications
  - Antacids
  - H2 receptor antagonists (e.g., famotidine)
  - Proton pump inhibitors (e.g., omeprazole)
- Prokinetic medications (e.g., metoclopramide, cisapride) may be used to increase LES pressure and gastric emptying and improve peristalsis; however, significant side effects may occur
- Annual upper GI endoscopy may be indicated to monitor for Barrett's esophagus and carcinoma

72. Hematuria

Hematuria is the intermittent or persistent excretion of red or brown urine that can occur with a variety of clinical symptoms. The amount of blood can be grossly evident or microscopic. About 2.5% of the general population has asymptomatic hematuria. It is important to evaluate the cause of hematuria, since gross painless hematuria is considered a urinary tract cancer until proven otherwise (even though a malignancy is found in only 10% of cases of hematuria in outpatient populations).

Differential Diagnosis

- Transient hematuria
  - Urinary tract infection/pyelonephritis
  - Nephrolithiasis (kidney or bladder stones)
  - Exercise
  - Trauma, instrumentation, catheterization, or foreign bodies
  - Endometriosis
  - Transient unexplained
  - Henoch-Schönlein purpura/HUS
  - Coagulopathy and excess anticoagulation
  - Prostatitis, epididymitis
- Persistent hematuria
  - Sickle cell anemia
  - Cancer (prostate, bladder, kidney)
  - Benign prostatic hypertrophy
  - Polycystic kidney disease
  - Intrinsic glomerular disease
- Other causes of red or brown urine (pseudohematuria)
  - Beeturia (14% population are susceptible after eating beets): Due to excretion of betalaine, a reddish pigment
  - Myoglobinuria: Rapidly filtered and excreted; source is usually due to rhabdomyolysis; look for increased elevation of plasma CPK levels
  - Hemoglobinuria: Occurs when the filtered load of unbound dimer exceeds resorptive capacity of the proximal tubules, generally at serum levels >100–150 mg/dL
- Urethral carbuncle
- Urethritis (e.g., *Chlamydia*)
- Porphyria
- Phenazopyridine (bladder analgesic): Produces an orange color in urine
- Postinfectious glomerulonephropathy
- Hereditary (Alport's syndrome)
- IgA nephropathy (Berger's disease): Often see gross hematuria without positive family history of disease
- Loin pain hematuria syndrome
- Thin basement membrane disease (benign familial hematuria): Usually see microscopic hematuria; gross hematuria or renal failure is rare
- Hypercalciuria or hyperuricuria
- Arteriovenous malformation
- Fistula
- Others include food dyes, phenolphthalein, rifampin, and porphyrins
- Excessive anticoagulation
- Trauma

Workup and Diagnosis

- History and physical examination
- Urinalysis in all patients (consider catheterization to distinguish vaginal bleeding from other sources)
  - Blood clots occur with extraglomerular sources
  - Glomerular source of bleeding results in RBC casts, large amounts of protein, dysmorphic RBCs
  - UTI results in pyuria, nitrates, leukocyte esterase
- Initial labs include BUN/creatinine, electrolytes, calcium, uric acid, CBC, and PT/PTT
- Centrifuge urine sample: Red sediment only suggests hematuria (RBCs in the urine); heme-negative red supernatant suggests hemoglobinuria; heme-positive clear supernatant suggests myoglobinuria
- Three-tube test: #1, collect first few mL of urine; #2, mid-stream; #3, last few mL
  - Hematuria in #1 suggests urethral lesion; in #3, bladder trigone lesion; equally in all three, diffuse lesion
- IVP (contraindicated in dye allergy), renal ultrasound, or spiral CT to evaluate for stones and renal masses
- Urine cytology and cystoscopy for patients at risk for bladder cancer (e.g., smoking, cyclophosphamide)
- Consider C3 level, ANA, ANCA, Anti-GBM, ASO, cryoglobulins, and hepatitis C antibodies
- Renal biopsy if persistent hematuria with negative workup and evidence of progression (increasing proteinuria, creatinine, and blood pressure)

Treatment

- Older patients with transient hematuria should always be evaluated due to increased risk of urinary tract cancers; refer to urologist for further evaluation and treatment
- UTI: Start appropriate antibiotics and follow up with urinalysis to see if hematuria resolves
- Glomerular sources (RBC casts, protein excretion >500 mg/dL, dysmorphic RBCs): Follow BUN/creatinine, blood pressure, creatinine clearance, and 24-hour urine protein, and refer for biopsy if worsening
- Nonglomerular source (no RBC casts or dysmorphic RBCs in the urine): Urologic consult if imaging indicates a lesion (renal, bladder, or urethral)
- Stones: Increase hydration, analgesics, urology referral for large or persistent stones
- Myoglobinuria/hemoglobinuria: Treat underlying cause
- Beeturia: Evaluate for iron deficiency or achlorhydria due to pernicious anemia, as treating these disorders may eliminate beeturia; eating foods high in oxalate (spinach, oysters) with beets can also cause beeturia

73. Hemiparesis & Hemiplegia

Hemiplegia (complete lack of motor function) and hemiparesis (decreased motor function) are almost always the result of a problem with the brain. The tempo of onset, past history, and associated findings on examination are usually helpful in localizing the problem and suggesting an etiology. Emergent stabilization and treatment are essential to save lives and decrease disability, but correct diagnosis is necessary to limit untoward risks of treatment, such as that of hemorrhagic stroke in a patient who receives thrombolytic therapy.

Differential Diagnosis

- Cerebrovascular disease is the most common cause of acute hemiparesis or hemiplegia
  - Infarction (thromboembolic)
  - Intracerebral hemorrhage
  - Transient ischemic attacks may produce a transient hemiplegia or paresis (though they are defined as cerebrovascular deficits that resolve within 24 hours, most TIAs last only minutes)
  - RINDs last 24–72 hours
- Chronic subdural hematoma
- Demyelinating disease (e.g., multiple sclerosis, Guillain-Barré syndrome)
- Trauma
- Congenital (e.g., cerebral palsy, congenital structural anomalies)
- Brain tumors (primary or metastatic)
- Cerebral abscess
- Complicated migraine
- Inflammatory conditions (e.g., cerebral vasculitis)
- Postictal (Todd's) paralysis
- Psychogenic or hysterical weakness
  - These patients usually lack associated physical findings such as hyperreflexia or Babinski's signs, and may also exhibit inconsistent or nonphysiologic patterns of weakness
- Amyotrophic lateral sclerosis
  - May present initially with asymmetric weakness, but more diffuse involvement develops over time
- Brown-Séquard syndrome (spinal cord hemisection)
  - Leads to weakness, upper motor neuron signs, and impaired proprioception and vibratory sensation ipsilateral to the lesion
  - Impaired pain and temperature sensation contralateral to the lesion
- Meningitis
- Syphilis
- Transverse myelitis
- Periodic paralysis

Workup and Diagnosis

- History and physical examination
  - Acute onset of hemiparesis or hemiplegia suggests a vascular cause until proven otherwise (although an exacerbation of multiple sclerosis may present relatively acutely)
  - More gradual onset of hemiparesis suggests a more slowly evolving process, such as a tumor
  - The pattern of weakness noted on exam and the associated deficits will help to localize the problem (e.g., right hemiparesis with greater weakness of the face and arm than the leg and associated aphasia suggest a cerebral infarction in the territory of the left middle cerebral artery; equal weakness of the face, arm, and leg without associated cortical deficits suggests a subcortical lesion (e.g., internal capsule); cranial nerve abnormalities and weakness of the contralateral limbs suggests a brainstem lesion)
- Initial laboratory studies may include CBC, electrolytes, calcium, glucose, BUN/creatinine, and PT/PTT
- MRI and/or CT scan are the imaging modalities of choice
- CSF examination is useful in suspected cases of multiple sclerosis (reveals oligoclonal bands and elevated IgG index)

Treatment

- Hemiplegia and hemiparesis are best managed by identifying and treating the underlying cause
- General measures, such as physical and occupational therapy, assistive devices, and orthotics, may be beneficial in improving the functioning of patients with hemiplegia or paresis
- Cerebral infarction is best managed medically
  - Thrombolytics within 3 hours of onset of symptoms in carefully selected patients improves the outcome of ischemic stroke patients
  - General measures include careful management of blood pressure, blood sugar, and avoiding infectious complications (e.g., pneumonia due to bedrest)
  - Identify underlying cause to direct long-term therapy (usually antiplatelet or anticoagulant therapy with risk factor management) to prevent recurrence
- Mass lesions affecting the brain, including tumors and hematomas, may require surgical management
- Multiple sclerosis: Steroids for acute exacerbations

74. Hemoptysis

Hemoptysis is defined as coughing up blood from a source below the vocal cords. Other potential sites of bleeding (nose, mouth, throat, GI system) must be eliminated; it can be particularly difficult to discern hemoptysis from hematemesis. Interestingly, bleeding occurs more commonly from the bronchial arteries than the pulmonary arteries (though the bronchial arteries have less blood flow, they are a higher-pressure system). Massive hemoptysis, although uncommon, may be fatal because of asphyxiation or respiratory failure.

Differential Diagnosis

- Other sources of bleeding (e.g., hematemesis, epistaxis, and other causes of upper airway bleeding)
- Airway disease is the most common cause of hemoptysis
  - Bronchitis (acute or chronic) causes more than 25% of cases
  - Cancers (metastatic and primary lung cancers) cause up to 25% of all cases
  - Bronchiectasis causes up to 10% of cases
  - Foreign body
  - Trauma
- Parenchymal disease
  - Infections: Tuberculosis (5%), pneumonia (5%), lung abscess, aspergilloma
  - Coagulopathy: Anticoagulant use, thrombocytopenia, DIC
  - Cystic fibrosis
  - Inflammatory: SLE, Wegener's granulomatosis, Goodpasture's syndrome
  - Iatrogenic: Transbronchial or percutaneous lung biopsy, bronchoscopy, intubation
  - Cocaine use
- Cardiovascular disease
  - Pulmonary infarction/embolism
  - Congestive heart failure
  - Mitral stenosis
  - AVM
  - Trauma to pulmonary artery (e.g., Swan-Ganz catheterization)
  - Aortic aneurysm
  - Osler-Weber-Rendu syndrome: Congenital telangiectasias
- Fistula formation between vasculature and airway
- Catamenial hemoptysis (intrathoracic endometriosis): Cyclic bleeding with menses
- Diffuse alveolar hemorrhage syndromes: ARDS, crack cocaine use, SLE, cytotoxic drug use
- Inflammatory
  - Behçet syndrome: Recurrent oral and genital ulcers, uveitis, and arthritis
  - Henoch-Schönlein purpura: Most common systemic vasculitis in children; presents with palpable purpura, abdominal pain, hematuria, and arthritis
  - Idiopathic pulmonary hemosiderosis
- Idiopathic in 20% of cases

Workup and Diagnosis

- Initial workup includes a chest X-ray; sputum for acid-fast stain, cytology and Gram stain/culture; pulse oximetry; PT/PTT; CBC; electrolytes; urinalysis; and BUN/creatinine
- Consider respiratory isolation until TB is ruled out
- Chest CT may show focal bleeding
- Minor hemoptysis: Bronchoscopy is required if any risk factors for cancer are present, such as age >40, abnormal chest X-ray, hemoptysis >1 week, tobacco use (>40 pack-years), anemia, and/or weight loss
- Major hemoptysis:
  - Active bleeding requires immediate bronchoscopy
  - Stable patients may undergo initial chest CT (if there is no active bleeding) followed by bronchoscopy
  - Bronchoscopy is both diagnostic and therapeutic—may localize bleeding and allow for balloon tamponade or vasoconstrictor injection at site of bleeding
- Consider immunologic tests (e.g., ANCA for Wegener's syndrome; anti-GBM antibodies for Goodpasture's; ANA, anti-dsDNA, and low complement for SLE; ASO titer for poststreptococcal glomerulonephritis)
- Arterial blood gas may be used to distinguish hemoptysis (alkaline serum pH) from hematemesis (acidic serum pH)

Treatment

- Minor hemoptysis: Treat the specific etiology
- Massive hemoptysis is a medical emergency
  - Attention to airway, breathing, and circulation
  - Administer supplemental O_2
  - Stabilize hemodynamics
  - Cough suppression (e.g., guafenesin, codeine)
  - Place bleeding side in dependent position to prevent blood from draining into the opposite lung
  - Intubation as needed for airway control (a double-lumen tube will preserve oxygenation if bleeding is persistent)
  - Control bleeding by bronchoscopic balloon tamponade, arteriography and embolization in persistent bleeding, or emergent thoracic surgery if embolization is not available and bleeding persists
- Treat underlying etiology as necessary
- Consider IV estrogen for massive hemoptysis

75. Hemorrhoids

Hemorrhoids are *not* protruding "varicose veins"—they are distinct from the rectal varices of portal hypertension. Rather, hemorrhoids are downwardly displaced anal cushions, which are normal vascular tissue (sinusoids) that protect the anal canal during defecation. The supporting tissue of the cushions deteriorates over time and, with increased anal pressure (straining), leads to sliding, engorgement, bleeding, and prolapse of the cushions. Hemorrhoids are common, affecting up to 50% of the population.

Differential Diagnosis

- External hemorrhoids
  - Located below the pectinate line
  - Typically painful
- Internal hemorrhoids
  - Located above the pectinate line
  - Typically not painful, unless thrombosis occurs
- Pregnancy
  - Up to 35% of pregnant females will develop hemorrhoids around the time of delivery, with most cases occurring after a vaginal delivery and/or a prolonged labor
- Condylomata acuminatum (genital warts)
- Rectal prolapse
  - External protrusion of the rectum
  - Complete prolapse versus partial full thickness prolapse versus prolapse of mucosa only
  - Partial rectal prolapse or mucosa-alone rectal prolapse is typically concentric, thus can be differentiated from internal prolapsing hemorrhoids that tend to have separation between cushions and inflammation
- Rectal polyp
- Rectal or anal cancer
- Hypertrophied anal papilla (polypoid structure at pectinate line)
- External skin tag
  - Redundant fold of tissue along the external anal margin
- Perirectal abscess
- Anal fissure or fistula
- Rectal varices
  - Develop secondary to portal hypertension
- Rectal cavernous hemangioma

Workup and Diagnosis

- History: The most common presenting complaints are bright red bleeding following defecation (in toilet or on paper), itching, and prolapse of a hemorrhoid
  - Hemorrhoids are usually *not* painful unless thrombosed, ulcerated, or gangrenous
  - Sudden onset of excrutiating perirectal pain with palpable mass usually suggests acute thrombosis of a hemorrhoid
- Physical exam: Evaluate for prolapse by having patient strain (may place them on a toilet to facilitate)
  - First-degree hemorrhoid: No prolapse
  - Second-degree: Prolapse during defecation followed by spontaneous return to anal canal
  - Third-degree: Prolapsed but manually reducible
  - Fourth-degree: Constant, irreducible prolapse
- Anoscopy and proctosigmoidoscopy are used to evaluate symptoms and bleeding
- Full colonoscopy is indicated in all patients over 50 years old or if diagnosis is inconclusive
- Rectal manometry is indicated if the patient complains of incontinence
- Biopsy is necessary for any rectal polyp or palpable lesion

Treatment

- Treatment is initially conservative: High-fiber diet, stool softeners, appropriate anal hygiene, sitz baths, and topical steroids
- Surgical options include rubber band ligation of internal hemorrhoids or surgical resection for large refractory hemorrhoids
- Acute thrombosis of a hemorrhoid may require incision and drainage

76. Hepatomegaly

Hepatomegaly, or enlargement of the liver, usually refers to a liver span of larger than 12 cm at the right midclavicular line or a palpable left lobe in the epigastrium. However, liver size on physical exam is only an approximation and should be accurately measured with an abdominal ultrasound, CT scan, or MRI. Abnormalities such as a low-lying liver or other abdominal masses must be considered.

Differential Diagnosis

- Right heart failure
- Inflammatory disorders, resulting in tender hepatomegaly
  - Hepatitis (viral or drug-induced): Associated with jaundice, fever, nausea, vomiting, fatigue, diarrhea, weight loss
  - Alcoholic liver disease: Associated with liver failure and portal hypertension (e.g., caput medusae, spider angiomata, hemorrhoids, testicular atrophy, ALT is more than two times higher than AST)
- Infiltrative disorders
  - Fatty liver (NASH): Predisposing factors include middle age, obesity, female gender, diabetes, and hyperlipidemia
  - Sarcoidosis: Associated with cough, hilar lymphadenopathy; more common in blacks, women, ages 30–40
  - Hemochromatosis: Iron overload resulting in bronzed skin color, diabetes, abnormal iron panel
  - Wilson's disease: Copper excess resulting in liver failure, lenticular degeneration, and Kayser-Fleischer rings in cornea
- Neoplasms present with focal enlargement, arterial bruit and/or hepatic rub, and constitutional symptoms (e.g., fever, night sweats, weight loss)
  - Metastatic cancer is more common than primary liver cancers (colon, lung, breast)
  - Hepatocellular carcinoma is most common primary liver cancer (often due to chronic hepatitis or cirrhosis)
  - Hepatic adenoma or hepatic cysts
  - Leukemia/lymphoma
- Liver abscess
- Less common causes ("zebras") include tricuspid regurgitation, Budd-Chiari syndrome, schistosomiasis, amyloidosis, kala-azar (visceral leishmaniasis), and HIV/AIDS

Workup and Diagnosis

- History should include past medical history, alcohol and drug use, medications (including herbal remedies), family history of liver disease, and presence of constitutional symptoms
- Physical exam should include palpation of liver surface for tenderness, consistency, nodularity, pulsations, bruits, rubs; skin examination (e.g., for jaundice, spider angiomata); cardiac exam; lymphadenopathy
- Liver function tests (ALT, AST, GGTP, albumin) and coagulation tests (PT/PTT/INR) to assess liver function
- Hepatitis serologies may be indicated, including hepatitis A, B, and C; CMV; and EBV
- Ultrasound will discriminate solid masses from cysts
- Abdominal CT to evaluate masses and fatty liver
- Doppler ultrasound to determine blood flow
- MRI of abdomen is useful to diagnose excess deposition of iron (hemochromatosis) or copper (Wilson's disease)
- Radionuclide scanning to characterize inflammatory and neoplastic lesions
- Angiography is the gold standard to differentiate hemangioma from solid tumor
- Iron panel (hemochromatosis) and ceruloplasmin (Wilson's disease)
- Consider gastroenterology consultation

Treatment

- Heart failure: Diuretics, inotropes, and afterload reduction
- Viral hepatitis: Supportive care and antivirals in some chronic cases
- Alcoholic liver disease: Abstinence from alcohol, steroids in severe cases, and possible transplant
- Fatty liver: Treat underlying obesity, diabetes, hyperlipidemia
- Sarcoidosis: Steroids
- Hemochromatosis: Iron removal by weekly phlebotomy for 2–3 years and/or deferoxamine chelation
- Wilson's disease: Copper chelation with D-penicillamine or trientine; may require liver transplantation
- Neoplasms: Resection and chemotherapy
- Abscess or cyst: Antimicrobials, percutaneous drainage, and/or surgical resection
- Amyloidosis: Prednisone and alkylating agents

77. Hoarseness

Hoarseness is any undesirable alteration of the voice. A rough sound of the voice, change in pitch, or increased effort of speaking can all be considered as hoarseness. "Acute" refers to hoarseness of sudden onset and/or a duration of fewer than 2 weeks. "Chronic" implies duration more than 2 weeks.

Differential Diagnosis

Acute (<2 weeks)
- Infections: Laryngitis, tracheitis, epiglottitis (accompanied by stridor and "thumb sign" on lateral neck X-ray), croup, upper respiratory infections, deep space face and neck infections (e.g., peritonsillar abscess, retropharyngeal abscess, parapharyngeal abscess)
- Voice abuse: Shouting, speaking, or singing loudly; may also cause chronic hoarseness if the abuse is recurrent
- Foreign body
- Trauma: Laryngeal trauma secondary to MVA, strangulation, assault, sporting injuries, intubation, arytenoid cartilage dislocation, or surgery (e.g., damage to recurrent laryngeal nerve following thyroid surgery)
- Irritants: Vomiting, chemical inhalation
- Anaphylaxis

Chronic (>2 weeks)
- Allergic rhinitis
- Irritants: Tobacco smoke, occupational
- GERD
- Chronic sinusitis
- Endocrine: Puberty, menopause, hypothyroidism
- Foreign body
- Aging
- Vocal cord problems: Polyps, nodules ("singer's nodules"), neoplasm (primary or metastatic), papilloma (infants and children), corditis (Reinke's edema or edema of vocal cords), vocal cord paralysis
- Malignancy: Laryngeal, esophageal, lung, and head and neck (e.g., tonsillar, tongue) cancers
- Iatrogenic: Medication side effect (e.g., pioglitazone, aerosolized steroids), postsurgical recurrent laryngeal nerve damage with vocal cord paralysis, radiation therapy
- Neurologic: Multiple sclerosis, amyotrophic lateral sclerosis, Parkinson's disease, muscular dystrophy
- Less common etiologies ("zebras") include hemorrhage into vocal folds, psychogenic (laryngeal conversion disorders), rheumatoid arthritis, sarcoidosis, and amyloidosis

Workup and Diagnosis

- History and physical exam
  - Assess prior history, onset, and duration; exposure to irritants, allergens, tobacco and/or alcohol, medications; voice use/abuse; trauma; associated symptoms (e.g., cold symptoms, heartburn, vomiting, weight loss, dysphagia); and past medical and surgical history
  - Focus on head and neck, thyroid, lung, and cardiac examinations, including an evaluation of voice quality
- Chest X-ray
- Lateral neck X-ray if history and physical suggest epiglottitis or foreign body
- Direct or fiber optic nasolaryngoscopy is the best way to assess the larynx; if suspect epiglottitis, must be done in operating room
- Biopsy if mass seen on direct laryngoscopy (usually refer to otolaryngoscopy for biopsy, if mass is visualized)
- If indicated by history or exam, consider upper GI endoscopy (EGD), upper GI series, CT of sinuses, thyroid function tests, and/or CT scan of head and neck (if suspect laryngeal or neck tumor that is not seen on nasolaryngoscopy and/or lymphadenopathy is present)

Treatment

- Evaluate airway, breathing, and circulation
- Trauma/obstruction: Cricothyrotomy or tracheostomy may be necessary to establish an airway
- Infections: Symptomatic measures (e.g., hydration, cough suppression, decongestants), antibiotics, voice rest, surgery for abscess
- Vocal abuse: Voice rest (whispering is *not* voice rest); if speaking is absolutely necessary, oral steroids may be used; voice therapy may be necessary in chronic voice abuse to correct faulty vocal habits
- GERD: H2 blockers or proton pump inhibitors, diet modification
- Allergic rhinitis/chronic sinusitis: Intranasal steroids and/or antihistamines (e.g., loratadine)
- Irritants: smoking cessation, protective clothing or masks
- Masses usually require surgical intervention
- Endocrine, neurologic, and rheumatologic etiologies should be treated appropriately

78. Hypercalcemia

Calcium is the most abundant mineral in the body, with 99% stored in bone. Calcium in the plasma is either protein-bound (mostly to albumin) or is ionized and readily available for use. Serum calcium is regulated by parathyroid hormone (PTH) and vitamin D metabolites (1,25-dihydroxyvitamin D, 25-hydroxyvitamin D). 90% of cases of hypercalcemia are secondary to an underlying malignancy (via bone metastases or PTH-related peptide secretion) or hyperparathyroidism (especially parathyroid adenoma).

Differential Diagnosis

- Primary hyperparathyroidism
  - Most commonly caused by an adenoma of one of the parathyroid glands (90% of cases of primary hyperparathyroidism)
  - Less commonly caused by parathyroid hyperplasia or carcinoma (may be associated with multiple endocrine neoplasia syndromes)
  - Symptoms may include weakness, confusion, polyuria, renal stones, nausea, and anorexia
  - Symptoms are usually only present when calcium rises over 12 mg/dL
- Drugs (e.g., thiazides, lithium)
- Malignancy (e.g., multiple myeloma, leukemia; lymphoma; breast, lung, and kidney cancers)
  - Most common cause in hospitalized patients
  - Hypercalcemia occurs due to stimulation of bone resorption by cytokines released from tumor cells or to the release of PTH-related peptide produced by the tumor
  - Symptoms are identical to primary hyperparathyroidism
- Renal failure
- Hyperthyroidism
- Addison's disease
- Familial hypocalciuric hypercalcemia
- Vitamin A or D intoxication
- Granulomatous disease (e.g., sarcoidosis, tuberculosis)
- Adrenal insufficiency
- Paget's disease
- Immobilization
- Hypophosphatemia
- Acromegaly
- Milk-alkali syndrome (due to excessive ingestion of milk or calcium supplements)

Workup and Diagnosis

- Complete history and physical examination
  - Most cases are relatively asymptomatic (fatigue and other nonspecific symptoms present)
  - "Stones, bones, abdominal groans, and psychic overtones" is the classic presentation; however, these are not common clinically
    * *Stones:* Renal stones in 50%
    * *Bones:* Bone pain, weakness, osteoporosis
    * *Groans:* Abdominal pain, nausea/vomiting, constipation, peptic ulcer disease, pancreatitis
    * *Psychic overtones:* Psychosis, depression, anxiety
  - Evaluate for increased urination or renal stones, GI upset, confusion, tiredness, mental status changes, hyporeflexia, hypertension, arrhythmias, and coma
- Initial laboratory studies include serum and urinary calcium, electrolytes, BUN/creatinine, parathyroid hormone, PTH-related peptide, CBC, albumin, magnesium, phosphate, alkaline phosphatase, vitamin D
  - The higher the plasma Ca^{2+}, the more likely it is due to a malignancy; it is generally more difficult to correct
  - Be sure to correct calcium level for serum albumin
  - Corrected calcium level = [0.8 × (normal albumin − serum albumin) + serum Ca^{2+}]
- ECG may show ST depression, wide T waves, short ST segment, QT shortening, bradyarrhythmias, heart block
- Further lab tests and/or imaging modalities may be indicated to evaluate for specific etiologies (e.g., CT scan to rule out nephrolithiasis, amylase/lipase)

Treatment

- Patients are often dehydrated; repletion of blood volume with normal saline may correct calcium level
- Severe hypercalcemia (calcium >13 mg/dL or symptoms) requires immediate intervention
  - IV rehydration with large volumes of normal saline
  - Loop diuretics to prevent volume overload and to augment renal calcium excretion
  - Bisphosphonates (e.g., IV pamidronate) inhibit bone resorption; full effect may not occur for 1–5 days
  - Calcitonin and mithramycin decrease bone resorption by osteoclast inhibition (note that mithramycin is cytotoxic and causes renal toxicity)
  - IV steroids may be used in vitamin D disorders, granulomatous diseases, and malignancy
  - Correct other electrolyte abnormalities as necessary
- Parathyroidectomy for primary hyperparathyroidism
- Treat malignancy according to established protocols

79. Hyperglycemia

Normal fasting glucose is <110 mg/dL, impaired fasting glucose is 111–125 mg/dL, and diabetes mellitus is defined as a fasting glucose >126 mg/dL. Several values above normal are indicated before making a diagnosis of impaired fasting glucose or diabetes.

Differential Diagnosis

- Impaired fasting glucose
- Medications
  - Corticosteroids are a common cause
  - Common medications include growth hormone, estrogen (including oral contraceptives), nicotinic acid, salicylates and NSAIDs, thiazide and loop diuretics, phenytoin, and epinephrine
- Diabetes mellitus type I
  - Diabetic ketoacidosis
- Diabetes mellitus type II
- Pancreatic disease
  - Acute or chronic pancreatitis
  - Pancreatectomy
  - Pancreatic carcinoma
  - Hemochromatosis
  - Cystic fibrosis
- Increased counter-regulatory hormones associated with acute disease
  - Myocardial infarction
  - Stroke or other neurologic disease
  - Renal insufficiency
  - Hepatic insufficiency
- Acromegaly
- Cushing's syndrome
- Pheochromocytoma
- Hyperthyroidism (thyroid storm)
- Glucagonoma
- Gestational diabetes
- Amyloidosis

Workup and Diagnosis

- History and physical examination
  - Symptoms of hyperglycemia include fatigue, polyuria, polyphagia, polydipsia, and stomach discomfort
  - Complete medication history is essential
  - Examination is most commonly normal, but patients occasionally present with acanthosis nigricans (hyperpigmented, velvety lesions commonly on the back of the neck and/or axilla), or necrobiosis lipoidica diabeticorum (atrophic, shiny, erythematous or pale macules on anterior shins)
  - Complicating problems of diabetes (end-organ dysfunction) involve many systems (e.g., diabetic retinopathy, peripheral neuropathy, diabetic nephropathy, hypertension, coronary artery disease)
- Initial presentation may be dramatic, with greatly elevated glucose and significant electrolyte abnormalities
- Both type I and type II result in elevated levels of insulin
  - In type I disease, exogenous insulin is often abnormally elevated
  - In type II disease, endogenous insulin is often abnormally elevated
- C-peptide is increased in type II and decreased in type I

Treatment

- IV fluids
- Acute treatment includes insulin administration (IV or subcutaneous) or oral hypoglycemic medications
- Remove offending medications if possible
- Treat the underlying etiology
- Acute treatment of diabetic ketoacidosis involves fluid repletion, correction of electrolyte disturbances, insulin administration, and very frequent monitoring of glucose and electrolytes (intensive care admission is often necessary for initial stages of treatment)
- Long-term management includes regular testing of Hb_{A1C}, glucose (home readings), blood pressure, lipid profile, renal function, and regular podiatric and ophthalmology examinations

80. Hyperkalemia

Hyperkalemia (plasma K^+ >5 mEq/L) causes increased extracellular potassium that leads to depolarization of the cell membrane and resulting cardiac arrhythmias, ventricular fibrillation, or asystole. Net K^+ absorption or excretion is determined by the actions of aldosterone and the effective plasma K^+ level on the collecting duct. Normally, potassium is excreted almost exclusively (90%) by the kidney, with some excretion by the colon.

Differential Diagnosis

Decreased renal excretion of potassium
- Acute or chronic renal insufficiency: Due to a decrease in distal solute (NaCl) delivery and a decrease in overall renal mass
- Impaired Na^+ reabsorption (common): Aldosterone deficit results in decreased K^+ excretion
  - Resistance to aldosterone: Drugs (e.g., potassium-sparing diuretics, trimethoprim, pentamidine), tubulointerstitial disease
  - Secondary hypoaldosteronism: Drugs (e.g., ACE inhibitors, NSAIDs, heparin), hyporeninemia, AIDS
  - Renal tubular acidosis, type 4
  - Primary hypoaldosteronemia
  - Gordon's syndrome
  - Postuterojejunostomy

Increased potassium release from cells
- Pseudohyperkalemia
  - Prolonged use of a tourniquet with or without repeated fist clenching
  - Hemolysis after blood is drawn
  - Marked leukocytosis and thrombocytosis: Cells release K^+ into the serum in the process of clotting; measure plasma K^+ rather than serum K^+ in these cases
- Tissue breakdown: Intravascular hemolysis, tumor lysis syndrome, excessive exercise, trauma, and rhabdomyolysis
- Metabolic acidosis: K^+ is shifted out of cells to buffer the increased H^+
- Hyperosmolar states (e.g., hyperglycemia): K^+ diffuses out of cells along with water
- Insulin deficiency
- Medications
  - α-adrenergic agonists
  - β_2 antagonists
  - Excessive supplementation in a patient with impaired renal function
  - Severe digitalis toxicity (paralyzes Na^+/K^+ ATPase)
  - Succinylcholine
- Hyperkalemic periodic paralysis
- Depolarizing muscle paralysis

Excess intake of potassium
- Oral or IV potassium replacement
- Dietary excess

Workup and Diagnosis

- History and physical examination
  - May be completely asymptomatic
  - May present with numbness, weakness (possibly leading to paralysis), decreased reflexes, or irritability
  - Hypoventilation is a late finding
  - Cardiac toxicity most likely will *only* be detected with ECG, unless the patient is hemodynamically unstable
- Rule out pseudohyperkalemia (e.g., hemolysis) by repeat measurement
- Initial laboratory tests may include electrolytes, calcium, magnesium, phosphate, and BUN/creatinine, cortisol, renin, and aldosterone levels
- ECG shows classic progressive changes, including peaked T-waves, prolonged PR and QT intervals, flattening of the P waves, and ST depression; QRS widening to a sine-wave pattern; Vfib may follow
- Assess K^+ secretion and calculate TTKG as follows: Urine K^+ concentration divided by ratio of urine to plasma osmolality (U_{osm}/P_{osm}); the ratio is finally divided by plasma K^+
  - TTKG >10 suggests hypovolemia or low protein intake
  - If TTKG <5, assess response to mineralocorticoids: An increase in TTKG to >10 suggests primary or secondary hypoaldosteronism; if TTKG is <10, assess the clinical picture; hypertension with low renin and aldosterone suggests chloride shunt (e.g., cyclosporine, RTA, Gordon's syndrome), whereas hypotension with high renin and aldosterone suggests aldosterone-resistant states (e.g., K^+ sparing diuretics)

Treatment

- Emergency intervention is necessary if K^+ exceeds 7.5 mEq/L, rise is sudden (e.g., less concern if patient has CRI, because these patients often live with K^+ levels of 5 to 5.5), or ECG changes are present
  - IV calcium to decrease cell membrane excitability
  - Sodium bicarbonate, insulin (add glucose to prevent hypoglycemia), and/or β_2 agonists (e.g., albuterol) are used to shift K^+ back into cells
- Removal of K^+ may be accomplished by ion exchange resins (e.g., sodium polystyrene sulfonate, retention enema), diuretics (loop and/or thiazide diuretics may be used if renal function is adequate), or dialysis (reserved for life-threatening hyperkalemia or renal failure)
- Treat underlying causes
  - Discontinue causative medications (e.g., NSAIDs, ACE inhibitors, K^+ supplements)
  - IV fluid administration if hypovolemic
  - Correct metabolic acidosis
  - Correct renal obstruction

81. Hypernatremia

Serum sodium may be increased by water deprivation, excessive water losses without sufficient repletion, or excessive sodium intake. The majority of cases of this common problem are due to free water deficit rather than sodium excess. When evaluating a patient with hypernatremia, the clinician must assess the volume status to determine the etiology and subsequent treatment.

Differential Diagnosis

- Increased water loss
  - GI losses (diarrhea, vomiting, intestinal fistula)
  - Drugs (e.g., diuretics, alcohol, amphotericin B, phenytoin, propoxyphene, lithium, demeclocycline)
  - Sweating
  - Burns
  - Fever
  - Hyperventilation
  - Diabetes insipidus (central versus nephrogenic)
  - Severe burns
  - Alcohol use
  - Hyperglycemia (resulting in osmotic diuresis)
  - Diuresis phase of acute renal failure
  - Peritoneal dialysis
  - Thyrotoxicosis
  - Hyperthermia
  - Adrenal or renal failure
- Decreased water intake
  - Poor oral intake (e.g., in the elderly)
  - Inability to swallow water due to physical limitation (e.g., coma, access/mobility problems, swallowing problems)
  - Inability to recognize the need for water due to a hypothalamic lesion (e.g., CVA)
  - Impaired thirst
  - Inappropriate IV fluids (e.g., renal failure)
  - Tube feeding with inadequate free water
- Excessive sodium intake
  - Endocrine causes: Cushing's syndrome, ectopic ACTH, primary aldosteronism
  - Iatrogenic (e.g., inappropriately administered hypertonic saline, administration of sodium bicarbonate)
  - Sea water ingestion/drowning
- Renal salt retention
  - Mineralocorticoid excess (Conn's syndrome)
  - Cushing's syndrome
  - Congenital adrenal hyperplasia
  - Multiple myeloma
  - Sjögren's syndrome
- Essential hypernatremia (reset osmostat)

Workup and Diagnosis

- Hypernatremia is defined as serum Na^+ >145 mEq/L; however, clinical signs and symptoms generally do not appear until serum Na^+ >158 mEq/L
  - Severity of symptoms relates to both the acuity and magnitude of rise in Na^+
- History should include questions about changes in thirst and urination, recent CNS surgery, administration of IV fluids, and history of mental status changes, seizures, polyuria, thirst, diarrhea, or vomiting
- Initial laboratory studies include electrolytes, BUN, creatinine, magnesium, calcium, serum and urine osmolarity, and urine Na^+
  - BUN/creatinine are elevated with diuretic use, glycosuria, fluid loss (e.g., GI, respiratory, skin), impaired thirst, adrenal deficiency, and DI
  - Normal in hyperaldosteronism (e.g., Conn's, Cushing's, CAH)
- Assess urine osmolality
  - Hyperosmolar urine (i.e., when the kidney reaction to hypernatremia is the excretion of a minimal volume of urine that is maximally concentrated) suggests an extrarenal etiology of the hypernatremia
  - Urine osmolarity is decreased in renal losses (e.g., diuretics and DI) and increased in GI, respiratory, and skin losses or poor intake
- Urine Na^+ is elevated in renal losses (>20 meq/L); decreased in GI, respiratory, and skin losses or poor intake (<10 meq/L); and normal in hyperaldosteronism

Treatment

- Patients with severe dehydration and hypotension should be treated emergently with IV fluids (lactated Ringer's or NSS)
- Calculate free water deficit:
  $0.6 \times$ weight (kg) $\times [(Na^+$ measured/140) $- 1]$
  - Correct free water deficit over 48–72 hours; give patient maintenance fluids and replacements for ongoing losses
  - Reduce serum Na^+ by no more than 10–15 mEq/L/day (0.5 mEq/L/hour) in chronic hypernatremia and 1 mEq/L/hr in acute hypernatremia
- Too-rapid correction of serum Na^+ can precipitate seizures or cerebral edema with ensuing herniation
- Isovolemic hypernatremia: Replace fluid with D_5W (replace half of fluid deficit in the first 24 hours)
- Hypovolemic hypernatremia: Replace fluid with NSS
- Hypervolemic hypernatremia: Administer D_5W and loop diuretics both to decrease hypertonicity by increasing Na^+ excretion and to add free H_2O while removing volume

82. Hyperpigmentation

Disorders of hyperpigmentation can be focal or diffuse. In diffuse hyperpigmentation, it is important to search carefully for an underlying endocrine or other systemic disease, or a history of medications or heavy metals that may explain the findings. See "Pigmented Lesions" entry for discussion of focal hyperpigmentation, which may be caused by hormonal influences (e.g., birth control pills, pregnancy)

Differential Diagnosis

- Acanthosis nigricans
  - Velvety, hyperpigmented thickening of skin folds (e.g., axillae, groin, neck, and inframammary regions)
  - Associated with insulin resistance (e.g., DM, Cushing's diseases, hypothyroidism, obesity, polycystic ovarian syndrome, and exogenous corticosteroids)
- Tinea versicolor
  - Mottled macular hyperpigmentation (and/or hypopigmentation) in rings and circles with little or no scale
  - Often on the upper trunk and shoulders
  - Caused by *Pityrosporum orbiculare and P. ovale,* which look like "spaghetti and meatballs" on KOH preparation
  - May be pruritic during acute phase, particularly in warm environments that encourage growth of the fungus
- Postinflammatory hyperpigmentation
  - Patchy, transient hyperpigmentation after resolution of inflammatory rashes
- Melasma (chloasma, "mask of pregnancy")
  - Gradual blotchy macular hyperpigmentation, especially of the malar surfaces, chin, and forehead
  - Occurs with oral contraceptives, pregnancy, or idiopathic
  - May fade postpartum or after discontinuing oral contraceptives, and recur if either occurs again
- Grey or blue hyperpigmentation
  - Medications: Amiodarone, minocycline, imipramine, chemotherapeutic drugs (e.g., bleomycin, doxorubicin), antimalarials, AZT
  - Heavy metal poisoning
- Incontinentia pigmenti
  - Genetic disorder with associated systemic abnormalities; the final stage of skin disease can present as linear and whorled streaks or hyperpigmentation
- Hemochromatosis
  - Diffuse hyperpigmentation
- Diabetic dermopathy
  - Hyperpigmented, round, atrophic lesions on shins of diabetics
- Mongolian spots

Workup and Diagnosis

- History and physical examination
  - Review the patient's medication list to rule out drug-induced pigmentation or melasma
  - Note whether rash, erythema, or scale preceded the hyperpigmentation
  - Heavy or irregular menses, hirsutism, and/or obesity may suggest PCOS
- Diffuse hyperpigmentation must be evaluated for underlying endocrine disorder; initial laboratory testing includes CBC, LFTs and iron profile (rule out hemochromatosis), fasting glucose (rule out diabetes), ACTH level (rule out Addison's disease), cosyntropin stimulation tests (rule out Cushing's disease)
- Trunk and chest lesions should have a KOH preparation performed (round "spores" and short nonbranching blunt hyphae to diagnose tinea versicolor)
- Age-appropriate malignancy screening is warranted in patients with acanthosis nigricans and no evidence of endocrine dysfunction

Treatment

- Acanthosis nigricans improves with adequate treatment of the underlying endocrine disorder; treatments may include weight loss, dietary/medication control of insulin resistance, and topical exfoliants (e.g., lactic acid, tretinoin, urea-based medications)
- Tinea versicolor: Treatment includes topical (e.g., ketoconazole) or oral antifungals (e.g., fluconazole); normalization of pigmentation may take many months; long-term maintenance therapy is necessary to prevent recurrence
- Melasma often improves spontaneously after pregnancy or discontinuation of oral contraceptives; sun avoidance and topical retinoids and hydroquinones facilitate normalization of pigment; chemical peels or laser procedures restore normal pigmentation
- Avoid offending medications; adjuvant laser therapy may be necessary to remove or destroy residual drug particles, hemosiderin, or excess melanin in skin

83. Hyperreflexia

Hyperreflexia is a finding that suggests upper motor neuron dysfunction; thus, it is usually associated with spasticity and a positive Babinski's sign. After an acute upper motor neuron lesion, hyperreflexia usually develops over a period of days to weeks, rather than appearing immediately. Hyperreflexia alone usually causes little specific disability; however, it is often associated with spasticity, which can be disabling.

Differential Diagnosis

- Cerebral lesions
  - Cerebral infarct or hemorrhage
  - Tumors or other mass lesions
  - Demyelinating disease (e.g., multiple sclerosis)
  - Congenital processes (e.g., cerebral palsy, neural tube defects, tethered cord)
  - Traumatic brain injury
- Brainstem lesions
- Cervical or thoracic myelopathy
  - Traumatic spinal cord injury
  - Compressive myelopathy from cervical spondylosis and/or osteoarthritis
  - Infectious or inflammatory causes [e.g., viral myelitis (consider HIV), vasculitis]
  - Syringomyelia: These patients frequently exhibit hyporeflexia at the level of the syrinx and hyperreflexia in segments below the level of the lesion; they may also exhibit a segmental area of sensory loss in the dermatomes involved by the syrinx
- Motor neuron disease
  - ALS: These patients have a combination of upper and lower motor neuron signs (e.g., hyperreflexia in a weak, atrophic limb with frequent fasciculations)
  - Primary lateral sclerosis: Hyperreflexia accompanied by slowly progressive weakness and spasticity
- Alcohol withdrawal
- Electrolyte disorders (e.g., hypocalcemia, hypomagnesemia)
- Tetanus
- Thyrotoxicosis
- Anxiety
- Lithium overdose
- Monoamine oxide inhibitor overdose
- Serotonin syndrome
- Less common etiologies ("zebras") include spinal cord infarction; syringobulbia; familial spastic paraparesis; spinocerebellar ataxia; HTLV-I associated myelopathy; and compressive myelopathy due to thoracic spondylosis, osteoarthritis, and/or epidural abscess

Workup and Diagnosis

- Hyperreflexia is an indication of upper motor neuron dysfunction; the etiology is usually suggested by the distribution of the hyperreflexia and associated physical findings
  - Hemihyperreflexia involving both the upper and lower extremities is most likely caused by a lesion of the brain or brainstem
  - Symmetric hyperreflexia involving only the lower extremities suggests a lesion of the thoracic or cervical spine
- CT is indicated for emergent evaluation of suspected intracranial lesions; however, MRI is a better choice for most suspected causes of hyperreflexia
- EMG/nerve conduction studies are helpful in cases of suspected ALS
- Laboratory testing may include electrolytes, calcium magnesium, drug screen, lithium level, serologies for HTLV-I, HIV, RPR, and DNA testing for many types of spinocerebellar ataxia
- CSF examination is indicated in suspected cases of multiple sclerosis (oligoclonal bands, elevated IgG index)

Treatment

- Hyperreflexia alone usually causes little specific disability; however, it is often associated with spasticity, which can be disabling; treat with antispasticity agents (e.g., baclofen, tizanidine, dantrolene)
- Replace electrolytes as needed
- Multiple sclerosis: Steroids for acute exacerbations, interferon, glatiramer acetate, mitoxantrone
- Compressive myelopathies usually require surgical intervention to relieve the compression
- Traumatic spinal cord injury frequently requires surgical stabilization; additionally, high-dose steroid infusion during the initial 24 hours following trauma has been shown to improve outcome
- Serotonin syndrome: Supportive care, cyproheptadine (a serotonin blocker)
- Syringomyelia may require surgical therapy
- HIV-related myelopathy: Antiretroviral therapy
- Some congenital conditions (e.g., neural tube defects, tethered cord) may be treated surgically

84. Hypersomnia

Hypersomnia is a symptom that may occur as a normal response to sleep deprivation, secondary to medications, or secondary to serious underlying brain pathology. It is also a common presenting symptom of many sleep disorders. A careful history of sleep habits, including the time spent in bed or trying to sleep elsewhere, bed mate, noise level, safety, and interruptions, is imperative for diagnosing and treating all sleep disorders.

Differential Diagnosis

- Sleep disorders
  - Poor sleep hygiene (e.g., going to bed too late, frequently changing sleep patterns secondary to shift work)
  - Sleep apnea
  - Narcolepsy: Characterized by attacks of irresistible sleepiness (REM sleep), cataplexy, hypnagogic hallucinations, and/or sleep paralysis
  - Periodic limb movements of sleep: Patients have repetitive movement of the extremities (usually legs) during sleep that may result in frequent arousals
  - Restless leg syndrome: Patients experience uncomfortable feelings in the lower extremities at rest that are improved with movement, causing difficulty in remaining still to fall asleep
- Depression
  - Frequently causes disturbances of sleep including hypersomnia, insomnia, and excessive daytime sleepiness
- Medications
- Encephalopathy
  - Metabolic (e.g., hepatic or uremic encephalopathy)
  - Toxic (e.g., sedating medications, alcohol, illicit sedating drugs)
- Structural brain lesions
  - Especially lesions involving the reticular activating system in the brainstem, large lesions, or bihemispheric lesions
- Infection
  - Mononucleosis
  - Encephalitis
  - Chronic meningitis (e.g., fungal)
- Complex partial status epilepticus
  - Frequently results in waxing and waning levels of alertness
- Idiopathic hypersomnia
  - Similar to narcolepsy, but with attacks of non-REM sleep
- Trypanosomiasis (African sleeping sickness)
  - A parasitic illness carried by the tsetse fly
- CO_2 retention

Workup and Diagnosis

- History and physical examination
  - Acute onset of hypersomnia suggests an acute illness or toxic effect
  - Chronic hypersomnia is more likely to be related to sleep disorders, depression, or chronic sedating medication use
  - Sleep diary may be useful
  - Review medication use
  - Physical examination should be directed toward identifying evidence of focal neurologic, psychiatric, and/or other organ system dysfunction (e.g., hepatic or renal failure)
  - Patients with obstructive sleep apnea are often obese
- Neuroimaging is indicated for patients with acute onset of hypersomnia without a clear cause or with focal neurologic abnormalities on examination
- Polysomnography is often used for sleep disorders
- Multiple sleep latency testing is especially useful for cases of suspected narcolepsy
- EEG
- CSF examination if an infectious cause is suspected
- Labs may include CBC, monospot, metabolic evaluation, and drug screen

Treatment

- Improve sleep hygiene: Maintain regular sleep hours; avoid caffeine, alcohol, and other substances that may interfere with natural sleep; avoid exertion at bedtime
- Correct metabolic abnormalities as necessary
- Treat infectious causes (e.g., acyclovir for herpes simplex encephalitis, appropriate antibiotics for bacterial meningitis, supportive care for mononucleosis)
- Obstructive sleep apnea: Nasal CPAP at night is very helpful but cumbersome to use consistently; weight loss often improves symptoms; surgical elimination of redundant tissue (uvulopalatopharyngoplasty)
- Narcolepsy may be treated with stimulants and antidepressants, which limit REM sleep
- Structural brain lesions may require surgical resection of other specifically directed treatment
- Periodic limb movements of sleep and restless leg syndrome may be treated with dopaminergic agents, benzodiazepines, or opiates

85. Hypertension

Elevated blood pressure is defined as diastolic BP $\geq$ 90 mmHg or systolic BP $\geq$ 140 mmHg. A diagnosis of hypertension requires three separate elevated blood pressure measurements. High normal: 130/85 to 139/89; stage 1: 140/90 to 159/99, stage 2–3: $\geq$ 160/100.

Differential Diagnosis

- Essential hypertension (95% of cases)
  - Associated with obesity, decreased physical activity, stress, and diets high in sodium or low in potassium, calcium, and/or magnesium
- Medications (e.g., oral contraceptives, pseudoephedrine, steroids, ephedrine, NSAIDs)
- Sleep apnea
- Secondary hypertension
  - Chronic renal disease
  - Renal vascular disease (e.g., renal artery atherosclerosis, fibromuscular dysplasia)
  - Cushing's disease
  - Pheochromocytoma
  - Primary hyperaldosteronism
  - Hyperthyroidism
  - Coarctation of aorta: Arm pulses are stronger than leg pulses and blood pressure is significantly higher in arms than in legs
- "White coat" hypertension
- Pain, stress (e.g., surgery, emotional), and post-exercise
- Isolated systolic hypertension
  - More common in elderly
  - Stronger risk factor for heart disease than diastolic hypertension in patients >50
- Excessive alcohol use
- Cocaine use
- Malignant hypertension
  - Markedly elevated blood pressure (diastolic BP >120–140 mmHg associated with papilledema)
- Preeclampsia/eclampsia
- Pregnancy-induced hypertension
- Congenital adrenal hyperplasia

Workup and Diagnosis

- History and physical examination, including evaluation of risk factors (e.g., history of diabetes, family history of heart disease, smoking, elevated cholesterol, drug use, stress, pain, obesity, body mass index)
- Evaluate for end organ disease (target organ damage): CAD symptoms, vascular disease, retinal hemorrhage, retinal venous crossing changes, heart exam (murmurs, gallops), lung exam (signs of CHF)
  - Labs may include urinalysis, basic metabolic panel (electrolytes, glucose, BUN/creatinine), calcium, lipids, ECG, echocardiogram, glomerular filtration rate measurement, and urinary albumin (albumin:creatinine ratio)
- Consider secondary causes of hypertension if sudden onset of hypertension, significant hypertension (>180/110), abnormally young (<30) or old (>50) patient, presence of end-organ symptoms, or poor response to treatment (not controlled with three medications)
  - Elevated creatinine suggests renal parenchymal disease
  - Abdominal bruits and hypokalemia suggest renal vascular disease
  - Cushing's disease is associated with osteoporosis, obesity, muscle weakness, moon facies, hirsutism, elevated lipids and sugar, low potassium
  - Pheochromocytoma is associated with extremely labile blood pressure (episodic or paroxysmal HTN), headaches, palpitations, and diaphoresis
  - Primary hyperaldosteronism is associated with isolated low potassium and non-anion gap metabolic alkalosis

Treatment

- Essential hypertension: Lifestyle changes are the initial interventions unless significant hypertension, end-organ damage, or diabetes is present (smoking cessation; dietary changes, e.g., DASH diet = low in sodium, rich in potassium and calcium; increased exercise)
- Pharmacologic therapy usually begins with a diuretic or β-blocker (ACE inhibitor in diabetics)
  - Diuretics are usually first-line agents, especially in CHF, diabetes, and risk of coronary artery disease
  - Use ACE inhibitors in patients with CHF, MI, renal disease, and diabetes
  - Use β-blockers in CAD, recent MI, angina, CHF, atrial fibrillation, migraines, hyperthyroidism
  - Additional drugs may include angiotensin receptor blockers (especially in patients with cough when using ACE inhibitors), calcium channel blockers, and β-blockers
  - Preferred drugs in pregnancy include methyldopa, β-blockers, and vasodilators (do not use ACE/ARBs)

86. Hypesthesia

Sensory loss (hypesthesia or decreased sensation, most commonly noticed in response to painful or touch stimuli) can occur secondary to a problem anywhere in the nervous system. It is often accompanied by paresthesias (an abnormal sensation such as numbness or tingling). The etiology of hypesthesia is usually suggested by the distribution of the finding and the associated symptoms.

Differential Diagnosis

- Peripheral neuropathy
  - Metabolic (e.g., diabetes mellitus)
  - Toxic (e.g., alcohol, heavy metal poisoning)
  - Inflammatory (e.g., chronic inflammatory demyelinating polyneuropathy)
  - Deficiency states (e.g., vitamin B_{12})
  - Inherited (e.g., Charcot-Marie-Tooth)
- Mononeuropathy (e.g., median nerve compression at the wrist, producing carpal tunnel syndrome; diabetic mononeuropathy)
- Radiculopathy
  - Results in dermatomal sensory loss in the territory of the affected nerve root
- Myelopathy
  - May result in sensory loss beginning at the dermatomal level of the lesion and progressing caudally
- Brainstem lesion
  - May cause both facial numbness (ipsilateral to the lesion) and hemicorporal sensory loss (commonly contralateral to the lesion)
- Subcortical lesions
  - Cerebrovascular infarct or hemorrhage
  - Multiple sclerosis
  - Tumor
- Cortical lesion (specific types of sensory loss, such as diminished graphesthesia or stereognosis, help to immediately localize the problem to the contralateral cerebral cortex, usually parietal lobe)
  - Cerebrovascular causes (e.g., cerebral infarct or hemorrhage)
  - Tumor
- TIA
- Syringomyelia: Results in a suspended area of sensory loss in the affected dermatomes with normal sensation elsewhere
- Cerebral abscess
- Paraneoplastic neuropathy
- Simple partial seizure
- Aura of migraine, producing transient numbness or paresthesias
- Plexopathy: Usually produces a polyradicular pattern of sensory loss in addition to motor findings
- Cauda equina syndrome

Workup and Diagnosis

- History and physical examination
  - Tempo of onset may help to suggest etiology (e.g., acute onset of sensory loss suggests a vascular event, migraine, or seizure)
  - Distribution of numbness or sensory loss will help to localize the lesion (e.g., distal symmetric sensory loss suggests peripheral neuropathy; sensory loss in the distribution of a single peripheral nerve or nerve root suggests a mononeuropathy or radiculopathy; a sensory level beginning at one dermatome and extending caudally suggests a spinal cord lesion; hemisensory loss suggests a brainstem or hemispheric cerebral lesion)
- EMG/nerve conduction studies are used to evaluate suspected peripheral neuropathy, mononeuropathy, or radiculopathy
- Labs may include screening for causes of neuropathy, including CBC, SPEP, ANA, RF, HIV, RPR, vitamin B_{12}, folate, thyroid function tests, Hb_{A1C}, heavy metals
- CT is a useful initial screen for suspected brain lesions
- MRI is usually the best imaging choice for suspected lesions of the brain or spinal cord
- Genetic testing is available for some forms of inherited neuropathy

Treatment

- Because few measures exist to restore feeling to numb areas, treatment generally consists of identifying and treating the underlying etiology
- General measures that may help to ameliorate painful dysesthesias include tricyclic antidepressants (e.g., amitriptyline), anticonvulsants (e.g., gabapentin), and topical preparations (e.g., capsaicin cream)
- Peripheral neuropathy: Treat the underlying etiology (e.g., treat thyroid disease, vitamin B_{12} deficiency)
- Mononeuropathies will frequently improve if the offending cause is alleviated (e.g., treat carpal tunnel syndrome with wrist splints or surgery)
- Radiculopathy may be treated conservatively with physical therapy and medications, more aggressively with epidural injections, or surgically
- Compressive myelopathies usually require surgical intervention to alleviate the compression
- Multiple sclerosis: Steroids, interferon, glatiramer acetate, or mitoxantrone

87. Hypocalcemia

Calcium is the most abundant mineral in the body, with 99% stored in bone. Calcium in the plasma is either protein-bound (mostly to albumin) or ionized and readily available for use. Decreased plasma Ca^{2+} stimulates PTH release; PTH counteracts the decreased serum Ca^{2+} by stimulating Ca^{2+} resorption from bone, renal phosphate excretion, and renal activation of vitamin D. Hypocalcemia is defined as a serum calcium level <8.5 mg/dL; however, "true" metabolic hypocalcemia requires a low level of free, ionized calcium.

Differential Diagnosis

- Hypoalbuminemia commonly results in a "pseudohypocalcemia"
  - Results in decreased total serum Ca^{2+} but normal free, ionized (active) Ca^{2+}
  - Does not result in sequelae of hypocalcemia
- Hypoparathyroidism
  - Often occurs after thyroidectomy or parathyoidectomy
  - Infiltrative diseases of the parathyroid gland (e.g., hemochromatosis, Wilson's disease, sarcoidosis, tuberculosis)
  - Pseudohypoparathyroidism (parathyroid hormone resistance)
  - Idiopathic (autoimmune)
- Medications (e.g., diuretics, heparin, foscarnet, cimetidine, glucagon, phosphates, aminoglycosides, theophylline, cisplatin)
- Vitamin D deficiency
  - Poor oral intake and/or absent sun exposure
  - Malabsorption
  - Hepatic and/or renal failure
  - Anticonvulsant use
- Pancreatitis
- Alkalosis (especially respiratory alkalosis)
- Sepsis
- Shock
- Burns
- Magnesium deficiency (often seen in alcoholism)
- Hyperphosphatemia
- Alcoholism (may directly suppress PTH and/or deplete magnesium)
- Postoperative (usually transient)
- Post-blood transfusion
- Malignancy
  - Medullary carcinoma of the thyroid
  - Osteoblastic metastases
- Familial hypocalcemia
- DiGeorge's syndrome (congenital absence of the parathyroid glands)
- Polyglandular autoimmune syndrome, type I (hypoparathyroidism, adrenal insufficiency, and mucocutaneous candidiasis)
- Rickets

Workup and Diagnosis

- History and physical examination
  - Severity of symptoms depends on rapidity of fall in serum calcium
  - Symptoms include weakness, fatigue, muscle cramping and spasm (difficulty speaking may indicate laryngeal spasm), paresthesias (perioral or fingertip), abdominal pain, nausea/vomiting, irritability, and depression
  - Severe hypocalcemia may cause delirium, psychosis, and seizures
  - Skin exam may reveal patchy hair loss, dry and/or scaly skin, hyperpigmentation, brittle nails, and mucocutaneous candidiasis
  - Trousseau's sign: Carpal spasms upon inflation of a blood pressure cuff for 2 to 3 minutes
  - Chvostek's sign: Tapping of cranial nerve VII (anterior to ear) causes twitching of facial muscles
  - Cardiac arrhythmias, decreased myocardial contractility (may lead to CHF), hypotension
- Initial labs include serum calcium, ionized calcium, albumin, magnesium, phosphorus, BUN/creatinine, CBC, and amylase/lipase
- Correct calcium for hypoalbuminemia: Serum Ca^{2+} decreases by 0.8 for each 1 g/dL drop in albumin (although ionized calcium is normal)
- Measure parathyroid hormone and vitamin D levels
  - Decreased in primary hypoparathyroidism
  - Elevated in renal failure, malabsorption, vitamin D deficiency, and pseudohypoparathyroidism
- ECG may reveal prolonged QT interval

Treatment

- Asymptomatic patients can be treated with oral calcium supplements plus vitamin D
- If severe symptoms are present, administer 10% IV calcium gluconate and recheck calcium levels frequently
- Change causative medications if possible
- Treat underlying diseases as necessary (e.g., sepsis, pancreatitis, renal failure)
- Correct other electrolyte abnormalities (e.g., hypomagnesemia)
- Hypoalbuminemia may improve with adequate nutrition; however, there is no need to correct serum Ca^{2+}, because the ionized calcium is normal
- Hypoparathyroidism: Calcium carbonate supplementation of 1–2 g per day plus vitamin D supplementation
- Vitamin D deficiency: Oral vitamin D or calcitriol (1,25-hydroxyvitamin D)

88. Hypoglycemia

Hypoglycemia causes release of glucagon, growth hormone, and catecholamines, which rapidly mobilize liver glycogen to provide fuel (elevated epinephrine causes the symptoms of hypoglycemia). Hypoglycemia rapidly causes neurologic dysfunction (may be irreversible), as glucose is the brain's primary source of energy. Hypoglycemia is a very common problem in diabetic patients. Patient education about coordinating the timing of hypoglycemic administration, diet, and exercise is the key to preventing repeated episodes of hypoglycemia.

Differential Diagnosis

- Exogenous insulin administration is the most common cause of hypoglycemia
  - Most commonly occurs in patients with known diabetes mellitus
  - May occur with inadequate food ingestion or excessive exercise after an insulin injection
  - May occur with delayed absorption of food (e.g., diabetic gastroparesis)
  - Rarely, may occur as part of attention seeking behavior (i.e., factitious)
- Oral hypoglycemic medications (e.g., sulfonylurea)
  - This is especially common with severe liver disease, which prevents gluconeogenesis
- Other medications (e.g., salicylates, sulfonamides, tetracyclines, warfarin, MAO inhibitors, phenothiazines)
- Reactive hypoglycemia occurs 2–4 hours after meals, due to delayed and exaggerated insulin release (associated with a family history of type II diabetes)
- Hypothyroidism
- Malnutrition/fasting
- Insulinoma/islet cell hyperplasia
- Alcohol consumption
- Sepsis
- Renal failure
- Sarcomas
- Pituitary or adrenal insufficiency
- Congenital hormone or enzyme defects
- Severe hepatic dysfunction (e.g., hepatitis, hepatic toxins, hepatic necrosis)

Workup and Diagnosis

- History and physical examination
  - Medication, diet, and exercise history
  - Associated symptoms include tachycardia, diaphoresis, tremor, anxiety, hyperventilation, and hyperthermia
  - CNS symptoms may include dizziness, headache, confusion, convulsions, mental status changes, abnormal behavior, and coma
- Immediately measure serum glucose in any patient with altered mental status—missed diagnosis may result in irreversible neurologic damage or unnecessary procedures (e.g., intubation)
- Clinical symptoms of hypoglycemia usually begin to occur when the blood glucose level reaches 50 mg/dL; however, in diabetes, symptoms may begin at higher blood glucose levels or not at all
- Initial laboratory studies include serum or finger-stick glucose level, CBC, electrolytes, BUN/creatinine, magnesium, and urinalysis
- Consider LFTs, urinalysis, chest X-ray, TSH, cortisol, alcohol level and drug screen, head CT, blood cultures, and lumbar puncture if etiology is unclear
- Measure C-peptide and insulin before glucose infusion
  - Serum insulin is elevated by insulinomas (insulin:glucose ratio >0.3) and sulfonylurea or exogenous insulin administration
  - C-peptide is produced during endogenous insulin production; thus, decreased after exogenous insulin use; increased in insulinoma, sulfonylureas
- CT/MRI may be necessary to evaluate for insulinoma

Treatment

- Glucose therapy (therapy goal is glucose >100 mg/dL)
  - Alert patients may be repleted with oral glucose (e.g., juice, glucose tablets) or IV D_{50}
  - Patients with altered consciousness require IV D_{50} solution
  - In children, use bolus of 25% dextrose
  - Frequently recheck blood glucose
- Glucagon may be used to increase glucose release from the liver if unable to obtain IV access and the patient cannot tolerate oral glucose; less effective in alcoholic and malnourished patients
- Octreotide may be used in cases of sulfonylurea-induced hypoglycemia to inhibit insulin release
- Thiamine must be given with glucose in any suspected case of alcohol abuse or nutritional deficiency to avoid Wernicke's encephalopathy
- Hydrocortisone should be administered if blood glucose remains persistently low to rule out adrenal insufficiency

89. Hypokalemia

Potassium is the major intracellular cation and is responsible for facilitating muscular contraction, including cardiac muscle function. Serum potassium concentration is mediated primarily by the actions of aldosterone. Hypokalemia is defined as plasma K^+ concentration less than 3.5 mEq/L. The possible etiologies are broadly divided into three categories: Decreased potassium intake, increased potassium losses (generally via renal or GI routes), and intracellular redistribution.

Differential Diagnosis

- Increased potassium loss (GI, urine, sweat)
  - Vomiting
  - Diarrhea
  - Laxative abuse
  - Drugs [e.g., diuretics, sodium polystyrene sulfonate (Kayexelate), penicillin, aminoglycosides, steroids]
  - Nasogastric suction
  - Hyperaldosteronism
  - Renal tubular acidosis types 1 or 2
  - Diabetic ketoacidosis
  - Magnesium deficiency
  - Bartter's syndrome
  - Cushing's syndrome
  - GI fistula
  - Excessive sweating
  - Geophagia
  - Liddle's syndrome (ureterosigmoidotomy)
- Intracellular redistribution (transcellular shifts of potassium may transiently decrease (or increase) plasma K^+ without altering total body K^+
  - Medications (e.g., insulin, catecholamines, β-adrenergic agonists, caffeine, vitamin B_{12})
  - Alkalosis
  - Hypokalemic periodic paralysis (familial disorder with recurrent acute hypokalemia and weakness)
  - Digibind therapy (for digoxin toxicity)
  - Barium or toluene ingestion
  - Anabolic states or conditions of rapid cell multiplication (e.g., thyrotoxicosis)
  - Hypothermia
  - Chloroquine overdose
- Decreased potassium intake (by itself, rarely causes hypokalemia, because the kidneys are very efficient at conserving K^+)
  - Starvation
  - Malabsorption
  - Postoperative
  - "Fad" diets (e.g., liquid protein)
- Pseudohypokalemia: Increased uptake of potassium by white cells in patients with marked leukocytosis (e.g., leukemia)

Workup and Diagnosis

- History and physical examination
  - Symptoms generally begin once K^+ <2.5 meq/L
  - Common symptoms include fatigue, weakness, myalgias, muscle cramps, constipation, and respiratory muscle weakness
  - Cardiac abnormalities may include hypertension, life-threatening arrhythmias (e.g., ventricular tachycardia, Vfib), potentiation of digoxin, and heart block
  - Other complications may include rhabdomyolysis, dehydration, hyperglycemia, ileus, hepatic encephalopathy, nephrogenic diabetes insipidus
- Initial labs should include electrolytes (may reveal associated hypomagnesemia or hypophosphatemia), glucose (rule out DKA), BUN/creatinine, calcium, magnesium, and CBC
- Check ABG (every 0.1 increase in pH causes a decrease in plasma K^+ of 0.5 mEq/L)
- Urine K^+ level and TTKG may aid in determination of underlying etiology
  - $$TTKG = \frac{(urine\ [K^+])\ (plasma\ Osm)}{(plasma\ [K^+])\ (urine\ Osm)}$$
- Consider urinary sodium, creatinine, and renin levels
- Progressive ECG changes occur as serum K^+ falls (however, changes do not correlate well with K^+ level): Low voltage and widening of QRS complexes, flattening of T waves, depressed ST segments, prominent P and U waves (U waves follow the T wave), prolonged PR and QT intervals, ventricular arrhythmias

Treatment

- Goal of treatment is to replace K^+ and minimize ongoing losses
- Replete potassium
  - Oral replacement may be attempted in patients who have minimal symptoms and can tolerate oral intake
  - IV replacement if severe sequelae (e.g., cardiac manifestations) are present; do not administer the K^+ in a dextrose solution (may worsen the hypokalemia by increasing insulin output)
  - Each 10 mEq of K^+ should increase serum K^+ by 0.1
  - Replete Mg^{2+} and Ca^{2+} concurrently, especially if the patient is on digitalis
- Volume-depleted patients require IV rehydration with normal saline plus K^+
- Estimation of the actual potassium deficit is imprecise because of redistribution between the plasma and intracellular space; thus, plasma potassium should be rechecked frequently during correction

90. Hyponatremia

Hyponatremia is classified on the basis of serum osmolality and volume status. Normal or increased osmolality suggests pseudohyponatremia. True hyponatremia causes a hypo-osmolar state. Once hypo-osmolality is demonstrated, evaluate the patient's volume status by clinical assessment (dry mucus membranes, decreased urine output, and skin tenting suggests hypovolemia; edema suggests hypervolemia). Correction rates should generally be slow in order to avoid severe complications, the worst of which is central pontine myelinolysis.

Differential Diagnosis

- Hypertonic hyponatremia (increased serum osmolality)
  - Pseudohyponatremia (decrease in Na^+ of 1.6 for every 100 mg/dL increase in glucose)
  - Iatrogenic hypertonic infusions
- Hypotonic hyponatremia (decreased serum osmolality)
  - Hypovolemic: Loss of both Na^+ and H_2O results in a total body water deficit plus a larger total body Na^+ deficit
    * Vomiting
    * Diarrhea
    * Third spacing (e.g., pancreatitis, burns)
    * Addison's disease
    * Renal tubular acidosis
    * Renal losses (e.g., diuretics, renal disease)
  - Euvolemic (e.g., SIADH, excess free water intake): Normal ECF volume with slightly decreased total body Na^+
    * SIADH is a very common cause of hyponatremia (six criteria must be present for diagnosis: Euvolemia; hypotonic hyponatremia; urine osmolality >200 mEq/L; urine Na^+ >20 mmol/L; normal organ function; and improves with water restriction)
    * Renal failure
    * Hypothyroidism
    * Psychogenic polydipsia
    * Drugs (e.g., thiazide diuretics)
  - Hypervolemic: Excess total body Na^+ plus a larger excess total body H_2O due to an impaired ability to excrete H_2O
    * Cirrhosis
    * CHF
    * Acute or chronic kidney disease
    * Nephrotic syndrome
    * Pregnancy
    * Hypoalbuminemia (secondary to malnutrition)
- Isotonic (normal serum osmolality) hyponatremia
  - Hyperlipidemia
  - Hyperproteinemia
  - Hyperglycemia without dehydration

Workup and Diagnosis

- History and physical examination
  - Clinical symptoms may include mental status changes, agitation, headache, ataxia, focal weakness, altered level of consciousness, seizures, and/or coma
  - Clinical symptoms of the underlying etiology may be present (e.g., pulmonary and pedal edema in CHF)
  - Symptoms and clinical signs become most apparent when serum Na^+ <120 mEq/L
- Initial laboratory testing includes serum electrolytes, osmolality, BUN/creatinine, calcium, magnesium, TSH, glucose, and urine sodium, creatinine, and osmolality
- Hypertonic (plasma osmolality >295): Check serum glucose
- Isotonic (osmolality 275–295): Check protein and lipids
- Hypotonic (osmolality <275): Assess volume status and check BUN/creatinine ratio, urine Na^+, and urine osmoles
  - Hypervolemic: Urine Na^+ <10 mmol/L in CHF, cirrhosis, nephrosis; urine Na^+ >20 mmol/L in renal failure
  - Hypovolemic: Urine Na^+ <10 mmol/L in extrarenal losses (e.g., GI, third spacing, hypotonic fluids); urine Na^+ >20 mmol/L in renal losses (e.g., diuretics, Addison's disease, salt-wasting nephropathy)
  - Isovolemic: Urine Na^+ is usually >20 mmol/L; in SIADH, urine osmoles >300 mOsm/L; in psychogenic polydipsia, urine osmoles <50 mOsm/L
- Calculate corrected sodium concentration to evaluate for pseudohyponatremia [corrected Na^+ = Na^+ × (glucose – 100) × 0.016]

Treatment

- Symptomatic patients require immediate Na^+ correction
  - Treat severe hyponatremia (serum Na^+ <120 mEq/L or rapid hyponatremia or hyponatremia with serious CNS symptoms) with 3% saline at 25–100 mL/hour
- Correct serum Na^+ gradually (especially in chronic cases) to prevent seizures, cerebral edema, or central pontine myelinolysis (CNS demyelination due to paradoxical dehydration of neurons)
  - Serum Na^+ should not rise faster than 0.5–1 mEq/L/hour or 12 mEq/L/24 hours (even if patient is symptomatic)
  - Na^+ deficit = (desired Na^+ – actual Na^+) × (0.6 × weight)
- Isotonic and hypertonic hyponatremia: Correct glucose, lipids, and protein abnormalities as necessary
  - Hypotonic, isovolemic hyponatremia: Restrict fluids (600– 800 mL/day) or administer saline plus a loop diuretic
- Hypotonic, hypovolemic hyponatremia: NSS
- Hypotonic, hypervolemic hyponatremia: Restrict Na^+ and H_2O and administer loop diuretics

91. Hyporeflexia

Hyporeflexia is a general indicator of lower motor neuron dysfunction, which may result from a lesion anywhere in the anterior horn cell, spinal motor nerve or nerve root, plexus, peripheral nerve, neuromuscular junction, or muscle. Diagnostic evaluation is usually suggested by associated findings on neurologic exam, and treatment must be individualized on the basis of an identified cause. Hyporeflexia alone in the absence of pathology generally causes no disability and requires no treatment.

Differential Diagnosis

- Peripheral neuropathy
  - Most common cause of symmetric hyporeflexia (polyneuropathy or mononeuropathy)
  - Patients usually present with symmetric sensory complaints and/or weakness with distal muscular atrophy
  - Most frequently associated with diabetes
- Isolated peripheral nerve injury/dysfunction
- Radiculopathy
  - Isolated loss of a single reflex may suggest dysfunction of that nerve root (ankle reflex = S1 nerve root; knee jerk = L2, 3, 4; brachioradialis = C5, 6; biceps = C5, 6; triceps = C7)
  - Other associated symptoms may include dermatomal sensory loss or pain and weakness of muscles in the territory of the affected root
- Guillain-Barré syndrome
  - Due to inflammatory demyelination (likely viral) of peripheral nerves
  - Results in a subacute onset of progressive weakness (over hours to days) and hypo- or areflexia
  - Patients may experience respiratory compromise or autonomic dysfunction
- Brachial or lumbosacral plexopathy
  - May be secondary to trauma or spontaneous
  - Usually associated with severe pain in the shoulder and arm (brachial plexopathy) or hip and leg (lumbosacral plexopathy)
- Obese patients or those with large muscle bulk may exhibit relatively quiet reflexes, without any associated pathology
- Lambert-Eaton myasthenic syndrome
- Multifocal motor neuropathy
  - May mimic ALS but without upper motor neuron signs
- Myopathy
  - These patients present primarily with weakness, but they may also exhibit hyporeflexia
- Motor neuron disease
- "Spinal shock"
  - Patients with acute CNS lesions (such as spinal cord injury) may initially exhibit hyporeflexia
- Cauda equina syndrome

Workup and Diagnosis

- Complete history, physical, and neurologic examination
  - The etiology of hyporeflexia will likely be identified by the associated signs on physical examination (e.g., symmetric stocking-glove territory sensory loss in association with hyporeflexia suggests peripheral neuropathy; isolated loss of an ankle jerk with associated weakness of ankle plantar flexion is suggestive of S1 radiculopathy)
- Nerve conduction studies and electromyography are useful in the evaluation of suspected peripheral polyneuropathy, single or multiple mononeuropathies, radiculopathy, or myopathy
- MRI of the spine may help to diagnose radiculopathy
- In cases of suspected Guillain-Barré syndrome or chronic inflammatory demyelinating polyneuropathy, CSF examination by lumbar puncture may show elevated protein levels
- For generalized peripheral neuropathy, laboratory testing should include CBC, glucose, calcium, SPEP, UPEP, ESR, ANA, RF, HIV, RPR, vitamin B_{12} levels, CPK, thyroid function tests, Hgb_{A1C}, and heavy metal screen

Treatment

- Although there may be no disability associated with hyporeflexia, treatment varies depending on the underlying identified cause
- Peripheral neuropathy: If a treatable cause is identified, specific therapy should be directed at that cause (e.g., treat thyroid disease, B_{12} deficiency, or syphilis)
- Guillain-Barré syndrome has improved outcomes if patients are treated with plasmapheresis or IVIG within 2 weeks of the onset of symptoms
- Radiculopathy may be treated conservatively with physical therapy and medications (e.g., NSAIDs), more aggressively with epidural steroid injections, or surgically
- Other causes of focal hyporeflexia (e.g., traumatic peripheral nerve injury) require individualized therapy, but usually the only option is supportive care while awaiting spontaneous recovery or surgical intervention

92. Hypotension

Chronic low blood pressure is generally not a serious problem. However, a sudden drop in blood pressure is a sign of an underlying condition and may result in serious consequences secondary to cerebral and renal hypoperfusion.

Differential Diagnosis

- Orthostatic hypotension
  - Most common in elderly
  - May result in syncope or near-syncope upon standing
  - Decrease of more than 20 mmHg in systolic blood pressure, or a decrease of 10 mmHg in diastolic blood pressure within 2–5 minutes of standing
- Hypotension secondary to medications is common in elderly patients (e.g., antihypertensives; vasodilators, including nitrates, calcium channel blockers, ACE inhibitors, angiotensin receptor blockers; hypoglycemic agents; antidepressants; opiates; alcohol)
- Volume depletion
  - Often due to hyperglycemia, dehydration, hemorrhage, occult bleeding, vomiting, diarrhea, or diuretic use
- Autonomic failure
  - Absence of reflex-induced increase in heart rate as blood pressure is decreased
  - Often due to Parkinson's disease, cerebellar disorders, neuropathies, or Shy-Drager syndrome
- Postprandial hypotension (within 75 minutes of eating)
  - Very common in elderly
- Adrenal insufficiency
  - ACTH stimulation test shows inadequate increase in serum cortisol from baseline
- Diabetic autonomic neuropathy
- Shock
  - Cardiogenic shock
  - Septic shock
  - Neurogenic shock
  - Hemorrhagic shock
- Anaphylaxis
- Splenic rupture
- Ectopic pregnancy
- Hepatitis

Workup and Diagnosis

- History and physical examination
  - Compare blood pressure to patient's usual values
  - The absence of reflex-induced increase in heart rate as blood pressure falls indicates autonomic failure, which may require a workup for suspected underlying neurologic or pharmacologic conditions
  - Cardiogenic shock is often accompanied by cool, clammy extremities
- Laboratory studies may include CBC, electrolytes, BUN/creatinine, glucose, calcium, urinalysis, and ECG
- Additional studies (e.g., blood cultures, echocardiogram, blood type and cross) may be indicated based on the underlying disorder
- Swan-Ganz catheterization (right heart catheterization) may be indicated to establish the etiology (e.g., cardiogenic versus noncardiogenic) and determine patient management
- For diagnosis of adrenal insufficiency, obtain baseline cortisol level and then administer 250 μg of ACTH (Cortrosyn); obtain serum cortisol levels 30 and 60 minutes after ACTH administration; if cortisol level increases by <7, then adrenal insufficiency is highly likely

Treatment

- Orthostatic hypotension: Increase salt and water intake; pharmacologic treatment for moderate to severe disease may include fludrocortisone acetate, sympathomimetic agents, NSAIDs, caffeine, and erythropoietin
- Volume depletion: Fluid replacement based on existing deficiencies (e.g., saline, dextrose, potassium, packed red blood cells)
- Remove offending medications, compensate for medication needs
- Adrenal insufficiency requires stress doses of IV hydrocortisone (100 mg IV every 6 hours)
- Patient education (e.g., rise slowly from sitting to standing)

93. Hypothermia

Hypothermia is defined as a core body temperature of 95°F (35°C) and can be further defined as mild (90–95°F, or 32–35°C), moderate (82–90°F, or 28–32°C), or severe (below 82°F, or 28°C). Accidental hypothermia is the most common cause of severe hypothermia. Return of spontaneous circulation has been documented from temperatures as low as 57.6°F (14.2°C) in infants and 56.7°F (13.7°C) in adults. For ventricular fibrillation due to hypothermia, bretylium is currently the ACLS agent of choice.

Differential Diagnosis

- Exposure
  - Alcohol intake is a common risk factor because it both alters thermoregulation and promotes risk-taking behavior
  - Shivering, amnesia, ataxia, and dysarthria occur with mild hypothermia (>89.6°F, or >32°C)
  - Stupor, absence of shivering, atrial fibrillation, and/or bradycardia occur with moderate hypothermia (82–90°F, or 28–32°C)
  - Coma, ventricular fibrillation, apnea, asystole, and/or areflexia occur with severe hypothermia (<82.4°F, or <28°C)
- Sepsis
  - Mild hypothermia is common in sepsis, especially in infection with gram-negative rods (e.g., *E. coli*), and in the elderly
- Hypothyroidism
  - Up to 10 times more common in females
  - May be of autoimmune, postsurgical, or pituitary etiology
  - Symptoms include hypothermia, hair loss, dry skin, pretibial myxedema, weight gain, constipation, and prolonged relaxation phase of deep tendon reflexes
- Stroke
  - Hypothermia may occur because of altered cerebral thermoregulation
- Hypovolemic shock
  - Poor peripheral perfusion often results in mild hypothermia
- Massive blood transfusion
  - Due to refrigerated blood that is rapidly transfused without warming
- End-stage liver disease
  - Consider spontaneous bacterial peritonitis and sepsis in patients with ascites

Workup and Diagnosis

- A complete history and physical examination are essential, especially if there is no definite history of exposure
  - Careful examination of the extremities and dependent body parts for signs of frostbite
  - Assess core temperature (rectal temperature is preferred) using a low-temperature thermometer
- ECG may reveal Osborne J waves if temperature is less than 91.4°F (33°C)
- Laboratory studies may include CBC, electrolytes, BUN/creatinine, glucose, calcium, liver function tests, coagulation studies, blood and urine cultures, TSH, free T$_4$, arterial blood gas analysis, creatine kinase, and urinalysis (evaluate for rhabdomyolysis)
- Chest X-ray may be indicated to assess for infection in cases of suspected sepsis
- Head CT scan to evaluate for altered mental status
- Blood cultures are indicated if infection and/or sepsis are suspected

Treatment

- "No person is dead until they are warm and dead"—this underscores the ability to resuscitate patients from profound hypothermia
- Exposure is treated by passive rewarming to prevent further heat loss (e.g., remove wet clothes, cover with blankets), active external rewarming (e.g., radiant warmers, heating blankets), and/or active core rewarming (e.g., warmed IV fluids, pleural lavage, cardiopulmonary bypass, dialysis)
- Hypothyroidism: Treat mild cases with levothyroxine, myxedema coma with IV thyroxine and IV hydrocortisone
- Sepsis: Administer appropriate antibiotics, vasopressors for hypotension, and fluids for resuscitation
- Shock: Volume expansion with crystalloid solutions (normal saline or lactated Ringer's) or blood products; vasopressors (e.g., norepinephrine, phenylephrine); positive inotropes (e.g., dopamine, dobutamine)

94. Incontinence

Incontinence, defined as the involuntary loss of urine, is one of the ten most common medical problems in the U.S. However, most patients do not seek treatment despite the significant effects on self-esteem and social interactions. Prevalence is estimated at 13–60 million Americans (men and women) and affects especially geriatric patients. Associated costs approach $16 billion per year.

Differential Diagnosis

Transient, acute incontinence (DIAPPERS)
- Delirium
- Infections of urinary tract
- Atrophic urethritis or vaginitis
- Pharmaceuticals [e.g., diuretics, sedatives, anxiolytics, alcohol, β-blockers (cause urethral relaxation), ACE inhibitors (chronic cough increases abdominal pressure), antidepressants, antipsychotics]
- Psychiatric conditions (e.g., depression)
- Endocrine disorders (e.g., hypercalcemia, hyperglycemia)
- Restricted mobility or (urinary)
- Retention
- Stool (fecal impaction)

Persistent, chronic incontinence
- Stress incontinence
    - Loss of urine upon increases in intra-abdominal pressure (e.g., laughing, coughing, change in position, exercise)
    - Women <60 years after vaginal births
    - Urethral trauma (e.g., prostate surgery)
- Urge incontinence ("overactive bladder")
    - Strong urge to urinate before reaching the toilet; usually in people >60
    - Commonly associated with reversible causes, increased fluid intake, or poor bladder contractility
    - Idiopathic causes, neurologic causes, hyperreflexia, neuropathies, poor bladder contractility, increased sphincter relaxation, and reversible causes (e.g., UTI, increased fluid intake)
- Overflow incontinence
    - Outlet obstruction: BPH, GU prolapse, tumors
    - Bladder contractility dysfunction: Neurologic disorder (e.g., diabetic or alcoholic neuropathy), sacral spinal cord lesions, anticholinergic medications
- Functional incontinence
    - Normal urinary system affected by external factors (e.g., age, mental status decline, poor mobility)
- Mixed incontinence
    - Combined elements of stress and urge incontinence is common in older females
    - Combined elements of overflow and urge incontinence are most common in men and frail nursing-home patients

Workup and Diagnosis

- History should include whether the patient has problems holding urine versus emptying bladder; leakage of urine with cough, exercise, sneezing, laughing, lifting; frequency of urination; nocturnal urination; strong urge to urinate; loss of urine before reaching toilet; hesitancy, dribbling, slow stream, incomplete voiding, dysuria; bowel habits (e.g., constipation); medications; fluid intake; and medical and surgical history
- Physical exam should include full neurologic and mental status examinations, assessment of physical frailness (e.g., use of walking aids, dysfunction secondary to stroke), abdominal exam (e.g., lower quadrant distension, pregnancy, fecal impaction), and genital and rectal exam (evaluate for cystocele, vaginal atrophy, strength of pelvic muscles in women; rectal tone, abnormalities of glans penis and prostate in men)
- Cough stress test: Immediate leakage indicates stress incontinence; delayed leakage indicates urge incontinence
- Voiding diaries may be used to track urinary habits
- Initial labs may include electrolytes, calcium, glucose, urinalysis, and urine culture
- Measurement of postvoid residual volume by catheterization and/or pelvic ultrasound (>100 mL of residual urine is abnormal)
- Specialized urodynamic tests are reserved for ambiguous results or treatment failure

Treatment

- Treat reversible causes appropriately (e.g., antibiotics for UTI, discontinue offending medications)
- Stress incontinence
    - Pelvic exercises (Kegel's) or electrical stimulation
    - α-adrenergic medications to increase urethral tone
    - Local estrogen replacement treatment
    - Pessaries prevent urine loss during stress maneuvers
    - Surgical therapy may be indicated
- Urge incontinence
    - Estrogen replacement therapy (local or oral)
    - Medications include oxybutynin and tolteridine
- Overflow incontinence
    - Improve bladder contractility
    - Remove outlet obstruction (enlarged prostate, defects in penis, prolapsed uterus or urethra)
    - Neuropathic conditions may require intermittent catheterization to improve symptoms
- Functional incontinence
    - Remove physical mobility barriers

95. Insomnia

Insomnia may be a primary diagnosis or a complaint or symptom secondary to an underlying acute or chronic disorder. Many patients have insomnia but do not tell their doctors, so questions about sleep quality should be asked during health maintenance visits. A careful history of sleep habits, including the time spent in bed or trying to sleep elsewhere, bed mate, noise level, safety, and interruptions, is imperative for diagnosing and treating all sleep disorders.

Differential Diagnosis

- Unnecessary concern about deviation from "normal" sleeping patterns
- Acute, transient insomnia (<4 weeks)
  - Situational stress (most common)
  - Acute illness or injury
  - Medications or drugs (e.g., cocaine)
  - Change in sleep environment or hours
- Chronic insomnia (>4 weeks)
  - Difficulty falling asleep: May be due to poor sleep hygiene, conditioned insomnia (initial acute insomnia progresses to chronic due to maladaptive distorted sleep cognitions), medications (e.g., sedatives, decongestants, oral contraceptive use, antidepressants, bronchodilators), drugs (including over-the-counter and herbal preparations, alcohol, nicotine, illicit drugs), and caffeine (e.g., coffee, soda, medications)
  - Difficulty staying asleep: May be due to sleep apnea, medications and drugs (e.g., alcohol), depression, anxiety, dementia, psychosis, mania, post-traumatic stress disorder, and various medical conditions (e.g., COPD, asthma, CHF, angina, GERD, peptic ulcer disease, IBD, BPH, UTI, pregnancy, uremia, diabetes mellitus, hyperthyroidism, menopause, pain, pruritus, seizures)
- RLS
  - "Creepy-crawly" unpleasant sensations in the legs and/or feet
  - Temporarily relieved by moving limbs
- Periodic limb movement disorder
  - Arms and/or legs jerk during sleep
  - May be a primary disorder or secondary to uremia, neuropathy, or iron deficiency
  - Often in the elderly
  - Often occurs with restless legs syndrome
- Narcolepsy
- REM-behavior disorder
  - Rare, mostly in elderly
  - Thrashing or seemingly purposeful behaviors during sleep
- Prion fatal familial insomnia

Workup and Diagnosis

- Sleep and medication/drug history, including bed partner history
- Sleep diary is the most effective specific assessment tool
  - Should be recorded each morning
  - Include time in bed, time asleep, awakenings, estimate of sleep quality, associated symptoms (e.g., pain, dyspnea, urinary frequency)
- A focused physical examination to evaluate cardiovascular, pulmonary, and neurologic systems and mental status will improve diagnostic accuracy
- Polysomnography (sleep study) is useful to evaluate sleep apnea, restless legs syndrome, periodic limb movement disorder, and REM-behavior disorder
- "Insomnia" is a self-reported condition; labs or other testing is often unnecessary unless underlying medical conditions are suspected
  - ECG, chest X-ray, echocardiogram, pulmonary function tests if suspect undiagnosed cardiac or pulmonary disease
  - EEG if suspect undiagnosed seizure disorder
  - TSH and free T_4 if suspect thyroid disease
  - Iron studies and BUN/creatinine if suspect restless legs syndrome or periodic limb movement disorder (iron deficiency and renal failure are risk factors for both)
  - Consider blood alcohol level, CBC and MCV, LFTs, and toxicology screen if suspect alcohol or illicit drug abuse

Treatment

- Acute transient insomnia: Reassurance, address stressors, treat identifiable underlying causes (e.g., pain), hypnotic agents for up to 7–10 days
- Chronic insomnia
  - Improve sleep hygiene (e.g., consistent bed/wake time, sleep environment, medications/drugs, daytime exercise, avoid naps, hot bath near bedtime)
  - Treat pain and underlying medical/psychiatric issues
  - Behavioral treatments: Relaxation therapy, sleep restriction therapy (curtail time in bed to improve sleep efficiency), stimulus control therapy (bed only for sleep), cognitive therapy (restructure negative thoughts about sleep/daytime functioning)
  - Medications are often used but none has demonstrated long-term efficacy nor safety
- Obstructive sleep apnea: Weight loss, CPAP, surgery
- RLS: Dopaminergic agents (e.g., carbidopa/levodopa, pergolide), benzodiazepines, opiates
- Narcolepsy: Modafinil, amphetamines

96. Irregular Heart Rhythms

The patient should be asked to describe the heart rhythm and to demonstrate it by either saying or tapping the speed and rhythm of the sensation. Additionally, teaching the patient to measure his or her pulse during the episode may give more clues as to the etiology of the sensation of an irregular rhythm. All complaints of irregular heart rhythms should be investigated to ensure that the arrhythmia is not life threatening.

Differential Diagnosis

- Atrial fibrillation
  - One of the most common causes of irregular rhythm
  - Narrow QRS complex without organized atrial contraction (no P waves)
  - Etiologies include infection, thyrotoxicosis, alcohol, cocaine, amphetamines, myocarditis, pericarditis, hypertensive crisis, ischemia, MI, CHF, hypoxia, PE, hypertension, valvular heart disease
- Atrial flutter with variable block
  - Narrow QRS complex
  - ECG: "Sawtooth" flutter waves
  - Atrial rate is typically 250–350 bpm
  - Ventricular rate is usually 1/2 or 1/3 of atrial rate (2:1 or 3:1 block)
  - Irregular when variable block is present
  - Result of a macro-reentrant circuit in atrium
- Premature atrial contractions
- Paroxysmal atrial tachycardia
- Multifocal atrial tachycardia
  - Multiple areas of atrial impulses (more than three P wave morphologies) followed by a narrow QRS complex
  - HR ≥ 100 bpm
  - Most often seen in patients with lung disease
- Wandering atrial pacemaker
  - Multiple areas of atrial impulses (more than three P wave morphologies) followed by a narrow QRS complex
  - HR ≤ 100 bpm
  - Often occurs in athletes and the very young (increased vagal tone)
- Premature ventricular contractions
- Sinus arrhythmia

Workup and Diagnosis

- History and physical examination
  - Associated symptoms may include lightheadedness, palpitations, dyspnea, chest pain, or syncope
  - Assess for hemodynamic instability
- ECG with rhythm strip is the key tool for establishing diagnosis
- Initial laboratory evaluation may include CBC, electrolytes, BUN/creatinine, calcium, pulse oximetry, chest X-ray, and possibly an ABG
- Consider cardiac enzymes, TSH, and toxicology screen
- Echocardiogram may be necessary to evaluate for underlying disease or the presence of thrombi
  - Transesophageal echocardiography is more sensitive than transthoracic echocardiography for detection of intracardiac thrombus (most commonly seen in left atrial appendage)

Treatment

- Ensure hemodynamic stability
- Administer supplemental O_2
- Rate control may be achieved via adenosine, digoxin, β-blockers, calcium channel blockers, and other pharmacotherapeutics
- Atrial fibrillation: Treated by rate control, anticoagulation for stroke prevention, and/or restoration/maintenance of sinus rhythm
  - Rate control: β-blockers, calcium channel blockers
  - Anticoagulation: Long-term coumadin in appropriate patients
  - Restoration/maintenance of sinus rhythm: Anti-arrhythmic medications, cardioversion
- Atrial flutter
  - Rate control is initial goal of therapy
  - Anticoagulation is controversial
  - Cardioversion to terminate rhythm
  - Radiofrequency ablation may be curative

97. Janeway Lesions

Janeway lesions are among the stigmata of infectious endocarditis. They are irregular, erythematous, flat, painless macules on the palms, soles, thenar, and hypothenar eminences of the hands, fingertips, and plantar surfaces of the toes. In acute endocarditis, the lesions may be hemorrhagic or purple. Infective endocarditis can be positively diagnosed by the Duke criteria (e.g., positive blood cultures, evidence of a cardiac vegetation, fever of unknown origin, vascular phenomena). Janeway lesions are considered a minor criterion in the category of vascular phenomena.

Differential Diagnosis

- Acute bacterial endocarditis
  - Presents with high fevers and chills with a new-onset heart murmur
  - Common organisms are *Staphylococcus aureus, Streptococcus pneumoniae,* and *Streptococcus pyogenes*
- SBE
  - Presents with low-grade fever, cough, dyspnea, weakness, fatigue, malaise
  - Most common organisms include *Streptococcus viridans,* enterococci, *Staphylococcus epidermidis,* and fungi
  - Cutaneous signs of bacterial endocarditis include Janeway lesions, conjunctival and palatal petechiae, subungual (splinter) hemorrhages, Roth spots (pale, oval areas surrounded by hemorrhage near the optic disc), and Osler nodes (painful lesions on the pulpy surface of the fingers and toes)
- Meningococcemia
  - Occurs in *Neisseria meningitidis* meningitis
  - Presents with headache, neck stiffness, photophobia, altered mental status, seizure
  - Positive Kernig's and Brudzinski's signs
- Systemic lupus erythematosus
  - May present with malar rash, discoid rash, arthritis, myalgias, photosensitivity, and oral ulcers
- Thrombotic thrombocytopenic purpura
  - Presents with splenomegaly, anemia, bleeding, jaundice
- Idiopathic thrombocytopenia purpura
  - Afebrile, mucosal bleeding, petechiae, and purpura
- Polyarteritis nodosa
  - Presents with fever, abdominal pain, and neuropathy
- Rocky Mountain spotted fever
  - Macular rash beginning on palms and soles that spreads centrally
- Secondary syphilis
- Erythema multiforme
- Disseminated intravascular coagulation
- Typhoid fever
- Cutaneous vasculitis
- Enterovirus infection (echovirus or coxsackievirus)

Workup and Diagnosis

- History and physical examination
  - Note history of infective endocarditis, IV drug abuse, heart valve injury/replacement, structural heart disease, family history of autoimmune disorders (e.g., SLE), recent head/neck or lung infection, HIV status, mucosal bleeding (e.g., epistaxis), tick exposure, and constitutional symptoms (fever/chills, night sweats)
  - Concentrate exam on cardiac (new-onset murmur suggests infective endocarditis), skin (malar rash suggests SLE), and musculoskeletal systems
- Initial labs may include CBC with peripheral smear, ESR, ANA, anti-dsDNA and anti-SM antibodies (specific for SLE), ASO, RPR, coagulation studies, UA
- Blood cultures (drawn at three different times from different body sites)
- Chest X-ray may reveal septic emboli
- Echocardiogram may reveal vegetations on heart valves
- Biopsy of lesions may reveal neutrophilic dermal microabscesses; organisms may or may not be found
- Infective endocarditis is diagnosed by Duke's criteria
  - Major criteria: Positive blood cultures from two different sites >12 hours apart, and echocardiogram showing endocardial involvement (e.g., vegetation, abscess, or new dehiscence of prosthetic valve)
  - Minor criteria: Predisposing heart condition, IV drug abuse, fever >100.4°F (>38°C), vascular or immunologic phenomena (e.g., Osler nodes, Janeway lesions), or positive culture that does not satisfy a major criterion

Treatment

- Bacterial endocarditis: Long-term antibiotic therapy [initiate broad-spectrum empiric therapy, then tailor to organism(s) found on culture]; valve replacement may be indicated if medical therapy fails; lifelong antibiotic prophylaxis is indicated before any dental work or minor surgery
- Meningococcemia: IV antibiotics; antibiotic prophylaxis (e.g., rifampin, minocycline) of all exposed individuals
- Treat other etiologies by established treatment protocols

98. Jaundice

Yellow skin pigmentation caused by elevated serum bilirubin level is termed jaundice. Bilirubin is the major breakdown product of hemoglobin that is released from dying or damaged erythrocytes. The normal serum bilirubin is less than 1 mg/dL, less than 5% of which is present in conjugated form. Jaundice cannot be detected until the bilirubin level rises above 2 mg/dL.

Differential Diagnosis

- Viral hepatitis
  - Fatigue, anorexia, fever, nausea, vomiting, dark urine, light-colored (acholic) loose stools, RUQ pain, hepatomegaly, and/or pruritis
- Alcoholic hepatitis
  - Associated with fever, leukocytosis, and AST:ALT ratio >2
- Nonalcoholic steatohepatitis or nonalchoholic fatty liver disease
  - Associated with obesity, diabetes, hyperlipidemia and medications
- Cholecystitis
  - RUQ pain, fever, leukocytosis
  - Female, fertile, fat, forty
  - Murphy's sign: Pain upon palpation of the gallbladder while taking a deep breath
- Drugs and toxins
  - Acetaminophen, alcohol, estrogens, isoniazid, chlorpromazine, erythromycin, nitrofurantoin, rifampin
- Gilbert's syndrome
  - Decreased conjugation of bilirubin, especially with dehydration, fasting, infection
- Sepsis
- Malignancy (liver, pancreas, gall-bladder/common bile duct, metastatic)
- Liver infiltration
  - Amyloidosis, lymphoma, sarcoidosis, tuberculosis
- Total parenteral nutrition (usually requires at least 2 weeks of therapy)
- Intravascular hemolysis
- Cholangitis
  - Charcot's triad of fever, RUQ pain, and jaundice
- Sickle cell disease
  - Chronic hemolysis, hepatic dysfunction
- Autoimmune hepatitis
  - May mimic viral hepatitis
  - Females >> males, often 10–30 years old
  - Associated with autoimmune disease (e.g., RA, UC, Sjögren's syndrome, thyroiditis)
- Intrahepatic cholestasis of pregnancy
  - Pruritus in third trimester
  - Resolves after delivery
- Hereditary cholestatic disorders (e.g., Dubin-Johnson syndrome, Rotor syndrome)
- Physiologic jaundice of newborn

Workup and Diagnosis

- History and physical examination
  - Duration, associated symptoms (e.g., abdominal pain, constitutional symptoms, pruritis), history of alcohol use or hepatotoxic medications, and/or personal/family history of liver disease
  - Jaundice is best seen in the periphery of ocular conjunctivae and oral mucous membranes
  - Yellow skin discoloration may occur with elevated serum carotene level without scleral icterus
  - Evaluate for hepatomegaly, splenomegaly, palpable gallbladder, and signs of chronic liver disease (e.g., gynecomastia, testicular atrophy, palmar erythema, spider telangiectasias)
- Initial laboratory evaluation includes total and unconjugated (indirect) bilirubin (cannot detect jaundice until serum bilirubin >2 mg/dL), AST, ALT, alkaline phosphatase (elevated with hepatocellular damage or cholestasis), albumin, HIV and hepatitis serologies (if risk factors present), reticulocyte count, LDH, haptoglobin (hemolysis), prothrombin time (to evaluate synthetic liver dysfunction or vitamin K deficiency), ANA (autoimmune hepatitis), and possibly antimitochondrial antibodies (primary biliary cirrhosis)
- Abdominal ultrasound or CT scan to evaluate for biliary obstruction, dilated ducts, pancreatic mass, or gallstones
- ERCP if extrahepatic obstruction on imaging tests
- Liver biopsy is generally not necessary

Treatment

- Discontinue and avoid potentially hepatotoxic medications
- Supportive care for viral hepatitis
- Rehydrate/refeed for Gilbert's syndrome
- Consider steroids in fulminant alcoholic hepatitis
- Cholecystectomy or ERCP with stone removal for obstructing gallstones
- Treat underlying causes of hemolysis or other disorders
- Antibiotics for cholangitis, sepsis
- Hydroxyurea and folate for sickle cell disease, prevent crises by adequate hydration, vaccinating against diseases, and try to prevent other infections

99. Jaw Pain/Swelling

Jaw pain is a common presenting or incidental complaint; its etiology is often identified by a careful history and physical examination. In many cases, consultation with a dentist will aid in the diagnosis and treatment. In older patients (>55), be sure to rule out serious causes (e.g., temporal arteritis, malignancy, angina, myocardial infarction). Note that cranial nerves V, VII, IX, and X and cervical nerves C2, C3, and C4 all have input to orofacial sensation.

Differential Diagnosis

- Dental or periodontal pathology
  - Associated with temperature sensitivity and pain upon biting
- TMJ disorders
  - Associated with unilateral or bilateral achy pain and diffuse tenderness of the masseter and temporalis muscles
  - Exaggerated by jaw use
  - Joint may be tender to palpation
  - "Clicking" sounds are often present
  - More common in females age <50
- Giant cell (temporal) arteritis
  - Unilateral pain in older patients
  - Headache, jaw claudication, and vision loss
- Mucosal lesions (buccal mucosa, hard and soft palate, floor of mouth, or oropharynx)
  - Aphthous ulcers
  - Herpes simplex or coxsackievirus B
  - Cancer
  - Tongue or lip lesions
- Paranasal sinus pathology
  - Most common pathology is maxillary sinusitis secondary to viral URI
  - Pain is often referred to the upper molars
- Salivary gland pathology, including inflammation (e.g., parotiditis), ductal stone, or neoplasm
- Headache with radiation to the jaw
- Referred pain from cardiac, cervical spine, pulmonary, or throat disease
- Neuralgias (e.g., trigeminal, glossopharyngeal)
- Neuropathies
  - Systemic neuropathies (e.g., HIV, diabetes)
  - Dental/alveolar neuropathies, usually subsequent to extrinsic trauma (e.g., blow to face, dental surgical intervention)
- Behavioral disorders
- Primary neoplasms of the maxilla, mandible, or major salivary gland
- Metastases to mandible, maxilla, or TMJ
- Herpes zoster or post-herpetic neuralgia
- Fibromyalgia
- Rheumatologic disease (e.g., Sjögren's syndrome)
- Systemic arthritis (e.g., rheumatoid arthritis)

Workup and Diagnosis

- History and physical examination, with focus on the head and neck
  - Review onset, character, and pattern of pain; past medical and surgical history; associated symptoms (e.g., weight loss, sinus pain, skin complaints); and complete review of systems, including screening for local and systemic pathology and a cervical evaluation for muscle, neural, or skeletal referred pain
  - Perform a thorough oral exam of the buccal mucosa, lips, hard palate, soft palate, posterior pharynx, floor of mouth, and the top, sides, and undersurface of the tongue
  - Perform a head, neck, ear, nose, cardiac, pulmonary, and lymphatic exam
  - Suspect dental pathology until proven otherwise
- Initial workup is aimed at assessing the mouth and jaw for dental, periodontal, or TMJ disorders
- Appropriate laboratory studies are based upon the suspected diagnosis (e.g., CBC and ESR for temporal arteritis)
- Imaging studies may include Panorex films, sinus X-ray, CT scan, and/or MRI
- Therapeutic trial of medications (e.g., NSAIDs)
- Temporal artery biopsy is indicated if ESR elevated
- Biopsy any suspicious lesion
- Referral to a dental or medical specialist may be necessary

Treatment

- Dental or periodontal pathology, oral lesions, salivary pathology, and oral neoplasms require specialized treatment by dental specialist or oral surgeon
- TMJ: Initial treatment includes pain management, bite block (night guard), cold/warm compresses, intra-articular steroid/lidocaine injections, and avoidance of jaw clenching and gum chewing
- Temporal arteritis: Temporal artery biopsy and high- dose steroids
- Headache: Pain relievers, stress reduction, migraine-specific therapy (e.g., triptans), and manipulation
- Neuralgia and neuropathies may be treated with NSAIDs, anticonvulsants (e.g., valproic acid, gabapentin), medical pain management and/or directed therapy (e.g., nerve block)
- Treat underlying systemic etiologies and behavioral disease as necessary

100. Jugular Venous Distension

Examination of the jugular venous pulse for abnormalities of the wave form or level of venous pressure is a critical component of the cardiovascular exam and can aid in the diagnosis of certain cardiac diseases.

Differential Diagnosis

- Congestive heart failure
- Constrictive pericarditis
- Cardiac tamponade
- Superior vena cava syndrome
- Tricuspid regurgitation
- Heart block (most often complete heart block)
- Atrial fibrillation
- Right ventricular infarction
- Tricuspid stenosis
- Right ventricular dilation
- Hypervolemia

Workup and Diagnosis

- History and physical examination
  - Best to evaluate the right internal jugular vein
  - Best seen in tangential light from foot of bed
  - Venous pulsation can be obliterated with compression, but arterial pulsation cannot
  - Right atrium lies 5 cm below the sternal angle (reference point)
  - Normal central venous pressure ≤ 8–9 cm
  - Hepatojugular reflex is a helpful adjunct in patients with normal central venous pressure suspected of having right heart failure
- ECG may reveal atrial fibrillation, ventricular tachycardia, right ventricular infarction, heart block, or other pathology
- Chest X-ray may reveal signs of congestive heart failure or cardiomegaly
- Echocardiogram is helpful to evaluate for valvular disease, myxomas, and right ventricular dysfunction
- Additional diagnostic testing depends on the suspected pathology

Treatment

- Treatment depends on the underlying disease process
- Atrial fibrillation
- Ventricular tachycardia: DC countershock in presence of hemodynamic instability; antiarrhythmic therapy with amiodarone or lidocaine; repletion of electrolytes with torsade de pointes; ICD to treat recurrences
- Constrictive pericarditis: Judicious management of volume status; pericardial stripping hemodynamic compromise is substantial
- Tricuspid regurgitation/stenosis: Surgical correction if symptomatic or severe enough
- Atrial myxoma: Surgical excision
- Heart block may require permanent pacemaker

101. Knee Pain/Swelling

Primary care physicians, rheumatologists, and orthopedists frequently encounter complaints about the knee. Because the range of illnesses affecting the knee varies greatly, a thorough history and physical exam are essential. Once a differential diagnosis is compiled, plain films of the joint are usually indicated.

Differential Diagnosis

- Degenerative joint disease (osteoarthritis)
- Ligamentous injury
  - ACL: Positive Lachman (more sensitive) and anterior drawer test
  - PCL: Positive thumb sign (more sensitive) and posterior drawer test
  - MCL: Pain and/or increased laxity with valgus stress
  - LCL: Pain and/or increased laxity with varus stress
- Meniscus tear
  - Patient may complain of pain and locking; positive McMurray circumduction test
- Patellofemoral syndrome
- Iliotibial band syndrome
  - Pain along the lateral aspect of the knee accompanied by a palpable or audible snapping
  - Occurs almost exclusively in runners
- Pes anserine bursitis
  - Patients complain of pain along the medial aspect of the knee (at pes anserinus insertion)
  - Caused by repetitive movement that creates an inflammatory response
- Joint effusion
  - May be secondary to osteoarthritis, inflammatory arthritis, ligament injury, gout, pseudogout, or infection
- Joint infection (septic joint)
  - *Staphylococcus aureus* is most common
  - *Neisseria gonorrhoeae* is common in adolescents and young adults
  - *Salmonella* is common in sickle cell patients
  - *Haemophilus influenzae* is common in children
- Osteochondritis dissecans (OCD)
  - Osteonecrosis of subchondral bone
  - Most commonly seen in the knee
  - Patient reports a gradual onset of pain
  - Exam reveals tenderness of the affected area with manipulation
- In the pediatric population, consider Osgood-Schlatter disease, physeal injury, and discoid meniscus
- Hip or foot/ankle disease with referred pain to the knee
- Malignancy
- Osteomyelitis

Workup and Diagnosis

- History and physical examination are often diagnostic
  - Inspect the patient's gait for limitations of motion or other abnormalities
  - Visually assess symmetry between the knees: Note swelling, deformity, erythema, and muscle atrophy
  - Palpate: Note tenderness, warmth, and crepitus
  - "Milk the joint" to elicit an effusion
  - Test for range of motion (active and passive)
  - Perform McMurray circumduction test and ligament testing (e.g., Lachman test, anterior/posterior drawer tests, thumb sign, varus/valgus stress tests)
- X-rays are often indicated
  - AP, lateral, and merchant or sunrise films of both knees
  - When possible, also obtain weight-bearing A/P films
  - Merchant and sunrise X-rays of the patella are used to evaluate alignment and injury to the patella
  - On occasion, tunnel views of the knee are useful (e.g., for OCD)
- Joint aspiration should be performed in patients with joint effusions; fluid analysis includes cell count with differential, crystals, Gram stain, and culture
- MRI may not be necessary during initial evaluation, but may help with confirmation of specific injuries and surgical planning (e.g., PCL tear, meniscus tear, OCD)
- Bone scan may be used to evaluate malignancy or infection
- In some cases, blood work may include CBC, ESR, C-reactive protein, alkaline phosphatase, and uric acid

Treatment

- Conservative therapy is usually sufficient
- OA: Lifestyle modification (e.g., weight loss, exercise); anti-inflammatory medications (e.g., NSAIDs, COX-2 inhibitors); joint injections may benefit some people (e.g. corticosteroids, hyaluronic acid); surgery may be necessary for those who fail conservative treatment
- Ligamentous injuries: ACL injuries may require definitive treatment via reconstructive surgery; PCL injuries are usually not repaired
- Meniscal tears may require repair or excision; however, most meniscus injuries are asymptomatic or mild and require no treatment
- Patellofemoral syndrome often responds to physical therapy and exercise
- Joint infection (e.g., septic arthritis) is a surgical emergency; irrigation, debridement, and antibiotic administration should be considered

102. Low Back Pain/Swelling

Low back pain is the second most common cause of doctor visits in the U.S. and is the most common cause of disability. Up to 90% of the population will experience back pain during their lives. Studies show that, at any given time, up to 20% of the population is experiencing low back pain. Most cases are due to mild muscle injury; however, "red flags" should be evaluated to rule out more serious disease.

Differential Diagnosis

- Lumbosacral muscle strain
  - Most common etiology of low back pain
  - Most common cause of disability in adults <45 years old
  - Aggravated by movement, better with rest
- Lumbar disc herniation
  - Especially of L4-L5 and L5-S1
  - Usually with unilateral radiation down the leg in a dermatomal pattern
  - Increased pain with sitting
- Spinal stenosis
  - Back and *bilateral* buttock and thigh pain in older patients relieved by rest (pseudoclaudication)
  - Increased pain with standing
- Sacral-iliac joint dysfunction
  - Especially in young, thin women or in pregnancy
  - Unilateral upper buttock pain, relieved with movement
- Vertebral fracture
  - Often associated with trauma or osteoporosis
- Spondylolisthesis
  - Especially in young athletes
- Secondary gain (e.g., drug seeking, disability or liability issue)
- Extraspinal causes (e.g., radiation from kidney stones)
- Systemic causes (<1%)
  - Inflammation (e.g., ankylosing spondylitis): Morning stiffness, limited mobility
  - Infection: Osteomyelitis, abscess
  - Abdominal aortic aneurysm
  - Cancer (especially metastases from prostate, lung, colon, and breast or myeloma); constant, worsening pain, wakes up from sleep
  - Cauda equina syndrome
  - Paget's disease

Workup and Diagnosis

- History and physical are the most important diagnostic tools
  - Evaluate for range of motion, sensation, strength, straight leg raise test, reflexes, and neurovascular status
- Imaging studies (e.g., X-ray, MRI, CT scan, myelogram, discogram) are indicated if "red flags" are present, if pain or limited function is refractory to treatment, or if trauma has occurred
- Evaluate for "red flags" that may indicate serious conditions—if present, further workup is necessary (e.g., lumbosacral X-ray, CBC, ESR, calcium, electrolytes, alkaline phosphatase, bone scan, metastatic workup)
  - Red flags that suggest fracture: Major trauma, minor trauma, or strenuous lifting in an older or osteoporotic patient
  - Red flags that suggest tumor or infection: Age >50 or <20, history of cancer, constitutional symptoms (weight loss, fever), IV drug use, immunosuppression, pain worse at night
  - Red flags that suggest cauda equina syndrome: Saddle anesthesia, recent onset of incontinence, severe or progressive neurological deficit in leg
- If red flags are absent, no imaging is necessary for 4–6 weeks; if pain persists, an MRI is the most useful study

Treatment

- In absence of red flag symptoms, return to activity as soon as possible; rest has not been shown to improve recovery
- Acetaminophen, NSAIDs, opioids, and/or muscle relaxants for pain; epidural corticosteroid injections may be indicated for resistant pain
- Patient education (weight loss, exercise, proper back biomechanics and ergonomics)
- Physical therapy, including pain relief modalities (ice, heat, ultrasound), stretching, strengthening, aerobic conditioning, and relaxation therapy
- Surgery may be indicated for refractory disease, large neurologic deficits, unbearable pain, or significant limitations

103. Lymphadenopathy

Lymphadenopathy refers to enlargement of the lymph nodes. Localized lymphadenopathy involves one lymph region, whereas generalized lymphadenopathy involves more than one region. More than two thirds of cases of lymphadenopathy in primary care are due to nonspecific causes or upper respiratory illnesses. Underlying malignancy must be ruled out; however, less than 1% of cases are due to an underlying malignancy.

Differential Diagnosis

Generalized lymphadenopathy (e.g., cervical, supraclavicular, axillary, and inguinal lymphadenopathy; hepatomegaly; splenomegaly)
- Infection
  - Tuberculosis
  - Secondary syphilis
  - Mononucleosis
  - HIV/AIDS
  - Kawasaki's syndrome
  - Typhoid fever
- Hypersensitivity reactions
  - Serum sickness
  - Drugs (e.g., hydantoin, phenytoin, hydralazine, allopurinol, primidone)
- Lymphoma
- Leukemia
- Connective tissue disorders (e.g., SLE, rheumatoid arthritis)
- Sarcoidosis
- Metastatic cancer [especially with left supraclavicular lymphadenopathy (Virchow's node) associated with abdominal malignancies, including stomach, pancreas, gallbladder, testis/ovary, kidney, and prostate cancers]
- Endocrine disorders (e.g., hyperthyroidism, hypoadrenalism)
- Amyloidosis
- Castleman's syndrome (angiofollicular lymph node hyperplasia)
- Kikuchi's disease

Localized lymphadenopathy
- Reactive hyperplasia, local inflammation (e.g., dermatitis, vaccination, trauma)
- Infection
  - Viral: Mononucleosis, CMV, HIV, rubella, mumps
  - Bacterial: *Streptococcus,* tuberculosis, salmonella, cat-scratch disease (due to *Bartonella henselae*); gonorrhea, *Chlamydia,* and other sexually transmitted diseases (inguinal)
  - Parasitic: Malaria, toxoplasmosis
  - Fungal: Histoplasmosis, coccidioidomycosis
- Lymphoma or metastatic disease (e.g. head and neck squamous cell cancer leads to cervical lymphadenopathy)

Workup and Diagnosis

- History and physical examination
  - Note extent of lymphadenopathy (localized or generalized), size of nodes, texture, presence or absence of nodal tenderness (tenderness suggests infection), signs of inflammation over the node, skin lesions, petechiae, splenomegaly, and hepatomegaly
  - Thorough ENT examination in adult patients with cervical adenopathy and/or a history of tobacco use
  - Supraclavicular and epitrochlear lymphadenopathy carry a high risk of malignancy or other abnormality and are rarely normal or reactive
  - Lymph nodes greater than 1 cm, and particularly greater than 2 cm, are likely to be pathologic
- Initial labs may include CBC, peripheral smear, ESR, CRP, uric acid, PPD, blood cultures, viral titers for specific organisms (e.g., HIV, CMV, toxoplasmosis, rubella), and serologies for brucellosis and typhoid
  - Atypical lymphocytes may indicate a viral illness
  - Immature leukocytes/blasts may indicate leukemia
  - Leukocytosis often indicates infection
- Chest X-ray and/or abdominal ultrasound may be used to evaluate for lymphadenopathy
- Biopsy is the gold standard for diagnosis
  - Strongly consider biopsy if node is >2.0 cm, associated with abnormal chest X-ray, and/or age >40 years
- Bone marrow aspiration may be necessary in some cases to rule out an underlying malignancy

Treatment

- Viral infections require supportive therapy in most cases
- Bacterial, parasitic, and fungal infections are usually treated with appropriate antibiotics, antiparasitics or antifungals, respectively
- Offending medication should be removed when possible
- Malignancies must be identified, staged, and treated as appropriate with chemotherapy, radiation, and/or resection as per the established oncology protocol

104. Murmurs - Diastolic

Diastolic heart murmurs are never normal and should always be further evaluated, in contrast to systolic murmurs, which are commonly benign or due to rapid flow rates. The part of the cardiac cycle that the murmur falls into (e.g. early, middle, or late) will help determine the etiology, as will the characteristics of the heart sounds and whether an opening snap is present.

Differential Diagnosis

- Aortic insufficiency
  - Decrescendo murmur heard best at the right second intercostal space
- Austin Flint murmur
  - Late diastolic rumble of severe aortic regurgitation
  - A result of aortic regurgitation so severe that it causes diastolic mitral regurgitation
- Mitral stenosis
  - Opening snap with mid-diastolic rumble, especially in the left lateral decubitus position
- Pulmonary insufficiency
  - Accentuated P2 and decrescendo murmur at the left second/third intercostal spaces
- Tricuspid stenosis
  - Mid-diastolic rumble at the left sternal border
  - Increases with inspiration
- Cervical venous hum (disappears upon pressure to the jugular vein)
- Hepatic venous hum (disappears with epigastric pressure)
- Mammary souffle (in pregnancy; disappears on compressing breast)
- PDA (continuous machinery sound)
- Coronary or pulmonary arteriovenous fistula
- Coarctation of the aorta
- ASD with left-to-right shunt
- Atrial myxoma ("tumor plop")
- Pericardial knock (constrictive pericarditis)
- Bronchial collaterals (congenital heart disease)
- Anomalous pulmonary venous drainage with left-to-right shunt
- Pulmonary artery branch stenosis
- Carey-Coombs murmur (mid-diastolic murmur that occurs in acute rheumatic fever)

Workup and Diagnosis

- Complete history and physical examination, including cardiac maneuvers
- ECG
- Echocardiogram
- Consider chest X-ray
- Laboratory studies may include CBC, electrolytes, glucose, BUN/creatinine, TSH, liver function tests, pulse oximetry, and/or arterial blood gas
- Consider cardiology consult

Treatment

- Attention to hemodynamic status
- Treat the underlying cause (e.g., anemia, infection, hyperthyroidism, MI)
- Serial examinations to track progression of underlying cause
- Valve repair or replacement may be indicated for severe valvular disease

105. Murmurs - Systolic

Systolic heart murmurs, in contrast to diastolic murmurs, may be normal or abnormal, although when coupled with a heave they are always abnormal. The part of the cardiac cycle that the murmur falls into (e.g., early, middle, or late) will help determine the etiology, as will the characteristics of the heart sounds and whether or not a click is present or absent.

Differential Diagnosis

- Innocent systolic murmur
  - Heard at left sternal border
  - Increased when supine
  - May be caused by increased flow states (e.g., anemia, hypovolemia, fever)
- Still's murmur
- Mitral valve prolapse
  - Midsystolic click with late systolic murmur that shifts with maneuvers
- Aortic stenosis
  - Right side at second intercostal space
  - Radiates to carotid arteries
- Aortic sclerosis
  - Right side at second intercostal space
  - Midsystole
- Hyperthyroidism
- Cervical venous hum
  - Disappears with jugular vein pressure
- Hepatic venous hum
  - Disappears with epigastric pressure
- Mammary souffle
  - Occurs in pregnancy
  - Disappears upon compression of breast
- Bicuspid aortic valve
  - Right side at second intercostal space
  - Little radiation
  - Possible early diastolic aortic murmur
  - Opening sound of aortic valve heard in early systole (systolic ejection click)
- Mitral insufficiency
  - Holosystolic murmur heard best in the left lateral decubitus position
  - S_1 is usually diminished in intensity
- Tricuspid insufficiency
  - Holosystolic murmur at second/third intercostal spaces
- Endocarditis
  - Abrupt onset of new murmur
- Peripheral pulmonary artery stenosis
- Atrial or ventricular septal defect
- Ventricular septal defect
- Patent ductus arteriosus (continuous machinery sound, second left intercostal space)
- Coarctation of the aorta
- Left ventricular outflow tract obstruction
- Pulmonary artery stenosis
- Prosthetic valve noises
- Pericardial friction rubs
- Papillary muscle dysfunction
- Pulmonic outflow obstruction
- Coronary/pulmonary arteriovenous fistula

Workup and Diagnosis

- History and physical examination
  - Family history of sudden cardiac death
  - Past medical history of heart disease, murmurs, or rheumatic fever
  - Evaluation for jugular venous distention, carotid upstroke, and/or bruits
  - Heart, lung, and abdominal examinations
  - Peripheral pulses and evaluation for peripheral edema
- ECG
- Chest X-ray
- Echocardiogram
- Laboratory studies may include CBC, electrolytes, BUN/creatinine, glucose, and TSH
- Consider cardiac enzymes
- Consider blood cultures
- Consider cardiology referral

Treatment

- Attention to hemodynamic status
- Treat the underlying cause (e.g., anemia, infection, hyperthyroidism, MI)
- Serial examinations to track progression of underlying cause
- Valve repair/replacement may be indicated for severe valvular disease

106. Myalgia

Myalgia, or muscle pain, is an extremely common complaint. Determine whether the pain is temporally related to trauma, exercise, associated illness, and/or medications.

Differential Diagnosis

- Acute muscle overuse/excessive physical exertion
  - Usually due to exercising poorly conditioned muscles
- Systemic febrile illness (e.g., influenza)
- Drugs/medications (e.g., statins)
- Electrolyte disturbances
  - Especially abnormalities of potassium, calcium, or magnesium
- Chronic overuse syndromes
  - Frequently related to occupational or vocational activities
- Myopathies
  - Metabolic: Usually result in muscle pain related to exercise
  - Dystrophies (e.g., mitochondrial myopathies)
  - Inflammatory (e.g., polymyositis, dermatomyositis)
  - Toxic (e.g., alcohol, cocaine, statins)
  - Infectious muscle disease (viral, bacterial, parasitic)
- Trauma
- Muscle ischemia (e.g., claudication in patients with peripheral vascular disease)
- Rheumatologic disorders
  - Polymyalgia rheumatica: Especially pain around the shoulders, back, and hips
  - Fibromyalgia: Diffuse muscle and soft tissue pain with many areas of point tenderness; regionally restricted areas of pain may be referred to as myofascial pain
- Endocrine disturbances
  - Thyroid disease
  - Parathyroid disease
  - Adrenal disease
  - Diabetes mellitus (muscle infarcts)
- Muscle pain must also be differentiated from pain of associated or nearby structures (e.g., tendons, ligaments, bone, connective tissue)
- Rhabdomyolysis

Workup and Diagnosis

- History and physical examination
  - History should focus on the temporal events surrounding the occurrence of myalgias (e.g., post-exercise, new vocational or avocational activities, onset of pain coinciding with initiation of new medications)
  - Focal versus generalized
  - Note abnormal urine (e.g., myoglobinuria causes tea-colored urine in rhabdomyolysis)
  - Physical exam should be directed at determining whether muscular weakness and features of systemic illness are present
- Labs may include electrolytes (including calcium), BUN/creatinine, glucose, creatine kinase, aldolase, creatinine, urinalysis, myoglobin, thyroid function tests, ESR, and CBC
- Electromyography may be helpful in identifying evidence of myopathy
- Imaging (usually MRI) may be necessary, especially in suspected focal muscle pathology
- Muscle biopsy may be useful in the evaluation of suspected inflammatory myopathies, muscular dystrophies, or metabolic myopathies

Treatment

- Remove offending drugs or identified toxins
- Correct electrolyte imbalance, especially sodium, potassium, calcium, or magnesium abnormalities
- Overuse injury is generally treated by rest, followed by gradual conditioning exercises
- Severe muscle trauma may require surgical treatment
- Fluids and other measures to protect renal function are necessary in rhabdomyolysis with myoglobinuria
- Appropriate treatment of an underlying endocrine disorder may improve muscle pain
- Treat infectious causes with appropriate antimicrobials
- Rheumatologic causes may respond to steroids or immunosuppressive therapy
- Inflammatory myopathies may be treated with steroids or other immunosuppressive therapies
- Claudication may be treated with exercise programs, medications such as pentoxifylline or cilostazol, or with endovascular or surgical procedures

107. Nail Disorders

Nail disorders are common and range from onycholysis (separation of the distal nail from the underlying nail plate, usually with nail thickening and subungual debris), to nail pitting, to paronychia (an abscess next to the nail plate that can be very painful). Various focal, skin, or systemic disorders must be considered in all cases, thus requiring a focused yet complete evaluation of the patient.

Differential Diagnosis

- Onychomycosis
  - Very common cause of nail thickening, yellowing, and subungual debris
  - Due to a dermatophyte infection
  - May affect one or all fingers and toenails
  - Patients often have coexisting tinea pedis or tinea manum
- Psoriasis
  - More than 50% of patients with psoriasis have associated nail changes, including pits, "oil spots," and onycholysis
  - Distinguishing nail fungus from psoriasis can be very difficult on clinical exam
  - Most patients with nail disease have some other skin manifestation of psoriasis (plaques of thick, silvery white, adherent scalp scale that overlies well-demarcated patches of erythema)
- Paronychia
  - Tenderness, erythema, and peeling around the nail
  - Very common and exquisitely painful
  - Often exacerbated by "wet-work" (e.g., dishwasher)
  - May have bacterial and/or yeast (candida) component
  - Occurs after minor cuticular trauma
  - Can cause nail dystrophy without treatment
- Nail trauma
  - Very common, especially great toenails and thumbnails
  - Easily misdiagnosed as fungal disease
  - Can cause separation of the nail from the nail plate
- Malignancy (e.g., subungual melanoma, squamous cell carcinoma)
- Endocrine disease (e.g., hyper- and hypothyroidism) can cause splitting, drying, and other nail changes
- Lichen planus and atopic eczema can affect the nail matrix and lead to nail dystrophy
- Alopecia areata (patchy autoimmune hair loss) can be associated with nail pits as well
- Several congenital disorders (e.g., ectodermal dysplasia) can cause nail dystrophy in association with other skin and systemic disorders
- Spoon-shaped nails may indicate iron deficiency

Workup and Diagnosis

- History and physical examination
  - Personal or family history of psoriasis
  - Full skin exam to assess for skin disease
  - Ask about the patient's work and hobbies
- Onychomycosis (nail fungus) is diagnosed by clipping the affected nail and curetting subungual debris for PAS (fungal stain) and/or culture
  - PAS stain is less expensive and quicker than culture
  - Cultures are more helpful when a patient is refractory to systemic therapy; certain nondermatophytes (e.g., *Aspergillus, Fusarium*) can act as nail pathogens and are difficult to eradicate with some antifungal drugs
- Paronychia requires incision and drainage for fungal and bacterial cultures to determine the appropriate topical or systemic treatment and to relieve pain
- Nail matrix biopsy is unnecessary unless a tumor may be the cause of a persistent, isolated, single nail dystrophy or deeply pigmented longitudinal band (>3 mm)
- Referral to dermatology is indicated in unusual, recalcitrant, or potentially malignant cases

Treatment

- Nail fungus can be treated with systemic antifungals (e.g., terbinafine, itraconazole, fluconazole)
  - Fingernail fungus often requires 6 weeks of systemic therapy, whereas toenail fungus requires 12 weeks of treatment to achieve a 70–80% cure rate
  - No absolute indication to treat nail fungus; if the patient is diabetic, nail fungus can compromise the integrity of the nail bed, thereby allowing bacterial pathogens to enter that may lead to extremity cellulitis
  - Topical paint-on ciclopirox has low success rate (17%)
  - Educate the patient that the risk of recurrence of onychomycosis is very high; modify lifestyles to prevent reinfection (antifungal powders on feet/shoes)
- Intralesional steroids in the nail matrix are very painful but offer long-term improvement in nail dystrophy due to lichen planus, psoriasis, atopic eczema
- Nail psoriasis may be treated topically with limited success; systemic antipsoriatic therapies (e.g., cyclosporine, methotrexate) are also used

108. Nasal Congestion

Nasal congestion is a common complaint in primary care. Although usually a sequela of an upper respiratory infection, it can also be a sign of acute or chronic illness. Regardless of its cause, the successful management of nasal congestion often significantly improves patients' quality of life.

Differential Diagnosis

- Upper respiratory infection
  - Most common cause of nasal congestion
  - Respiratory droplet spread, 1–2 day incubation, duration 7–14 days
  - Cough, rhinorrhea, fever, malaise
  - Viral etiology (adenovirus, rhinovirus)
- Perennial allergic rhinitis
  - Family history of allergy
  - Onset <20 years
  - Persistent watery nasal discharge
  - No variation with season
  - Pale, bluish, watery, nasal mucosa
- Seasonal allergic rhinitis
  - Itchy, teary eyes
  - Sneezing
  - Watery nasal discharge
  - Varies with season
  - Exposure to allergen (dust, mold, pollen)
  - Pale, bluish, watery, nasal mucosa
- Perennial nonallergic rhinitis
  - No variation with season
  - Obstruction may alternate nares
  - Swollen nasal mucosa
- Sinusitis (acute or chronic)
  - Patients often have a history of sinusitis
  - Craniofacial discomfort
  - Sinus headaches
  - Pain with percussion of teeth in maxillary sinusitis
  - Retro-orbital pain upon coughing or sneezing in cases of ethmoid sinusitis
  - Mucopurulent nasal drainage
- Rhinitis medicamentosa (rebound rhinitis)
  - Prolonged use of intranasal decongestants
- NARES
- Nasal polyps
- Vasomotor rhinitis
- Foreign body in nose
- Intranasal cocaine use
  - May see nasal septum perforation
- Medication side effects (e.g. aspirin, β-blockers, NSAIDs, oral contraceptives, reserpine, and thioridazine)
- Idiopathic rhinitis
- Less common etiologies include cystic fibrosis, Wegener's granulomatosis, folliculitis of nasal hair, congenital abnormality, sarcoidosis

Workup and Diagnosis

- History and physical examination with attention to head and neck
  - Onset, duration, recurrence pattern, associated symptoms (e.g., cough, fever, itchy palate or eyes), medication/illicit drug use, and family history
  - Examine the eyes, ears, sinuses, nares, oral mucosa, tongue, posterior pharynx, neck, chest, and heart in all cases
- Allergy (skin prick) testing to common inhaled antigens will be positive in patients with perennial and seasonal allergic rhinitis (perform only if chronic or recurrent)
- Nasal lavage with identification of cell type
  - Increased eosinophils in NARES and perennial and seasonal allergic rhinitis
  - Increased PMNs in infectious etiologies
- Rhinoscopic exam/flexible nasopharyngolaryngoscopy may reveal polyps, deformity, mucosal inflammation, or discharge draining from sinus meatus
- CT scan of the sinuses is usually reserved for patients who are resistant to medical therapy for 6–8 weeks
  - May see opacification and air fluid levels in sinusitis
- Nasal cultures have low specificity and are of little clinical value

Treatment

- Initial symptomatic treatment with intranasal saline lavage may provide short-term symptomatic relief
- Intranasal decongestants (e.g., oxymetazoline, phenylephrine) or oral decongestants (e.g., pseudoephedrine, phenylephrine, ipratropium)
- Treat sinusitis (but never viral URI) with antibiotics
  - First-line agents include amoxicillin, trimethoprim-sulfamethoxazole, or doxycycline
  - Amoxicillin plus clavulanic acid is indicated if a β-lactamase-producing strain is suspected
  - Surgery may be indicated for recurrent disease
- Allergic rhinitis
  - Intranasal steroids: Budesonide, fluticasone
  - First- or second-generation antihistamines
  - Cromolyn sodium
  - Allergen avoidance
- Perennial nonallergic rhinitis is treated with decongestants and intranasal steroids for symptoms

109. Nausea & Vomiting

Vomiting is an involuntary forceful extrusion of stomach contents. It is a mediated by a complex reflex that is located in the vomiting center of the medulla oblongata. Reflex vomiting results when afferent fibers of the inner ear, meninges, or gastrointestinal tract fire; central vomiting results from direct stimulation of the vomiting center. Vomiting of blood (hematemesis) requires immediate workup and possible resuscitation and identification of the source of bleeding (see "GI Bleeding—Hematemesis" entry)

Differential Diagnosis

- Central nausea/vomiting
  - Pregnancy (hyperemesis gravidarum)
  - Uremia
  - Hypercalcemia
  - Drugs (e.g., chemotherapy agents)
  - Carbon monoxide poisoning
- Gastrointestinal disease
  - Infection (e.g., gastroenteritis, appendicitis, cholecystitis)
  - Obstruction (e.g., pyloric stenosis, small bowel obstruction, large bowel obstruction, gastroparesis, Ogilvie's syndrome)
  - Inflammation (e.g., pancreatitis, peptic ulcer disease)
  - Food poisoning
- Toxic ingestions
  - Syrup of ipecac
  - Alcohol
  - Salicylates: Result in tachypnea, tinnitus, and metabolic acidosis/respiratory alkalosis
  - Iron: Causes profound gastritis
  - Arsenic
- Middle ear disease (e.g., Ménière's disease, labyrinthitis, benign positional vertigo)
- Post-tussive emesis (especially in children)
- Motion sickness
- CNS disease
  - Increased intracranial pressure due to brain tumor, CNS infection (e.g., meningitis, abscess), head trauma, hydrocephalus, subarachnoid hemorrhage, vestibular neuritis, or intracerebral hemorrhage
  - Migraine headache
- Acute myocardial infarction (especially inferior MI)
- Ovarian torsion
- Testicular torsion
- Malingering: Relatively common, but should be a diagnosis of exclusion until more serious causes are excluded
- Intussusception: Classically causes colicky abdominal pain, vomiting, and currant jelly stools
- Pyelonephritis or other abdominal process

Workup and Diagnosis

- Complete history and physical examination is the most useful diagnostic aid
  - Neurologic examination looking for clues to CNS lesions
  - Ear examination to evaluate for middle ear disease
  - Ophthalmologic examination to evaluate for nystagmus in labyrinthitis or benign positional vertigo
  - Abdominal examination including stool guaiac to evaluate for GI pathology
- Labs may include CBC, electrolytes, liver function tests, amylase, lipase, urinalysis, calcium, magnesium, salicylate level, hepatitis serologies, toxicology screen, and CSF analysis (for meningitis or bleeding)
- ECG and cardiac enzymes may be indicated to evaluate for cardiac ischemia
- Abdominal CT scan with oral and IV contrast if history and physical examination suggest abdominal pathology
- Plain KUB X-rays may be indicated to evaluate for bowel obstruction or perforation
- Abdomen/pelvic ultrasound is especially helpful in cases of lower abdominal pain in female patients or in suspected gallbladder disease
- Endoscopy is indicated for suspected peptic ulcer disease
- Head CT with and without contrast if CNS lesion is suspected

Treatment

- Fluid resuscitation is a mainstay of therapy, because vomiting may cause significant dehydration
- Antiemetics (e.g., metoclopramide, ondansetron, prochlorperazine) may be administered to control symptoms
- Treat reversible causes as necessary (e.g., uremia, hypercalcemia, CNS infections, toxic exposures)
- Treatment of underlying etiologies generally eliminates vomiting
- Inner ear causes of vomiting may respond to treatment with anticholinergics (e.g., meclizine)
- Endoscopy/colonoscopy may be used diagnostically and therapeutically in cases of peptic ulcer disease or large bowel obstruction

110. Neck Masses

Indications for surgical resection of a neck mass include cancer or suspected cancer, hyperthyroidism not responsive to medical therapy, hyperparathyroidism, substernal extension, symptoms of pressure or choking, and cosmetic disfigurement.

Differential Diagnosis

- Inflammatory/infectious (enlarged lymph nodes are the most common neck mass)
  - Abscess
  - Acute lymphadenitis (bacterial, viral, fungal)
  - Tuberculous scrofula
  - Atypical mycobacterium
  - Mononucleosis
  - Cat-scratch disease
  - Sarcoidosis
  - HIV
- Congenital
  - Thyroglossal duct cyst
  - Branchial cleft cyst
  - Laryngocele
  - Cystic hygroma
  - Hemangioma
- Thyroid
  - Cancer (papillary, medullary, follicular/Hurthle cell, anaplastic)
  - Thyrotoxicosis (Graves', toxic multinodular goiter, toxic thyroid nodule)
  - Thyroiditis (Hashimoto's, acute, subacute, Riedel's)
- Parathyroid
  - Hyperplasia
  - Adenoma
  - Carcinoma
- Primary tumor
  - Thyroid (see above)
  - Parathyroid (see above)
  - Salivary gland (parotid tumor most common)
  - Soft tissue tumor (lipoma, sebaceous cyst, inclusion cyst, carbuncle)
  - Carotid body tumor
  - Neurofibroma
  - Schwannoma
  - Angioma
  - Laryngeal tumor (chondroma)
  - Sarcoma
  - Skin cancer (melanoma, squamous cell carcinoma, basal cell carcinoma)
  - Lymphoma
  - Upper aerodigestive tract tumor
- Metastasis

Workup and Diagnosis

- History should include age (congenital in young, cancer in elderly), recent growth (malignant lesions are fast-growing), localized symptoms (pain, dysphasia, hoarseness), radiation exposure (risk of thyroid cancer), social history (tobacco, alcohol), and family history (thyroid cancer)
- Physical exam (including direct laryngoscopy) should evaluate for size, color, location and symmetry, consistency, and tenderness of the mass
- Initial labs may include CBC, chemistries, BUN/creatinine, TSH, free T4, parathyroid hormone, ESR, calcium, phosphorus, and monospot test
- Imaging
  - Chest X-ray to rule out lung metastasis
  - Ultrasound to determine whether mass is solid or cystic
  - CT/MRI
  - Angiography
  - Barium swallow
  - Radioactive iodine uptake scan
- Fine needle aspiration and/or open biopsy may be necessary for definitive diagnosis

Treatment

- Antibiotics
- Incision and drainage (abscess)
- Antithyroid medications (PTU, methimazole)
- Thyroid ablation with radioactive iodine (I^{131} therapy)
- Surgery
  - Parotidectomy
  - Parathyroidectomy
  - Thyroid lobectomy
  - Subtotal or total thyroidectomy
  - Neck dissection
  - Excisional biopsy
- Chemotherapy
- Radiation therapy
- Immunotherapy

111. Neck Stiffness/Pain

Neck stiffness may be caused by inflammation, infection, or trauma. True nuchal rigidity is characterized by the inability to actively or passively touch the chin to the chest and is due to inflammation of the brain and spinal cord. A positive Brudzinski's sign is spontaneous flexion at the hips in response to passive neck flexion. A positive Kernig's sign is an inability to extend at the knee with the hip in flexion.

Differential Diagnosis

- Trauma
  - Paraspinal neck stiffness: Commonly due to motor vehicle collisions ("whiplash") or abnormal sleep posture
  - Cervical spine fracture with spasm of neck muscles
  - Subarachnoid hemorrhage: Most commonly due to ruptured cerebral aneurysm
  - Epidural hematoma
  - SCIWORCA: Spinal Cord Injury Without Radiographic Abnormality occurs in pediatric patients with ligamentous laxity and hypermobility of the cervical spine
  - Rotary atlantoaxial subluxation: Subluxation of the cervical spine at C1-C2 level, resulting in sternocleidomastoid spasm with tilting of the head toward the affected side and chin pointed toward the ipsilateral side
- Infection
  - Meningitis: Often bacterial (e.g., *Neisseria meningitidis, Streptococcus pneumoniae*) or viral (e.g., HIV, Epstein-Barr virus, enterovirus, herpes simplex virus)
  - Cervical lymphadenitis
  - Tonsillopharyngitis
  - Epiglottitis
  - Retropharyngeal abscess
  - Epidural abscess
  - Discitis
- Torticollis: Idiopathic sternocleidomastoid spasm, resulting in tilting of the head toward the affected side with the chin pointed to the contralateral side
- Inflammatory
  - Rheumatoid arthritis
  - Ankylosing spondylitis
  - Degenerative joint disease
- Tumors (especially leptomeningeal metastases)
- Dystonic reaction: Idiosyncratic drug reaction, often to psychiatric medications (e.g., haloperidol, prochlorperazine)

Workup and Diagnosis

- History and physical examination focusing on evidence of trauma and infection
  - All patients with possible traumatic injury should be maintained in a cervical collar and backboard until diagnostic workup is complete
- Initial labs may include CBC, electrolytes, BUN/creatinine, calcium, glucose, and ESR
- Blood cultures are indicated if infectious etiologies are suspected
- Lumbar puncture with CSF analysis is useful in cases of suspected infection or subarachnoid hemorrhage
- Cervical spine radiographs are indicated in trauma or neck infection (may reveal prevertebral soft-tissue swelling)
- Head CT scan without contrast may show bleeding in cases of subarachnoid hemorrhage (fails to reveal subarachnoid blood in 10% of cases)
- Neck CT scan may be indicated in suspected soft tissue disease (e.g., retropharyngeal abscess) or occult vertebral fracture if not adequately visualized on plain films
- MRI of the spine may be indicated in suspected epidural abscess or epidural hematoma

Treatment

- Trauma: Soft-collar immobilization is no longer routinely recommended
  - Cervical spine fractures may be treated with surgical fixation, halo brace immobilization, or careful observation
  - Soft-tissue injuries to the neck and torticollis are treated symptomatically with NSAIDs and muscle relaxants (e.g., benzodiazepines, cyclobenzaprine)
  - Subarachnoid hemorrhage is often treated surgically
- Infection
  - Bacterial meningitis requires immediate broad-spectrum antibiotics (e.g., ceftriaxone and vancomycin); steroids may decrease the morbidity associated with the inflammatory response to infection
  - Viral meningitis is treated supportively (IV fluids, NSAIDs)
  - Abscess requires antibiotics and drainage
- Inflammatory arthropathies typically respond to NSAIDs, steroids, or antirheumatic agents

112. Night Sweats

Night sweats are a common complaint in primary care medicine. Different authors define night sweats variably, but this term generally pertains to drenching sweats at night that are not caused by excessive room temperature or clothing/covering.

Differential Diagnosis

- Infections
  - HIV
  - Tuberculosis
  - Infectious mononucleosis
  - Fungal (e.g., histoplasmosis, coccidioidomycosis)
  - Lung or other abscess
  - Endocarditis
  - Osteomyelitis
- Neoplasms
  - Leukemia
  - Hodgkin's disease and other forms of lymphoma
  - Solid tumors (e.g. prostate, adrenal, renal, testicular)
- Menopause/premature ovarian failure
- Hyperthyroidism
- Diabetes mellitus (nocturnal hypoglycemia)
- GERD
- Obstructive sleep apnea
- Chronic fatigue syndrome
- Anxiety
- Pregnancy
- Drugs [e.g., antipyretics (most common), antihypertensives, phenothiazines, antiretroviral agents]
- Substance abuse (including alcohol)
- Orchiectomy
- Endocrine tumors
  - Pheochromocytoma
  - Carcinoid
- Chronic eosinophilic pneumonia
- Prinzmetal's angina
- Temporal arteritis
- Takayasu's arteritis

Workup and Diagnosis

- Complete history and physical examination
  - Note associated symptoms, such as flushing, pain, and tachycardia
  - Review full past medical and social history; review of systems
  - Complete physical with focus on endocrine, lymphatic, and dermatologic systems
- Laboratory testing depends on the presumed etiology; a reasonable initial workup includes CBC with differential, eosinophil count, electrolytes, BUN/creatinine, calcium, magnesium, TSH, urinalysis and culture, and ESR
- Consider the following testing if indicated: FSH (peri-menopause), PPD, chest X-ray, HIV viral load/antibody, blood cultures, monospot, 3 AM glucose level to assess for nocturnal hypoglycemia, sleep study, free T4, 24-hour urinary catecholamines, 5-hydroxyindoleacetic acid, echocardiogram, and/or CT of chest/abdomen/pelvis

Treatment

- Treatment depends on etiology, although identifying the correct diagnosis is usually the most difficult aspect of the disease
- Treating the appropriate condition if amenable to therapy will relieve the night sweats
- Antipyretics (e.g., ibuprofen, acetaminophen)
- Cessation of substance abuse
- Appropriate antimicrobials if infectious cause
- Cessation or decreased dose of causative medication(s), if possible

113. Nodular Lesions

A palpable lesion <1 cm is described as a papule. A nodule is a nodular lesion ≥ 1 cm. Nodules can be on the skin (exophytic), within the skin (intraepidermal or dermal), or beneath the skin (subcutaneous). The differential diagnosis of skin nodules is enormous. Color, rapidity of appearance or growth, symptomatology, and the underlying medical condition of the patient will guide you in determining the correct diagnosis.

Differential Diagnosis

- Epidermoid or epidermal inclusion cyst
  - These may change in size, become intermittently tender and erythematous, or even have a central punctum with extrusion of caseous or "cheesy" material
  - Although they may become secondarily infected, they are completely benign
- Pilar cyst
  - Usually on the scalp
  - Usually asymptomatic
- Dermatofibroma
  - Flesh colored or hyperpigmented, fibrous lesions that dimple when pinched
  - May occur after minor trauma
  - Common on lower extremities
- Pyogenic granuloma
  - Erythematous, papular, friable lesion due to capillary proliferation
  - May occur after minor trauma
- Ganglion cyst
  - Somewhat mobile lesions that appear most frequently on the dorsal wrist or over the joints of the hands
- Lipoma
  - Common, usually nontender, and freely mobile, very soft, and pliable
- Many benign neoplasms of the skin present as indolent dermal nodules
- Dermal or subcutaneous neoplasms can arise from the hair follicle, sweat glands (i.e., sebaceous adenomas), blood vessels (i.e., hemangiomas), nerves (i.e., neurofibromas) and eccrine sweat ducts
- Subcutaneous nodules on the extensor surface of joints may be tender, which may indicate gout, calcification of the bursa or calcinosis cutis (seen in renal failure), or rheumatoid nodules
- Nodular melanomas, metastatic tumors, and lymphomas can present as isolated skin nodules that appear suddenly and/or grow rapidly in size
- Hypertrophic scars and keloids can appear as pink, tender skin nodules
- Yellow skin nodules such as xanthomas may portend an underlying lipid disorder
- Red skin nodules may indicate bacillary angiomatosis or other infection
- Kaposi's sarcoma may present as purplish skin nodules and tumors
- Erythema nodosum

Workup and Diagnosis

- History and physical examination
  - Note whether lesion is changing in appearance or increasing in size
  - Note whether lesion is tender or symptomatic
  - Note medical history of cutaneous or systemic malignancies, arthritis (e.g., gout, rheumatoid disease)
  - Note immunosuppression, which makes patients more vulnerable to malignant skin nodules
  - Note family history of melanoma and/or lipomas
- When in doubt, biopsy to ascertain the true nature of the lesion
  - Shave biopsy is sufficient for exophytic lesions
  - Punch biopsy, excisional biopsy, or incisional biopsy may be warranted for intradermal or subcutaneous nodules
  - Excisional, full-thickness biopsy allows full staging when melanoma is in the differential diagnosis
- Appropriate cultures should be obtained from tender or suppurative lesions

Treatment

- Treatment depends on the diagnosis, and includes excision, in most cases, for symptomatic and/or cosmetic purposes
- Epidermoid cysts
  - Lesions that are actively inflamed must "cool down" before excision can be successfully performed
  - Intralesional steroids and/or oral first-generation cephalosporins will cause the inflammatory reaction to subside more quickly
  - Incision and drainage are indicated for tense and painful inflamed cysts
  - Once the infection and or inflammation has resolved, the cyst can be excised
  - It must be marsupialized (i.e. the entire cyst contents and its complete lining must be removed) to prevent recurrence

113

114. Nystagmus

Nystagmus is defined as involuntary, rhythmic, biphasic oscillation of eyes. It is characterized as horizontal, vertical, rotary, or a combination; fast or slow; symmetric or asymmetric; and pendular (equal speed in either direction) or jerk (slow in one direction followed by fast in the opposite direction). By convention, nystagmus is named in the direction of the fast phase. Usually results from a defect in the slow eye movement system (visual fixation, vestibular system, smooth pursuit, vergence, optokinetic, and neural integrator pathways).

Differential Diagnosis

- Vestibular
  - Peripheral (horizontal rotary nystagmus, slow phase toward hypoactive side, latency, fatigability, and accompanied by vertigo, tinnitus, or deafness): Etiologies include labyrinthitis, vestibular neuronitis, Ménière's disease, migraine, BPV
  - Central (asymmetric, rotary nystagmus that changes direction in different gazes, no latency, not fatigable): Etiologies include lesions of cerebellum, pons, or cerebello-pontine angle
  - Horizontal
- Gaze-evoked
  - Physiologic: Fixing on objects with eyes when head is turned (e.g., ballerinas)
  - Pathologic (asymmetric): Etiologies include toxic-metabolic lesions, cerebellar or pontine lesions
- Dissociated (different nystagmus between eyes): Etiologies include internuclear ophthalmoplegia of multiple sclerosis or cerebral disease
- Periodic alternating nystagmus (cervicomedullary junction)
- Downbeat (cervicomedullary junction, characteristic of syringobulbia)
- Upbeat (brainstem or cerebellum when present in primary gaze; drug effect if only present in upgaze)
- Drug-induced (e.g., anticonvulsants, sedatives, alcohol)
- Monocular visual loss (ipsilateral slow vertical oscillation)
- Head nodding, head turn (due to motor or sensory deficits)
  - Latent nystagmus (occurs only when one eye is viewing, and is always associated with strabismus)
  - Nystagmus blockage syndrome (convergence, esotropia, and head turn)
  - Spasmus nutans: Onset 4–14 months, resolves by age 5; head nodding, torticollis, see-saw

Workup and Diagnosis

- History and physical examination
  - Note age of onset, associated symptoms (e.g., oscillopsia, decreased vision, nausea/vomiting, vertigo, hearing loss, tinnitus, diplopia, dysarthria, facial numbness, dysphagia), medications, and drug use
  - Complete ocular exam: Eye movements in primary gaze and all positions of gaze; iris transillumination (albinism), dilated fundus exam, careful refraction, vestibulo-ocular reflex
  - Dix-Hallpike maneuver (for positional vertigo, peripheral versus central)
  - Caloric stimulation
  - Complete neurologic examination
  - Nystagmus is asymptomatic, unless acquired after age 8, at which time the patient may have oscillopsia (a sense that the surroundings are oscillating)
- Consider drug, toxin, and dietary screen of urine/serum
- Consider MRI of brain
- Consider visual field exam
- Consider neurology and/or ophthalmology consultation
  - Eye movement recording
  - Electronystagmogram
  - Visual evoked response
  - Electroretinography

Treatment

- Treat the underlying etiology if possible
- Remove offending medications/toxins if possible
- Medications to treat the nystagmus (e.g., meclizine for BPV) have varying success
- BPV: Otolith repositioning maneuvers (Epley's, Semont's)
- Botulinum toxin injection to the appropriate extraocular muscles may be used for severe disabling nystagmus
- Congenital nystagmus: Maximize vision by refractive lenses, treat amblyopia ("lazy eye") if indicated, prism, and/or eye muscle surgery
- Vestibular: Vestibular suppressant (meclizine, diazepam), vestibular adaptation exercises
- Baclofen may be useful in periodic alternating nystagmus and some congenital nystagmus
- Clonazepam for downbeat nystagmus

115. Oral Lesions

Recurrent oral erosions are most often secondary to herpes simplex virus or idiopathic aphthous stomatitis. A thorough review of systems and complete skin exam are the best tools to assure diagnostic accuracy, particularly in light of the fact that serious medical conditions may manifest first as oral lesions. Referral to an oral surgeon, otorhinolaryngologist, or dermatologist is necessary if a definitive diagnosis cannot be determined.

Differential Diagnosis

- Aphthous stomatitis
  - Idiopathic
  - Recurrent, shallow, painful, spontaneously resolving oral ulcers
- Herpes stomatitis
  - Due to a primary outbreak of HSV-1
  - Severe gingivostomatitis with pain, redness, and erosions around the gum line
  - Recurrent oral HSV ("cold sores") often occur at the lip border
  - Stress, sun exposure, and many other factors contribute to flare-ups
- Self-limited viral disease (e.g., herpangina, hand-foot-mouth disease)
  - Most often seen in children
  - Prodrome of malaise and fever followed by a 5–10 day outbreak of oropharyngeal erosions or vesicles is common
- Chemotherapy drugs (especially 5-FU and methotrexate)
- Squamous cell carcinoma should always be considered if a nonhealing ulcer or oral erosion is noted
- Bullous diseases (e.g., pemphigoid, pemphigus, lichen planus)
  - Recurrent painful oral ulcers and erosions
  - Evaluate for other skin rashes suggestive of these disorders
- Behçet syndrome
  - Uncommon but well-known cause of oral ulcers
  - Patients must exhibit other symptoms (e.g., uveitis, CNS problems, GI complaints, genital ulcers) before this diagnosis can be made
- Allergic contact dermatitis to amalgams in dental work may result in buccal tenderness
- Erythema multiforme (Stevens-Johnson syndrome)
  - Characterized by oral ulcers, ocular involvement, and simultaneous targetoid, erythematous, or bullous skin lesions
  - May be triggered by HSV infection, *Mycoplasma infection,* or drugs (e.g., phenytoin, sulfonamides)
- Primary syphilis
  - Painless chancre
- Agranulocytosis or leukopenia
- Histoplasmosis (especially in immunosuppressed patients)

Workup and Diagnosis

- Detailed history and physical examination
  - Associated symptoms (e.g., fever, prodrome)
  - Review the patient's past medical history and medication list
  - If ulcers occur in the same location with every episode, oral HSV is likely
  - Is the patient sexually active (consider HIV, immunosuppression, or syphilis)
  - Perform a thorough skin exam to evaluate for rashes or other mucosal lesions (ocular, urethral, or perianal)
  - Lacy white plaques on the tongue or buccal mucosa may suggest lichen planus
  - Ocular or anogenital complaints can be suggestive of Behçet syndrome, pemphigus, or pemphigoid
- Initial evaluation includes a viral swab for culture and/or serum for HSV-1 IgG detection to diagnose HSV, and consider an RPR and CBC to rule out syphilis and leukopenia, respectively
- Consider a punch biopsy of the *edge* of an ulcer/erosion to determine if there are viral changes or cytologic atypia; or evidence of an autoimmune bullous disease
- Recurrent aphthous stomatitis is a diagnosis of exclusion, but is also the most common diagnosis of recurrent painful oral ulcers after HSV

Treatment

- Orabase^R compounded with high-potency topical steroids (e.g., clobetasol) may offer symptomatic relief and increase speed of healing
- "Magic mouthwash" may be used to swish and spit as necessary for relief (these may contain lidocaine, diphenhydramine, antacids, and even liquid tetracycline)
- Aphthous stomatitis: Intralesional triamcinalone injections are painful but very helpful
  - Lesions spontaneously resolve within 2 weeks
- Recurrent herpes stomatitis: Episodic treatment with 1–7 day courses of oral antivirals (e.g., acyclovir) can shorten the duration of the episode and speed healing
  - These are efficacious only if started within 24 hours of the onset of the prodrome (often tingling or pain at the site of eruption occurs hours before onset)
  - Chronic suppressive therapy with oral antivirals may be indicated if recurrences are frequent
- Bullous diseases: Corticosteroids (topical or oral), cyclosporine, and even thalidomide

116. Orthopnea

Orthopnea is defined as difficulty breathing (dyspnea) while in the recumbent position. The dyspnea is due to increased venous return to the lungs while recumbent, resulting in increased pulmonary venous and capillary pressures. Elevating the head/chest toward an upright position relieves the dyspnea. Orthopnea implies left-sided heart failure in about 95% of cases.

Differential Diagnosis

- Congestive heart failure is the most common cause of orthopnea
  - Etiologies include uncontrolled HTN, pulmonary embolus, endocarditis, hyperthyroidism, pericardial disease, endocardial disease (e.g., valvular stenosis, insufficiency, rupture, endocarditis), and myocardial disease (e.g., MI, ischemia, arrhythmias)
- Aortic regurgitation
  - Most commonly due to rheumatic fever
- Cardiomyopathies
- Pleural effusion
  - Common causes: CHF, pneumonia, cancer, pulmonary embolus, connective tissue disease (e.g., SLE, rheumatoid arthritis), pancreatitis, renal or liver disease
- Aortic stenosis
  - Associated with angina, syncope, and CHF
- Mitral stenosis
  - Usually secondary to rheumatic heart disease (after 15–40 years)
  - Advanced cases result in pulmonary hypertension and right heart failure
  - Dyspnea is the most significant symptom
  - Classic triad: Diastolic rumble, opening snap, and loud first heart sound
- Congenital heart disease
  - May see failure to thrive, progressive CHF symptoms, cyanosis, and/or murmur
- Severe COPD and asthma
- Severe bilateral apical lung disease
- Bilateral diaphragmatic paralysis

Workup and Diagnosis

- Thorough history and physical exam
  - Note onset (sudden or chronic, progressive)
  - Timing (persistent or intermittent)
  - Associated symptoms (e.g., chest discomfort, syncope)
- Initial labs should include CBC, electrolytes, thyroid function tests, pulse oximetry (resting, ambulatory, and nocturnal), and chest X-ray
- Arterial blood gas will identify barriers to oxygen diffusion (increased A-a gradient), hypoxemia, and chronic hypercapnia
- ECG may reveal evidence of MI, right ventricular strain (e.g., due to mitral stenosis), left ventricular hypertrophy (e.g., aortic stenosis), low voltage (cardiomyopathy), and dysrhythmias
- BNP may be useful if the etiology is uncertain to distinguish CHF from other causes of dyspnea
- Pulmonary function tests may be indicated to identify restrictive or obstructive disease and barriers to diffusion
- Echocardiogram to establish a diagnosis of structural heart disease, valve disease, and LV dysfunction
- Consider cardiac catheterization to evaluate valve disease, cardiomyopathy, and congenital heart disease

Treatment

- Attention to airway, breathing, and circulation
- Administer supplemental O_2 as needed
- CHF: Decrease preload by venodilation and afterload by arteriodilation and volume removal, to improve forward blood flow and decrease symptoms; give nitrates (sublingual/IV), loop diuretics, IV morphine, ACE inhibitors, digoxin, spironolactone; treat refractory respiratory distress with CPAP, BiPAP, or intubation
- Valvular disease: Reduce blood pressure with an ACE inhibitor or β-blocker; surgery (balloon valvuloplasty, valve repair, or valve replacement) for severe disease
- Pleural effusion: Treat underlying cause; thoracentesis may be indicated; pleurodesis for recurrent effusions
- Asthma: Avoid triggers; bronchodilation with inhaled $β_2$ agonists (e.g., albuterol) and anticholinergics (e.g., ipratropium); inhaled, oral, and/or IV steroids
- COPD: Inhaled bronchodilators (e.g., albuterol, ipratropium); systemic corticosteroids; antibiotics in severe exacerbations; mechanical ventilation

117. Osler Nodes

Osler nodes are small, tender, nodular or papulopustular, violaceous, cutaneous lesions in the pads of the fingers or toes. They are most characteristic of subacute bacterial endocarditis. The exact pathogenesis of Osler nodes (septic emboli versus immune complex formation) is controversial.

Differential Diagnosis

- Acute bacterial endocarditis
  - Associated with high fever, chills, and new onset heart murmur
  - Most common organisms include *Staphylococcus aureus, S. pyogenes,* and *Streptococcus pneumoniae*
- Subacute bacterial endocarditis
  - Associated with low-grade fever, cough, dyspnea, weakness, fatigue, malaise
  - Most common organisms are *Streptococcus viridans, Enterococcus, Staphylococcus epidermidis,* and fungi
  - Other cutaneous signs include conjunctival and palatal petechiae, subungual (splinter) hemorrhages, and Roth's spots (pale oval retinal areas surrounded by hemorrhage)
- Meningococcemia
  - Caused by *Neisseria meningitidis*
  - Associated with signs of meningitis (e.g., headache, neck stiffness, photophobia, altered mental status, seizures)
  - Positive Kernig's and Brudzinski's signs
- Systemic lupus erythematosus
  - Associated with malar rash, discoid rash, arthritis, myalgias, photosensitivity, and oral ulcers
- Thrombotic thrombocytopenic purpura
  - Associated with splenomegaly, anemia, bleeding, and jaundice
- Idiopathic thrombocytopenia purpura
  - Autoimmune disorder associated with mucosal bleeding, petechiae, and purpura
  - Afebrile
- Polyarteritis nodosa
  - Associated with fever, abdominal pain, neuropathy, hematuria, proteinuria
- Rocky Mountain spotted fever
  - Associated with macular rash beginning on palms and soles and spreading centrally
- Disseminated intravascular coagulation
- Typhoid fever
- Cutaneous vasculitis
- Enteroviral infection
- Syphilis (secondary)

Workup and Diagnosis

- History and physical examination
  - New-onset murmur suggests infective endocarditis
- Initial labs should include CBC, peripheral smear, coagulation studies, urinalysis, ESR, ANA, anti-dsDNA and anti-SM antibodies
- Blood cultures must be drawn at three different times and from different body sites
- Chest X-ray (septic emboli) and echocardiogram (vegetations on heart valve) are indicated if suspect infective endocarditis
- Biopsy of lesions
- Infective endocarditis is diagnosed by Duke's criteria: If two major *or* one major and two minor *or* five minor criteria are present, endocarditis is considered definite
  - Major criteria include positive blood cultures from two different sites >12 hours apart and echocardiogram showing endocardial involvement (e.g., vegetation, abscess, or new dehiscence of prosthetic valve)
  - Minor criteria include predisposing heart condition or IV drug abuse, fever >100.4°F (>38°C), vascular phenomena or immunologic phenomena (e.g., Osler's nodes, Janeway lesions), or a positive blood culture that does not satisfy a major criteria
- TTP presents with schistocytes on peripheral blood smear, increased LDH, and increased indirect bilirubin
- ITP is diagnosed by platelet-associated IgG test
- Polyarteritis nodosa: Biopsy shows areas of necrosis

Treatment

- Bacterial endocarditis: Long-term antibiotic therapy [initiate broad-spectrum empiric therapy, then tailor to organism(s) found on culture]; valve replacement may be indicated if medical therapy fails; lifelong antibiotic prophylaxis is indicated before any dental work or minor surgery
- Meningococcemia: IV antibiotics; antibiotic prophylaxis (e.g., rifampin, minocycline) of all exposed individuals
- Treat other etiologies by established treatment protocols

118. Otorrhea

Otorrhea, or ear discharge, usually results from an inflammatory process in the ear canal, middle ear, or mastoid. A thorough cleaning of the ear canal (with suction if possible) is essential to determine the source of the otorrhea. Ear lavage should be avoided in the presence of otorrhea, because of possible injury to the inner ear if the tympanic membrane is perforated, commonly from otitis media. CSF otorrhea must always be considered in patients with recent face or head trauma or surgery.

Differential Diagnosis

- Otitis externa (swimmer's ear)
  - Most common source of otorrhea
  - Usually associated with water contamination or cotton swab abuse
  - Pain with movement of pinna
  - Usually secondary to *Pseudomonas* or *Staphylococcus* infection
- Malignant otitis externa
  - Also known as necrotizing external otitis and skull base osteomyelitis
  - Suspect in patients with diabetes or immunosuppression who present with persistent otorrhea, ear pain, and granulation tissue in the ear canal
  - Usually secondary to *Pseudomonas*
- Foreign body
  - Frequently a retained cotton swab
  - Often occurs in toddlers
- Otitis media (acute or chronic) with perforated tympanic membrane
- Cholesteatoma
  - A skin-lined cyst of the middle ear or mastoid that occurs secondary to chronic otitis media
  - In most cases there is fullness, bulging, or a white mass of the tympanic membrane (may easily be confused with ear wax)
- Mastoiditis
  - Tenderness or bogginess over mastoid
- Cerebrospinal fluid otorrhea
  - Clear, colorless discharge through a tympanic membrane perforation or tympanostomy tube
  - Patients usually have a history of trauma or surgery, but CSF otorrhea may occasionally be spontaneous

Workup and Diagnosis

- History should focus on onset, duration, appearance of discharge, associated symptoms, activity history (e.g., swimming), and past history (e.g., frequent otitis, tympanostomy tubes, diabetes)
- A thorough cleaning of the ear canal under direct visualization (with magnification is ideal) with a curette or suction is necessary to determine the source of discharge
  - The presence or absence of tympanic membrane pathology must be determined
  - The absence of tympanic membrane pathology usually signifies that the source of otorrhea is limited to the external ear canal
  - Unless the ear canal is cleaned with suction, many pathologies will not be identified
  - Ear lavage should be avoided in the presence of otorrhea
- Ear cultures from the canal may be helpful in persistent cases; however, contamination by normal ear canal flora usually decreases their value
- If CSF otorrhea is suspected, an assay for β_2 transferrin will identify CSF from other fluids
- CT of the temporal bones is helpful in evaluation of patients with suspected cholesteatoma, mastoiditis, and CSF otorrhea
- Gallium and technetium scans may be helpful in patients with malignant external otitis

Treatment

- Otitis externa is treated with antibiotic drops; alternatively, acidification of the ear canal with acetic acid is also effective; patients should follow water precautions and abstain from the use of cotton swabs
- Otomycosis of the ear canal is also treated with topical antifungal preparations as well as acidification
- Otitis media with tympanic membrane perforation should be treated with systemic antibiotics; precautions should be taken with topical antibiotics because many are known to be ototoxic (only ofloxacin is approved for usage in the middle ear)
- Foreign bodies in the ear can be removed with alligator forceps under direct visualization, or the patient can be referred to an otolaryngologist emergently
- Patients with cholesteatoma, mastoiditis, and cerebrospinal fluid leak should be emergently referred to an otolaryngologist

119. Palpitations

Palpitations are the subjective sensation of the heart beating rapidly, strongly, or irregularly. It often means that a rapid heart rate is occurring, but it can also be seen even when the heart rate is normal, such as in anxious patients. The patient should be asked to describe the palpitations and to demonstrate them by saying or tapping the speed and rhythm of the palpitation sensation. Additionally, teaching the patient to measure his/her pulse during the palpitations may give further clues as to the etiology of the sensation.

Differential Diagnosis

- Premature atrial contractions
- Premature ventricular contractions
- Sinus tachycardia
    –Regular heart rhythm at 100–140 bpm
- Atrial fibrillation
    –Irregularly irregular heart rate
- Atrial flutter
    –Regular heart rhythm at about 150 bpm
- Drugs leading to tachyarrhythmias
  (e.g., aminophylline, amphetamines, alcohol,
  atropine, cocaine, coffee, epinephrine,
  ephedrine, MAO inhibitors, tea, thyroid
  extract, tobacco)
- Psychiatric disorders (anxiety, panic reactions)
- Anemia (with exertion)
- Heart failure (with exertion)
- Menopausal syndrome (with hot flashes)
- Paroxysmal atrial tachycardia
- Re-entry tachycardias, including
  Wolff-Parkinson-White syndrome
- Ventricular tachycardia
- Atrioventricular heart blocks
- Junctional tachycardia
- Mitral valve prolapse
- Myocardial ischemia
- Hyperthyroidism-associated arrhythmias
- Severe deconditioning (with exertion)
- Hypoglycemia
- Postural hypotension
- Atrial septal defect
- Adrenal tumor
- Pheochromocytoma

Workup and Diagnosis

- History and physical exam
    –Note duration, frequency, and precipitating factors
    –May be associated with chest pain, dyspnea, diaphoresis,
     or lightheadedness/syncope
    –Heart rhythm may be regular or irregular
    –May have family history of prolonged QT syndrome,
     hypertrophic cardiomyopathy, syncope, arrhythmias, or
     sudden death
- ECG
- 24-hour Holter monitor may be indicated
- Event monitor (if events are infrequent)
- Echocardiogram
- Exercise stress test if exercise-related
- Laboratory studies normally include CBC, electrolytes,
  glucose, TSH, calcium, magnesium
- Consider drug screen
- Consider cardiology consult
- Electrophysiologic studies may be necessary if symptoms
  suggest sustained arrhythmia

Treatment

- Attention to airway, breathing, and circulation
- Treat the underlying cause
- Discontinue offending drugs
- Anxiolytics may be needed for significant anxiety
- Administer adenosine, amiodarone and/or other anti-
  arrhythmics, β-blockers, diltiazem, digoxin as indicated for
  rate control, suppression, or cardioversion
- Electrophysiologic intervention (radiofrequency ablation of
  re-entrant pathway) may be necessary for symptomatic
  patients

120. Papilledema

Papilledema is defined as swelling or edema of the optic discs; it is usually bilateral and is due to increased intracranial pressure. Clinically, the disk appears elevated and the margins appear indistinct or blurred with obscuring of some small and medium vessels. Patients may present with transient visual loss (lasting seconds), often precipitated by changes in posture. Papilledema is also commonly associated with headache, double vision, nausea, and vomiting. Patients very rarely have decreased visual acuity.

Differential Diagnosis

Optic disc swelling due to increased ICP
- Pseudotumor cerebri (idiopathic intracranial hypertension)
    - Most common cause of papilledema
    - Young, obese, or pregnant females
    - Associated with vitamin A overdose, OCPs, tetracycline, steroid withdrawal
- Cerebral tumor (primary or metastatic)
- Hydrocephalus (e.g., tumor, Arnold-Chiari malformation, aqueductal stenosis, postinfectious)
- Intracranial hemorrhage (papilledema may not be seen acutely because it takes about 24 hours to develop after the ICP increases)
    - Subdural hematoma
    - Subarachnoid hemorrhage
    - Hemorrhagic stroke
    - Epidural hematoma
- Intracranial infection
    - Brain abscess
    - Encephalitis (e.g., herpes)
    - Neurosyphilis
    - Toxoplasmosis
- Meningitis (e.g., bacterial, viral, TB)
- Malignant hypertension
- Pre-eclampsia

Optic disc swelling not due to increased ICP
- Pseudopapilledema (the vessels traversing the disk margins are obscured, as in true papilledema): Optic disc drusen or congenitally anomalous disc
- Papillitis: Unilateral, painful, vitreous cells
- Papillophlebitis: Mild visual loss and disk swelling in young, healthy patient
- Central retinal vein occlusion: Unilateral, associated with an acute loss of vision
- Diabetic papillopathy: Disk edema with minimal visual loss, resolves spontaneously
- Optic-disc vasculitis/ischemic optic neuropathy (giant cell/temporal arteritis)
- Orbital optic-nerve tumors
- Graves' ophthalmopathy: History of thyroid dysfunction; may be associated with lid lag, proptosis, increased intraocular pressure
- Uveitis: Associated with pain, photophobia, and scleral injection
- Atypical optic neuritis

Workup and Diagnosis

- Papilledema is considered a medical emergency caused by increased intracranial pressure until proven otherwise
- Complete neurologic and ocular exam, including a color vision assessment, slit lamp exam, posterior vitreous evaluation for WBCs, and a dilated fundus exam
    - True papilledema presents as bilaterally swollen, hyperemic discs with blurring of the disc margin that often obscures the blood vessels
    - True papilledema is due to increased ICP; if spontaneous venous pulsations are present, then ICP is normal
- Noncontrast CT and/or MRI of the head/orbit will identify cerebral tumors, hydrocephalus, and intracranial hemorrhage
    - Pseudotumor cerebri have normal CT/MRI
    - Cerebral tumors appear as space-occupying lesions
    - Hydrocephalus appears as enlarged ventricles
- Lumbar puncture (if CT/MRI negative)
    - Opening pressure for pseudotumor cerebri
    - Definitive diagnosis of meningitis and encephalitis
    - CSF CBC, Gram stain, cultures (bacterial, viral, VDRL if neurosyphilis is suspected, and fungal), cryptococcal antigen, protein, glucose,
    - Bloody tap in subarachnoid hemorrhage
- Further laboratory studies may include CBC, thyroid tests (e.g., TSH, T_3, T_4), and blood glucose

Treatment

- Pseudotumor cerebri may be self-limited with weight loss, discontinuation of offending medications; diuretics may be used (e.g., acetazolamide) to decrease CSF production, lumboperitoneal shunting or optic nerve sheath decompression may be indicated in some cases
- Intracranial tumors may require resection
- Hydrocephalus: Surgical correction of anatomic abnormalities, with or without VP shunt
- Intracranial hemorrhage: Conservative management versus surgical evacuation depends on size and location
    - Acute subdural hematoma: Control elevated ICP with osmotic and loop diuretics and mild hyperventilation; emergent craniotomy for evacuation of hematomas that result in significant mass effect
    - Epidural hematoma: Usually does not require surgery; hyperventilation and mannitol to decrease ICP
- Intracerebral infections require appropriate antibiotics
- Encephalitis: Control ICP by hyperventilation, diuresis
- Malignant hypertension: Aggressive IV pressure control

121. Papulosquamous Lesions

Papulosquamous is a term used for skin lesions that are papular and present in the superficial skin layer (the squamous layer). Papulosquamous rashes are defined as exanthems that have palpable epidermal changes with scale. The diagnoses within the papulosquamous categories are quite broad and must be considered systematically on the basis of history and physical examination, and only occasionally with a biopsy. The distribution of the lesions is a key characteristic that helps with a correct diagnosis.

Differential Diagnosis

- Allergic and irritant contact reactions and drug-induced rashes are included in the papulosquamous diseases
- Psoriasis
  - Affects 2% of the U.S. population
  - May acutely present as guttate (drop-like), round plaques with minimal scale
  - More common is the variant called psoriasis vulgaris: Presents as thick plaques of silvery adherent scale on an erythematous base on the extensor joints
- Seborrheic dermatitis
  - An inflammatory "dandruff" that manifests as light scale on a greasy and/or erythematous background around the hairline, upper lip, nasolabial creases, chin, external ears, eyebrow areas, scalp
  - Due to overgrowth of *Pityrosporum ovale*
- Pityriasis rosea
  - A common exanthem that is self-limited; the etiology is unclear
  - Presents with initial "herald patch," with subsequent scaly pink papules/plaques over the trunk in a "Christmas tree" distribution
  - May be very itchy and is often confused with guttate psoriasis
- Atopic dermatitis
  - Common among children with a history of asthma, hay fever, or seasonal allergies
  - Manifests as itchy eczematous plaques on the antecubital and popliteal fossae; often becomes secondarily lichenified (i.e., thickened with chronic rubbing changes)
  - 60% of patients have initial symptoms before 1 year of age
  - The disease often lasts 15–20 years
- Fungal infections of the skin caused by dermatophytes often present as itchy, scaly papulosquamous rashes that can mimic nummular eczema
- Nummular eczema
  - An idiopathic disease that affects many patients mostly in the winter months
- Lichen planus
  - Present with flat topped, polygonal, and purplish papules that may have white streaks or "Wickham's striae"
- Eczematous diseases (e.g., eczema craquelé, lichen simplex chronicus)
- Infection (e.g., secondary syphilis meningococcemia, RMSF)

Workup and Diagnosis

- Perform a focused history and physical examination
  - Evaluate for family history of psoriasis or other skin disease
  - Look for fingernail pitting, subungual debris, distal separation of the nail plate from the nail bed (called onycholysis), and "oil spots" (extravasated proteins under the nail) that are characteristic of psoriasis; always consider psoriasis if the scale is markedly silver and very thick/adherent to the skin
- Seborrhea of the face and scalp is far more common than psoriasis of these areas, and it has a much thinner and lighter scale
- Pityriasis rosea presents in healthy young adults after a viral prodrome; observe carefully for the larger, thicker herald patch to confirm the diagnosis; patients can often point the first patch out to you, because it appeared several days before the more diffuse eruption
- Consider atopic dermatitis in a young patient with allergic rhinitis or asthma and a very itchy, chronic, or subacute rash that is often symmetric on the flexural skin
- A KOH preparation and examination by light microscope can quickly establish the diagnosis of a dermatophyte infection
- Patch testing to potential allergens and review of a patient's chemical exposure can help rule in allergic contact or irritant dermatitis, respectively

Treatment

- Psoriasis can be effectively controlled
  - Topical calcipotriene is a nonsteroidal, long-term agent used to control the cutaneous disease
  - Topical steroids, tar, and anthralin preparations; intralesional steroids; salicylic acid and ultraviolet light therapy; methotrexate; acitretin; cyclosporin; and newer biologic therapies such as alefacept and etanercept are used as well
  - Avoid using systemic steroids whenever possible, because a severe flare is common upon their completion
- Pityriasis rosea is managed symptomatically with oral antihistamines, topical steroids, topical antipruritics (e.g., sarna, calamine), and, in severe cases, with oral steroids, erythromycin or phototherapy
- Atopic dermatitis
  - Must be approached as a disease of skin barrier function; it is crucial to repair that function with the use of gentle cleansers, emollient creams/oils, topical steroid ointments

122. Paraplegia

Paralysis is the total loss of voluntary motor function of an affected area and most frequently indicates a serious neurologic problem in the site of distribution of the affected area. The key to correct diagnosis of paralytic syndromes is knowledge of the neurologic pathways and dermatomes, so the site of the problem can be defined anatomically, after which a focused imaging examination can define the specific etiology.

Differential Diagnosis

- Myelopathy
  - Compressive (e.g., spondylitic, spinal epidural abscess or hematoma)
  - Traumatic
  - Metabolic (e.g., vitamin B_{12} deficiency)
  - Infectious (e.g., HIV or other viral myelitis, botulism)
  - Inflammatory (e.g., multiple sclerosis, SLE, vasculitis, transverse myelitis)
  - Vascular (spinal cord or cerebral infarct)
  - Neoplastic
- Congenital
  - Dysraphism: Spina bifida, tethered cord
  - Cerebral palsy
- Syringomyelia
- Cauda equina syndrome
  - Caused by compression of the cauda equina, often by a central disc herniation
  - Variable presentation with lower extremity weakness, sensory loss, pain, lower motor neuron findings on examination, and bowel/bladder disturbances
- Polyradiculopathy
- Peripheral neuropathy
  - Usually results in a chronic or insidious onset of lower extremity weakness (except Guillain-Barré syndrome, which may result in weakness over hours to days)
  - Guillain-Barré syndrome: Also results in upper extremity weakness
  - Myasthenia gravis
  - Eaton-Lambert syndrome
  - Amyotrophic lateral sclerosis
- HTLV-I associated myelopathy
- Hereditary spastic paraparesis
- Spinocerebellar or Friedreich's ataxia
- Myopathies (e.g., muscular dystrophy) may result in paraparesis, but usually also result in upper extremity weakness
- Parafalcine meningioma
  - May result in bilateral lower extremity weakness by compressive effects on the medial frontal lobe bilaterally
- Bilateral anterior cerebral artery infarction
- Medications (e.g., pancuronium)
- Periodic paralysis (secondary to hyper- or hypokalemia)
- Tick paralysis
- Lyme disease
- Psychogenic (e.g., conversion disorder)

Workup and Diagnosis

- History and physical examination
  - Determine whether the weakness is more likely secondary to an upper or a lower motor neuron disorder (e.g., symmetric lower extremity weakness with hyperreflexia, positive Babinski's signs, and a dermatomal area of sensory loss suggests a myelopathy, whereas symmetric lower extremity weakness with areflexia and flexor plantar responses suggests a peripheral neuropathy; difficulty with bowel and/or bladder control suggests a myelopathy or cauda equina syndrome)
- MRI is the usually the best imaging modality
  - Acute paraplegia/paraparesis is suggestive of an acute myelopathy or polyradiculopathy, and prompt imaging is required to identify surgically treatable lesions
- EMG/nerve conduction studies to evaluate for possible neuropathy, polyradiculopathy, or myopathy
- CSF examination may show signs of infection, elevated protein in Guillain-Barré syndrome, or findings consistent with multiple sclerosis (e.g., oligoclonal bands)
- Laboratory testing may include CBC, electrolytes, calcium, glucose, ESR, vitamin B_{12}, folate, ANA
- DNA testing is available for many of the inherited ataxias
- Genetic testing

Treatment

- Paralysis or paraplegia is best managed by identifying and treating the underlying cause
  - In cases of compressive lesions of the spinal cord, cauda equina, or nerve roots, surgical therapy is usually required
  - Traumatic spinal cord injury often requires surgical stabilization; also, acute high-dose steroid treatment is effective in improving outcomes of traumatic myelopathy
- Spinal dysraphism is often treated surgically
- Infectious myelopathies: Antimicrobial agents
- Multiple sclerosis: Acute exacerbations may be treated with steroids; prevent exacerbations with interferons, glatiramer acetate, and mitoxantrone
- Guillain-Barré syndrome: Plasmapheresis or IVIG within 2 weeks of onset of symptoms
- Physical therapy, assistive devices, orthotics, and wheelchairs may all be beneficial in improving the functional abilities of patients with paraplegia/paresis

123. Paresthesias

Paresthesias are abnormal sensations, such as numbness or tingling, that may occur secondary to lesions anywhere in the nervous system. They may be accompanied by hypesthesia (decreased sensation), most commonly noticed in response to painful or tactile stimuli. The etiology of paresthesias are usually suggested by the distribution of the finding and the associated symptoms.

Differential Diagnosis

- Nerve compression or entrapment neuropathy
  - Lumbosacral disc herniation with nerve root compression
  - Posterior tibial nerve compression (tarsal tunnel syndrome)
  - Peroneal nerve compression (foot drop)
  - Cervical spine spondylosis/disc herniation with nerve root compression
  - Median nerve compression (carpal tunnel syndrome, often seen in hypothyroidism and pregnancy)
  - Ulnar nerve compression
  - Long thoracic nerve compression (winged scapula)
- Infections (e.g., HIV/AIDS, herpes zoster, Lyme disease)
- Diabetic neuropathy (bilateral symptoms)
- Alcoholic neuropathy
  - Bilateral symptoms
  - Due to thiamine deficiency (vitamin B_1) and/or direct toxic effect of alcohol
- Vitamin B_{12} deficiency
- Uremia
- Vasculitis or collagen vascular disease
- Tumor (including hematologic malignancy)
  - Carcinomatous infiltration or direct compression
  - Paraneoplastic syndrome (especially lung cancer)
- Toxins
  - Industrial exposures (e.g., lead, mercury, pesticides)
  - Medications (e.g., pyridoxine, isoniazid, vincristine, cisplatin, antiretrovirals, hydralazine)
- Guillain-Barré syndrome (usually bilateral)
- Hereditary motor or sensory neuropathies
- Amyloidosis
- Porphyria
- Paraproteinemias (e.g., multiple myeloma)
- Amyotrophic lateral sclerosis
- Alcohol withdrawal (sensation of "crawling bugs")
- Trigeminal neuralgia

Workup and Diagnosis

- A complete history and physical examination is necessary to determine the etiology of most cases
  - Time course of onset
  - Anatomic distribution (focal, unilateral, bilateral)
  - History of trauma, diabetes, alcohol abuse, cancer, or collagen vascular disease
  - Associated weakness, cramping, pain, or loss of position or temperature sense
  - Comprehensive neurologic exam with a focus on cervical or lumbosacral nerve patterns
- Initial tests may include fasting CBC, electrolytes, calcium, magnesium, TSH, glucose, BUN/creatinine, hemoglobin A_{1C}, ESR, vitamin B_{12}, thiamine level, and chest X-ray
  - Additional tests may be indicated based on history (e.g., lead level, SPEP and UPEP to rule out paraproteinemia, Lyme titers)
- Electromyography may be used to differentiate neuropathic versus myopathic causes of muscle atrophy
- Nerve conduction studies
- Nerve biopsy (usually the sural nerve) is reserved for proof of histologic processes that have an impact on management (e.g., amyloidosis)

Treatment

- Compression or entrapment neuropathy
  - Avoid aggravating activities and repetitive trauma
  - Immobilization/splinting of affected limb
  - Physical therapy and proper ergonomics/biomechanics
  - NSAIDs and/or acetaminophen
  - Epidural steroids in severe cases
  - Surgical release of entrapped nerve/herniated disc if conservative measures fail and symptoms persist
  - Surgical removal of compressive tumors
- Treat and control underlying diseases (e.g., diabetes, alcoholism, HIV, renal disease, vasculitis)
- Treat underlying infections (e.g., zoster treated by acyclovir or famciclovir for 7 days)
- Supplement vitamin deficiencies
- Discontinue offending medications or toxic exposures
- Painful peripheral neuropathies (diabetic, alcoholic) may be relieved by amitriptyline or desipramine, phenytoin or carbamezapine, or topical capsaicin cream

124. Paroxysmal Nocturnal Dyspnea

Paroxysmal nocturnal dyspnea is defined as severe difficulty breathing or air hunger that awakens the patient from sleep (usually 1–3 hours after lying down) and forces them to a sitting or standing position. The patient may gasp and proceed to an open window for fresh air. The dyspnea tends to resolve in 10–30 minutes. PND almost always implies heart failure.

Differential Diagnosis

- CHF is the most common cause
  - Etiologies include uncontrolled HTN, pulmonary embolus, endocarditis, hyperthyroidism, pericardial disease, endocardial disease (e.g., valvular stenosis, insufficiency, rupture, endocarditis), and myocardial disease (e.g., MI, ischemia, arrhythmias)
- Mitral stenosis
  - Almost always secondary to rheumatic heart disease (after 15–40 years)
  - Advanced cases result in pulmonary hypertension and right heart failure
  - Dyspnea is the most significant symptom
  - Classic triad: Diastolic rumble, opening snap, and loud first heart sound
- Aortic regurgitation
  - Most commonly due to rheumatic fever
- Cardiomyopathies
  - Abnormal myocardium, resulting in impaired cardiac output and CHF
- Aortic stenosis
  - Due to senile valve degeneration, rheumatic disease, or congenital
  - Associated with angina, syncope, and CHF
- Congenital heart disease
  - May see failure to thrive, progressive CHF symptoms, cyanosis, and/or murmur
- "Cardiac asthma"
  - Bronchospasm secondary to pulmonary congestion and interstitial edema that compresses small airways
  - Standing decreases lung congestion
- Anxiety
- Severe COPD and emphysema
- Asthma
- Obstructive sleep apnea
- Obesity/hypoventilation
- Tropical pulmonary eosinophilia (filariasis)

Workup and Diagnosis

- Complete history and physical exam with special attention to cardiac and respiratory systems
- Initial laboratory studies may include CBC, pulse oximetry, electrolytes, BUN/creatinine, glucose, and calcium
- Chest X-ray to evaluate for effusion and heart size
- Echocardiogram may be used to evaluate valves, chamber size, and ventricular function
- ECG
- Consider cardiology consult
- Cardiac catheterization may be indicated for valvular disease, cardiomyopathies, and congenital heart disease

Treatment

- Attention to airway, breathing, and circulation
- Administer supplemental O_2
- Many patients feel relief with cold air blowing in face
- CHF: Mainstay of therapy is to decrease preload (by venodilation) and afterload (by arteriodilation and volume removal) to improve forward blood flow and decrease symptoms; nitrates (sublingual and IV), loop diuretics, IV morphine, ACE inhibitors, and spironolactone; treat refractory respiratory distress with CPAP, BiPAP, or intubation
- Valvular disease: Blood pressure reduction with an ACE inhibitor or β-blocker is first-line therapy; surgical intervention (balloon valvuloplasty, valve repair, or valve replacement) is needed for severe disease

125. Pelvic Masses - Female

Pelvic masses are most common in women, but they do occur in men. Obvious causes, such as bladder distension and pregnancy, must be ruled out prior to a full workup. Malignancy must be considered in all cases, particularly as the age of the patient increases or in patients with a past history of malignant disease.

Differential Diagnosis

- Postmenarche/premenopause
  - Ovarian: Follicular and corpus luteum cysts (most common), endometrioma, polycystic ovarian syndrome, neoplasms (benign or malignant)
  - Infectious: Tubo-ovarian abscess (secondary to PID), hydrosalpinx
  - Pregnancy: Uterine, ectopic, or molar
  - Leiomyomas (fibroids)
  - Retroperitoneal tumors
  - Constipation
- Postmenopause (increased risk of malignant neoplasms)
  - Ovarian fibromas
  - Ovarian cysts
  - Leiomyomas (fibroids)
  - Diverticular abscesses
  - Enlarged bladder
  - Hernia (femoral or inguinal)
  - Primary ovarian carcinoma
  - Metastatic disease from uterus, breast, or GI tract
  - Colorectal cancer
- Newborns/children
  - Functional ovarian cysts
  - Germ cell tumor: Dermoid (benign cystic teratoma), dysgerminomas
  - Wilms' tumor
  - Lymphoma
- Sacral promontory can occasionally be confused with a pelvic mass by inexperienced clinicians
- Less common etiologies ("zebras") include ovarian torsion, leiomyoma torsion, congenital obstructive genital lesion (e.g., imperforate hymen, blinded uterine horn), bicornuate uterus, pelvic kidney, and cervical cancer
- Males
  - Lymphoma
  - Colorectal cancer
  - Diverticular abscesses
  - Metastatic disease from colorectal cancer
  - Bladder distension (often secondary to BPH)
  - Hernia (femoral or inguinal)
  - Retroperitoneal tumors
  - Constipation

Workup and Diagnosis

- History and physical examination
  - Note whether mass is painful (constant or intermittent, cyclic or noncyclic, dyspareunia) or associated with menstrual disturbance (dysmenorrhea and menorrhagia are associated with endometriosis and leiomyomas) or other symptoms (e.g., fever, weight loss/gain, nausea, vomiting, dyspepsia, early satiety, abdominal bloating, constipation, diarrhea, change in stool caliber)
  - Full abdominal, breast, lymph node, and pelvic/genital exams, including bimanual and rectal
- Laboratory evaluation may include urine pregnancy test, urinalysis, BUN/creatinine, CBC with differential, Pap smear with culture for gonorrhea and *Chlamydia,* hemoccult testing, and liver function tests
- Pelvic ultrasound for adnexal/uterine masses to determine size, location, and composition of mass
- Pelvic/abdominal CT
- Colonoscopy to rule out colorectal cancer
- Consider bladder catheterization if bladder distension is considered
- Tumor markers are indicated if abnormal ultrasound
  - β-hCG (nongestational choriocarcinomas)
  - α-fetoprotein (endodermal sinus tumors)
  - LDH (dysgerminomas)
  - Serum CA-125

Treatment

- Treat the underlying etiology
- Ovarian masses
  - Premenarchal: Immediate gynecologic referral because of high malignancy potential
  - Premenopausal: If simple ovarian cyst <10 cm, observe 4–6 weeks, attempt to suppress with OCP; if persists, consider diagnostic laparoscopy; surgical evaluation is indicated if ovarian solid mass, complex cyst, or ascites is present
  - Postmenopausal: If <3 cm, asymptomatic, and normal exam, follow with serial ultrasounds; if persists, consider surgical evaluation; laparoscopy if cyst is >3 cm, symptomatic, or solid
- Leiomyoma
  - Hypoestrogenic medications (e.g., Depo-Provera, leuprolide)
  - Minimally invasive procedures: Hysteroscopic laser myomectomy, uterine artery embolization
  - Surgical: Myomectomy versus hysterectomy

126. Pelvic Pain - Female

Pelvic pain is a common primary care complaint that should be distinguished as acute (<6 months) versus chronic (>6 months), and cyclic, noncyclic, or pregnancy-related. Gynecologic, urologic, and intestinal etiologies are common, but psychological, oncologic, and other causes must also be carefully considered.

Differential Diagnosis

Acute pain (<6 months)
- Pregnancy-related
  - Ectopic pregnancy
  - Threatened abortion
  - Incomplete abortion
  - Septic abortion
  - Ruptured corpus luteal cyst
- Gynecologic (noncyclic)
  - Ovarian cyst
  - Pelvic inflammatory disease
  - Tubo-ovarian abscess
  - Vaginitis/cervicitis
  - Ovarian torsion
  - Uterine fibroids
  - Pelvic (ovarian, uterine, urinary) neoplasm
  - Pelvic floor prolapse (cystocele/rectocele)
- Gynecologic (cyclic pain)
  - Primary dysmenorrhea
  - Endometriosis
  - IUD
  - Mittelschmerz (midcycle ovulation)
- Nongynecologic
  - Irritable bowel syndrome
  - UTI/pyelonephritis
  - Nephrolithiasis
  - Appendicitis
  - Diverticulitis
  - Sexual abuse/trauma
  - Abdominal aortic aneurysm
  - Mesenteric ischemia/infarction

Chronic pain (>6 months)
- Very difficult to diagnose; differential includes gynecologic and nongynecologic etiologies (above), as well as the following
  - Pelvic adhesions
  - Interstitial cystitis
  - Inflammatory bowel disease
  - Adenomyosis
  - Leiomyoma (fibroids)
  - Hernia (femoral or inguinal)
  - Depression
  - Irritable bowel syndrome
  - Diverticulosis or diverticular abscess
  - Lymphoma
- Less common etiologies ("zebras") include pelvic congestion syndrome, mesenteric adenitis, surgical adhesions, Asherman's syndrome, foreign body (e.g., tampon), abdominal wall nerve entrapment, and porphyria

Workup and Diagnosis

- History and physical examination
  - Note the nature, severity, onset, radiation, duration of pain; relation to menstrual cycle, intercourse, or other activities; chronic versus acute; chance of pregnancy
  - Note associated symptoms: Fever, nausea, vomiting, dysuria, frequency, vaginal bleeding/discharge, abdominal or back pain
  - Screen for domestic violence and sexual abuse
  - Full abdominal and pelvic exams, including speculum, bimanual, and rectal exam
- Laboratory studies may include urine pregnancy test, urinalysis, urine Gram stain and culture, cervical cultures for *Chlamydia* and gonorrhea, and wet mount of vaginal smear
- Consider ultrasound if ovarian cyst, torsion, or mass is suspected, or to evaluate for intrauterine versus ectopic pregnancy
- Diagnostic laparoscopy for acute abdomen or endometriosis

Treatment

- Primary dysmenorrhea: NSAIDs; consider oral contraceptives to suppress ovulation in severe disease
- Positive pregnancy test: Determine last menstrual period; obtain quantitative β-hCG; confirm intrauterine pregnancy
- In patients at high risk for STDs, treat empirically for PID (to cover gonorrhea and *Chlamydia*)
  - Ofloxacin 400 mg PO BID for 14 days plus metronidazole 500 mg PO BID for 14 days, or
  - Ceftriaxone 250 mg IM single dose plus doxycycline 100 mg PO BID for 14 days
- Endometriosis: Treat with hormonal medications or surgical laparoscopy
  - Oral contraceptives for 3–4 months, or
  - Provera 39 mg QD for 2 months, or
  - Danazol 200–800 mg QD for 6 months, or
  - GnRH agonist (e.g., leuprolide)

127. Penile Discharge

Penile discharge is a common complaint that requires a thorough history, including a complete and accurate sexual history and a thorough physical examination that includes cultures and evaluation for common sexually transmitted diseases. Less commonly, nonsexually transmitted diseases are the etiology of penile discharge.

Differential Diagnosis

- Infection
  - *Neisseria gonorrhoeae:* Profuse, purulent, thick yellow or gray discharge; presents as urethral discharge and dysuria, ± urinary urgency or frequency; untreated primary gonorrhea may progress to disseminated gonococcal infection [clinical triad includes tenosynovitis (asymmetric, involving small joints), dermatitis (erythematous macules that progress to pustules with a hemorrhagic component), and arthritis]
  - *Chlamydia trachomatis:* Most common cause of nongonococcal urethral discharge; thin, scant, and mucoid (watery)
  - *Trichomonas vaginalis:* Usually asymptomatic in men but may present with penile discharge and dysuria; female partner tends to be symptomatic, with pelvic pain, itching, and vaginal discharge
- Nonspecific urethritis
- Prostatitis
- Carcinoma of the urethra
  - Presents with bloody penile discharge
- Foreign body in the urethra
  - Presents with pain and bloody discharge
- Reiter's syndrome
  - Triad of urethritis, conjunctivitis, and arthritis ("can't see, can't pee, can't climb a tree") is associated with *Chlamydia* infection
  - Skin lesions involve the palms and soles, begin as vesicles, and become hyperkeratotic
- Lack of circumcision may increase the risk of HIV, gonorrhea, and ulcerative chancres (syphilis)

Workup and Diagnosis

- History and physical examination, including sexual history and genital exam
  - Note onset, duration, and character of discharge (thin versus thick; color; presence of blood or odor)
- Urethral cultures are the gold standard for diagnosis of gonorrhea and *Chlamydia*
  - Obtain cultures by holding the penis up and carefully inserting the tip of the culture swab into the meatus about 1/2 inch; twirl, remove, and place in culture medium
- Urinalysis and urine culture
- Wet mount to evaluate for trichomonads
  - To express penile discharge, have the patient "milk" the penis from the base up to the tip
- Further STD workup may include HIV, RPR, hepatitis B studies, and hepatitis C antibody
- Obtain blood cultures, CBC, and joint fluid aspiration in suspected disseminated gonococcal infection
- If foreign body is suspected, obtain plain film X-rays of the penis and pelvis
- Urologic consult if diagnosis is unclear or foreign body is identified and needs to be removed

Treatment

- Penile discharge without dysuria or frequency should be treated as an STD until proven otherwise
- Begin empiric antibiotic therapy upon clinical suspicion
  - Gonorrhea: Single-dose ceftriaxone IM (give in office for 100% compliance) or PO cefixime or ciprofloxacin
  - *Chlamydia:* PO azithromycin single dose, doxycycline (7 days), ofloxacin (7 days), or erythromycin (7 days)
  - Trichomonas: Metronidazole single dose or for 7 days
- If cultures are positive, obtain test of cure 6–8 weeks after initiating antibiotic treatment
- Encourage patient to inform sexual partners of disease so that they can be treated also, and inform the health department if required
- Use this visit with the patient to educate about safe sex and the use of barrier methods to decrease STD transmission, and to test for other STDs
- Emergent urology consult is required for foreign bodies or carcinoma of the penis

128. Pericardial Rubs

A pericardial friction rub is a "creaking leathery" or sandpaper-like sound usually heard best with the diaphragm over the left sternal border (but can be very localized and repeat with the cardiac cycle). It can be a three- (more common), two-, or one-component sound and implies pericarditis. The clinician must distinguish etiologies that produce rub from other sounds that mimic rub and those etiologies.

Differential Diagnosis

- Pericarditis
  - Most common cause of pericardial rub
  - Often presents with pulsus paradoxus
  - Diffuse ST and T wave elevations and electrical alternans (alternating higher and lower voltage QRS complexes) on ECG
- Ischemia/myocardial infarction
- Viral (e.g., CMV, coxsackie virus)
- Myocarditis
- Cardiac tamponade
- Uremia
- Rheumatic fever
- Tuberculosis
- Collagen vascular diseases (e.g., SLE, rheumatoid arthritis, scleroderma, dermatomyositis, vasculitis)
- HIV
- Toxoplasmosis
- Trauma
- Mediastinal radiation
- Neoplasm
- Leukemic infiltration
- Sarcoid
- Amyloidosis
- Familial Mediterranean fever
- Parasitic (amebic) infection
- Pulmonary embolism
- Means-Lehrman scratch (thyrotoxicosis)
- Mediastinal emphysema ("crunching" noise that may be heard with systole after open cardiac surgery)
- Pleuropericardial rub (between inflamed pleura and parietal pericardium)
- Sail sound of Ebstein's anomaly
- Movement of balloon catheter or transvenous pacing catheter across tricuspid valve
- Sounds that may mimic a pericardial rub
  - Ventricular septal defect
  - Mitral regurgitation
  - Tricuspid regurgitation
  - Diaphragm or intercostal muscle twitch during artificial pacing (scratchy sound unrelated to cardiac cycle)
  - Mill wheel murmur (air in right ventricle, "slushing" during systole and diastole)
  - Combined aortic regurgitation and stenosis
  - Patent ductus arteriosus
  - Ostium primum atrial septal defect

Workup and Diagnosis

- History and physical examination
  - Include past medical history, family history, exposures (e.g., HIV, TB), recent viral or other illness, fever, or trauma
  - Evaluate for exaggerated pulsus paradoxus
- ECG evaluates for myocardial ischemia/infarction, pericarditis, and other pathology
- Echocardiogram may be indicated to evaluate for pericardial effusion and other pathology (e.g., valvular abnormalities, atrial septal abnormalities, ventricular septal abnormalities)
- Chest X-ray may reveal cardiomegaly
- Myocardial enzymes to rule out MI
- CBC with differential
- ESR, ANA, rheumatoid factor, BUN/creatinine, PPD, blood cultures, viral titers (acute and convalescent), and ASO titers may be indicated

Treatment

- Ensure hemodynamic stability
- Administer supplemental O_2 as needed
- Emergent pericardiocentesis for drainage of pericardial effusions may be necessary for cardiac tamponade
- Pericarditis: NSAIDs; avoid steroids unless the patient is in critical condition and all other measures fail (steroids may suppress the immune system and aid viral replication)

129. Periorbital Edema

Periorbital or eyelid edema has many possible etiologies, including mechanical, hemodynamic, infectious, inflammatory, and neoplastic causes. A careful history and physical examination are necessary to determine whether the problem is localized or generalized, and treatment should be directed at the underlying etiology.

Differential Diagnosis

- Conjunctivitis
- Allergy
  - Systemic (e.g., reaction to medication, urticaria/angioedema)
  - Local (e.g., insect bite)
- Contact dermatitis/dermatitis medicamentosa
- Chalazion
  - Zeis or Meibomian gland obstruction of eyelid
- Orbital disease (see "Proptosis/Exophthalmos" entry)
- Preseptal/periorbital cellulitis
- Acute dacryocystitis (infection of the lacrimal ducts)
- Orbital fat herniation through attenuated or dehiscent orbital septum and/or orbicularis oculi muscle (aging changes)
- Herpes simplex/zoster
- Blepharitis/dermatitis
- Trauma/postsurgical (e.g., orbital fracture)
- Dermatomyositis/polymyositis
  - Associated with a heliotropic (violet colored) rash on the upper eyelids
- Chemical, ultraviolet, or thermal burn
- Cardiac failure (generalized edema)
- Renal failure
- Nephrotic syndrome
- Blepharitis/rosacea
- Dacryoadenitis
- Hypothyroidism
  - Associated with fatigue, pretibial edema, and delayed relaxation of reflexes
- Superior vena cava syndrome
- Sebaceous gland carcinoma
- Squamous or basal cell carcinoma
- Discoid lupus
- Ocular cicatricial pemphigoid (symblepharon)

Workup and Diagnosis

- History should include symptom course, exposure history (allergens, irritants, chemicals, ultraviolet, or thermal injury), associated symptoms, past medical and family history, and medication history
- Physical exam, including a full ophthalmologic exam for erythema, tenderness, cutaneous vesicles, discharge, proptosis, vision changes, and conjunctival injection or chemosis
- Initial laboratory evaluation may include CBC with differential, electrolytes, BUN, creatinine, TSH, ESR, ANA, albumin, and urinalysis
- Culture and Gram stain of eye discharge if infection is considered
- Consider CT/MRI of orbits, neck, and/or chest as appropriate
- Consider biopsy of suspicious or persistent lesions
- Consider echocardiogram if heart failure is being considered
- Consider ophthalmology consultation

Treatment

- Treat underlying cause
- Lid hygiene and bland antibiotic ointment for blepharitis (e.g., erythromycin ophthalmic ointment)
- Topical and/or systemic antibiotics for infectious causes
- For allergic causes, remove the inciting allergen or medication; use oral antihistamines and cool compresses; and consider topical steroids for local process or systemic steroids for systemic processes
- Cold compresses and chilled, preservative-free artificial tears are generally helpful for allergic or inflammatory conditions
- Blepharoplasty for herniated orbital fat if interfering with vision or cosmetically indicated

130. Peripheral Edema

Chronic venous insufficiency affects up to 25% of the general population and is the most common cause of edema or swelling of the lower extremities. Normal venous blood return to the heart requires competent venous valves, intermittent muscle contraction of the legs, and the force of respiration; venous hypertension, leading to insufficiency and edema, results when one of these components fail. Edema can be described as pitting (an indentation left after pressing in with a finger, which indicates fluid movement with pressure) or nonpitting (edema caused by swelling of tissue rather than fluid in the tissue, as occurs with lymphedema or myxedema).

Differential Diagnosis

- Venous insufficiency
  - Caused by incompetent venous valves
  - Skin characteristically has superficial varicose veins associated with a reddish-brown pretibial discoloration ("venous stasis skin changes")
  - Swelling is typically worse after legs are held in a dependent position and is least noticeable after a night's sleep
- Congestive heart failure
  - Associated with pitting peripheral edema
  - Other signs of heart failure include a third heart sound, cardiomegaly, and hepatomegaly
- Cellulitis
  - Usually unilateral
  - Edematous legs are typically red, warm, and inflamed
  - The patient may exhibit signs of systemic toxicity with fever and leukocytosis
- Deep venous thrombosis
  - Typically unilateral swelling
  - May exhibit a palpable cord representing a thrombosed vein
  - Homan's sign (pain in the calf with passive dorsiflexion of the foot)
  - Virchow's triad (hypercoagulable states, venous stasis, and vessel injury) are risk factors
- Cirrhosis
  - Advanced liver disease results in hypoalbuminemia and poor venous return through cirrhotic liver tissue
  - Other stigmata of chronic liver disease include caput medusae, ascites, and spider angiomata
- Nephrotic syndrome
  - Glomerular damage results in protein loss and decreased oncotic pressure
- Less common etiologies ("zebras") include filariasis (lymphatic infection by *Wuchereria bancrofti* worm), myxedema (seen in patients with severe hypothyroidism), Milroy's disease (congenital lymphedema), chronic lymphedema (e.g., lymphatic damage due to surgery, such as vein harvesting for CABG), and gout

Workup and Diagnosis

- History and physical examination should focus on time course, associated symptoms (e.g., dyspnea, urinary changes, fever), unilateral versus bilateral involvement, pitting versus nonpitting edema, and risk factors for DVT
- Initial labs may include CBC, electrolytes, BUN/creatinine, urinalysis, coagulation studies, LFTs, serum albumin, and thyroid function tests
- Chest X-ray may reveal signs of pulmonary edema or cardiomegaly
- Duplex ultrasound of the legs is useful in diagnosing deep venous thrombosis
- Echocardiography may reveal a depressed ejection fraction in cases of congestive heart failure
- Blood cultures are often indicated in immunocompromised or systemically ill patients
- Renal or liver biopsy may be necessary to diagnose cirrhosis or renal pathology leading to nephrotic syndrome

Treatment

- Venous insufficiency: Mild cases should respond to leg elevation, avoidance of standing for prolonged periods, and compression stockings; surgical stripping of varicosities may relieve pain in severe cases
- Congestive heart failure: Dietary salt restriction, diuretics, digoxin, ACE-inhibitors, β-blockers to improve cardiac function and control fluid overload
- Cellulitis: Elevation of extremity, antibiotics to cover skin flora (streptococci, staphylococci)
- Deep venous thrombosis: Anticoagulation with unfractionated heparin, low molecular weight heparin or warfarin for 3–6 months
- Cirrhosis: Liver disease is typically progressive; symptoms may respond to diuretics and low salt diet; hepatic bypass procedures (e.g., TIPS) or transplantation may be necessary
- Nephrotic syndrome: 80% of cases in children are caused by minimal change disease and treated with steroids; adults tend to have progressive illness; dialysis or renal transplant may be necessary

131. Photophobia

Photophobia is ocular pain or discomfort upon exposure to light. It may be a symptom of a primary ocular disorder or underlying central nervous system disorder and should always be evaluated, unless a known etiology (e.g., migraine headache) is present.

Differential Diagnosis

- Corneal abrasion
- Conjunctivitis
  - Viral: Watery discharge; adenovirus most common, also herpes simplex
  - Allergic: Usually bilateral
  - Chemical: History of exposure
  - Bacterial (rare): Purulent discharge
- Migraine headache: Normal eye and neurologic exam, headache, phonophobia
- Idiopathic anterior uveitis/iritis (often associated with a triad of pain, photophobia, and blurred vision)
  - Ankylosing spondylitis
  - Reiter's syndrome
  - Inflammatory bowel disease
  - Psoriatic arthritis
  - Sarcoidosis
  - Infections (e.g., Lyme disease, herpes simplex/zoster, tuberculosis, syphilis)
  - Postoperative reactions
- Meningitis/encephalitis
- SAH
- Influenza
- Lightly pigmented eye
- Mydriatic use
- Keratoconjunctivitis sicca, or dry eye syndrome
- Less common etiologies ("zebras") include albinism, total color blindness, vitamin A deficiency, measles, posterior uveitis, congenital glaucoma, sinusitis, mononucleosis, influenza, Colorado tick fever, babesiosis, botulism, and acute viral hepatitis (A, B, or E)

Workup and Diagnosis

- History and physical examination
  - Focused history for exposure to foreign bodies (e.g., woodworking or other flying debris), allergens, exposure to others with URI and/or conjunctivitis, systemic symptoms (e.g., arthritis)
  - Physical exam should include a detailed neurologic exam, ocular exam (including dilated fundoscopic and slit-lamp exam if possible), eyelid eversion to rule out foreign bodies, fluorescein staining of the cornea to rule out abrasion, and intraocular pressure measurement
- Head CT scan without contrast if subarachnoid hemorrhage is suspected
- Lumbar puncture if subarachnoid hemorrhage or meningitis is suspected
- CBC and/or blood cultures if suspect meningitis
- Further workup is based on examination
  - If anterior uveitis is suspected, targeted testing may include CBC, ESR, ANA, ACE level (sarcoidosis), RPR (syphilis), PPD, chest X-ray (TB/sarcoidosis), Lyme titers, *Chlamydia* cultures (Reiter's syndrome), HLA-B27 assay, sacroiliac spine films (ankylosing spondylitis), and colonoscopy (inflammatory bowel disease)
  - If optic neuritis is diagnosed, an MRI of the brain and orbits is indicated to evaluate for multiple sclerosis

Treatment

- Corneal abrasion: Topical antibiotics with or without cycloplegic agents; NSAIDs; patching may be the preferred treatment, depending on the size of the abrasion and the patient's level of discomfort
- Bacterial conjunctivitis: Topical antibiotics
- Allergic conjunctivitis: Topical antihistamine/mast cell stabilizers
- Chemical conjunctivitis: Copious irrigation, topical cycloplegics, and topical antibiotics
- Anterior uveitis: Cycloplegic agents, topical steroids, treat secondary glaucoma and underlying disorder
- Migraine: Abortive therapy (triptans), oral pain medication, antiemetics
- Meningitis: IV antibiotics
- Episcleritis: Topical steroids in moderate to severe cases
- Subarachnoid hemorrhage: Emergent neurosurgical consult

132. Pigmented Lesions

Pigmented lesions are very common. The more common lesions are benign, but the physician must accurately rule out a malignant lesion or biopsy the lesion for definitive diagnosis. Nevi, seborrheic keratoses, and dermatofibromas are common benign lesions that often require evaluation by a physician. Dermatofibromas have a positive "dimple sign"; that is, when squeezed between two fingers, this firm subcutaneous pink, gray, or brown lesion puckers down into the skin.

Differential Diagnosis

- Benign mole (nevus)
  - Junctional (flat, pigmented), compound (raised, pigmented), and dermal (raised, usually not pigmented)
- Seborrheic keratosis
  - Very common and benign
  - Pink to dark brown, appear "stuck on" skin, usually waxy and rough
- Freckle (also known as ephilides)
- Solar lentigo ("liver spot" or "sunspot")
  - Very common on the face and hands
  - Light to dark brown macules, up to 2 cm
  - If more than one color/abnormal borders, consider diagnosis of lentigo maligna melanoma
- Dermatofibroma
  - Firm, nodular, asymptomatic or slightly pruritic, often hyperpigmented lesion, most often on the lower extremities
  - Dimples when pinched
  - May result from minor trauma such as a scratch or insect bite
- Dysplastic nevus
  - "ABCD" changes: Asymmetry, Borders (irregular, jagged, streaked or "faded" edges), Color (more than one color; gray or black pigment or loss of pigment within the borders of a lesion), and Diameter (consider biopsy if >5 mm in diameter)
- Blue nevus
  - Usually benign
  - Deep dermal pigmentation gives blue color
- Malignant melanoma
  - Look for "ABCD" changes (see above)
  - Superficial spreading type most common
  - Acral lentiginous, nodular, and lentigo maligna are other subtypes
- Café au lait macule
  - Light brown, present at birth/toddlerhood
  - Consider neurofibromatosis if five or more café au lait and axillary freckling
- Less common lesions include Spitz nevus (tan/pink, more common in children), nevus spilus, pigmented actinic keratosis, pigmented basal cell carcinoma, Becker's nevus [acquired in childhood or teens , usually large (>8 cm) and near shoulder], and Mongolian spot (benign, blue-gray, sacral area, congenital; fade/resolve in 1–2 years)

Workup and Diagnosis

- History and physical exam
  - Note changes in the appearance of the lesion, pruritis, increase in size, or frequent bleeding/irritation
  - Moles newly acquired after the age of 40 should be closely examined for dysplasia/malignancy
  - Note family history of malignant melanoma and personal history of skin cancer or abnormal moles removed in the past
  - Patients with light skin and blue eyes have a higher risk of abnormal moles and malignant melanoma
- When in doubt, it is wise to perform a biopsy
  - Shave biopsy is adequate for suspected actinic keratoses or seborrheic keratoses
  - Deep scoop shave biopsy, excisional biopsy, or punch biopsy are indicated if dysplastic nevus or melanoma are considered, to sample the entire depth of the lesion
- Referral to a dermatologist or plastic surgeon should be considered if an appropriate differential diagnosis cannot be made or if melanoma is being considered

Treatment

- Sunscreen is indicated in all patients to prevent malignant and nonmalignant sun-induced lesions
- Pigmented actinic keratoses and seborrheic keratoses can be successfully removed with topical cryotherapy
- Solar lentigines and freckles can be treated with reassurance, or they can be removed with lasers and intense pulse light sources
  - Solar lentigines may be lightened by topical hydroquinones and retinoids
- Patients with dysplastic nevi or prior malignant melanoma require at least annual full skin exams and close follow up of their nevi with body mapping if possible

133. Pleural Rubs

A pleural friction rub is a "creaking leathery" or grating lung sound, usually inspiratory and expiratory, heard best with the stethoscope diaphragm. It is caused by inflamed visceral and parietal pleural linings that rub over each other during respiration. The sound tends to be localized and does not change with deep breaths or coughing. This is pathognomonic for pleurisy (pleuritis) and tends to be associated with an exudative pleural effusion with sharp chest pain upon breathing.

Differential Diagnosis

- Distinguish pleural rub from pericardial rub (varies with cardiac cycle, does not vary with respiration)
- Viral pleurisy (e.g., coxsackievirus B, influenza)
  - Associated with upper respiratory tract symptoms (e.g., runny nose, earache, low grade fever)
- Pneumonia
  - "Typical" pneumonia (e.g., *Streptococcus pneumoniae, Haemophilus influenzae,* influenza/parainfluenza viruses) is character-ized by acute or subacute onset of fever, dyspnea, fatigue, pleuritic chest pain, and productive cough
  - "Atypical" pneumonia (e.g., *Mycoplasma, Legionella, Chlamydia*) is characterized by more gradual onset, dry cough, headache, fatigue, and minimal lung signs
- Pulmonary infarct secondary to pulmonary embolus
  - Risk factors (Virchow's triad) include venous stasis (e.g., immobility, pedal edema), hypercoagulability (e.g., malignancy, hypercoagulable states, obesity, pregnancy, estrogen replacement therapy, or OCPs), and endothelial damage (e.g., recent trauma or surgery, burns, indwelling catheters)
- Tuberculosis
- Rheumatic pleural effusion
- Trauma (e.g., rib fracture, electrical burn, thoracic surgery)
- Connective tissue disease (e.g., SLE)
- Pancreatic pleurisy (enzymes leak into pleural space)
- Hemothorax
- Drug-induced pleural disease (amiodarone, nitrofurantoin, bromocriptine)
- Uremia
- Radiation therapy
- Pulmonary metastases
- Subphrenic/intra-abdominal abscess
- Less common etiologies ("zebras") include Meigs' syndrome, mesothelioma, asbestos-related pleural disease, amebic empyema, bronchiectasis, chylothorax, esophageal rupture, lymphoma, and sarcoidosis

Workup and Diagnosis

- Complete history and physical exam
  - May present with localized pain over the affected area that worsens with deep breathing or coughing and is relieved by pressure on the chest wall or abdomen
  - Respirations tend to be fast and shallow with decreased breath sounds and decreased motion on affected side
- Initial labs include CBC with differential, electrolytes, BUN/creatinine, glucose, calcium, and pulse oximetry
- Chest X-ray may show pleural effusion and/or reveal evidence of the underlying etiology (e.g., pneumonia, tuberculosis, tumor)
- Consider blood and sputum cultures if pneumonia or tuberculosis is suspected
- Spiral CT, V/Q scan, pulmonary angiography, arterial blood gas, and/or D-dimer assay if pulmonary embolus is suspected
- Diagnostic thoracentesis may be indicated
  - WBC count >100,000 suggests tumor or infarct
  - WBC 10,000–100,000 suggests parapneumonic effusion, pancreatitis, malignancy, or tuberculosis
  - Red cell count >100,000 suggests malignancy
  - Glucose <50% of serum suggests bacterial infection or connective tissue disease
  - LDH and total protein to distinguish transudate from exudate
  - Fluid pH <7.2 may necessitate chest tube insertion
  - Gram stain and culture
  - Cytology for malignant cells

Treatment

- Immediate airway stabilization and possible intubation are necessary with airway distress signs (e.g., cyanosis)
- Administer supplemental O_2
- NSAIDs, narcotics, and/or chest wraps for pain
- Isolation is necessary if suspect tuberculosis or influenza
- Identify and treat the underlying disease
  - Community-acquired pneumonia: Oral (macrolide, doxycycline, or quinolone) or IV antibiotics (third-generation cephalosporin and a macrolide; or a second-generation quinolone)
  - Pulmonary embolus: Anticoagulation (e.g., unfractionated heparin or low molecular weight heparin) in all patients unless contraindicated; institute warfarin concomitantly with heparin and continue for at least 6 months; inferior vena cava filter may be indicated if anticoagulation is contraindicated, recurrent embolus occurs while on adequate anticoagulation, massive PE has occurred, or patient has poor baseline cardiac/respiratory status
  - Discontinue offending medications

134. Polyuria

Polyuria is defined as urine output greater than 3 L per day. The output of a large volume of dilute urine leads to extracellular dehydration, which stimulates the thirst centers to influence the patient to increase fluid intake; thus, this condition may also lead to polydipsia.

Differential Diagnosis

- Diuretic use
- Primary polydipsia
  - Usually in middle-aged, anxious women
  - Psychiatric illnesses due to increased water intake (e.g. psychogenic polydipsia)
  - May be due to hypothalamic lesions in the thirst centers (e.g., sarcoidosis)
- Chronic lithium use
  - 20% of patients develop polydipsia
- Central diabetes insipidus
  - Due to decreased output of antidiuretic hormone
  - May be idiopathic, familial, autoimmune, or due to head trauma, infiltrative diseases (e.g., sarcoidosis, granulomas, Langerhans cell histiocytosis), pituitary tumors (intrasellar, suprasellar), or ischemic or hypoxic encephalopathy
- Nephrogenic diabetes insipidus
  - Due to decreased response of the kidneys to antidiuretic hormone
  - May be idiopathic, familial, or due to drugs (e.g., colchicine, fluoride, phenothiazine), chronic renal disease, hypercalcemia, hypokalemia, sickle cell disease
- Uncontrolled diabetes mellitus
  - Patients have polydipsia and subsequent polyuria secondary to high sugar levels

Workup and Diagnosis

- Complete history and physical exam with corroboration from caretakers and family if available
- Initial laboratory studies include serum and urine fasting glucose, creatinine, electrolytes, osmolality, and serum BUN
- Water deprivation test
  - Give no fluids for 12–18 hours and measure body weight, plasma and urine osmolarity, blood pressure, and urine specific gravity every 2 hours
  - Stop test if severe dehydration or drop in BP occurs (indicates diabetes insipidus likely)
  - A normal response is a drop in urine output to 0.5 mL/min, and urine osmolarity > plasma osmolarity
  - Maintenance of dilute urine with specific gravity <1.005 indicates diabetes insipidus (central or nephrogenic)
  - Continue test until plateau phase (hourly increase UOP <30 mOsm/kg for 3 consecutive hours)
  - Then give 5 mg ADH SQ and measure urine osmolarity 1 hour later
- Measure ADH and osmolarity levels during water test
  - Nephrogenic diabetes insipidus: Normal or slightly increased ADH; urine osmolality increases <50% after ADH given
  - Complete central diabetes insipidus: Decreased levels of ADH; urine osmolarity > plasma osmolarity
  - Primary polydipsia: Serum and urine osmolarity are decreased before the test and increase during the water deprivation test

Treatment

- Central diabetes insipidus: Intranasal or oral DDAVP (a synthetic analog of ADH); must measure serum osmolarity and sodium levels regularly
- Nephrogenic diabetes insipidus: Control the underlying cause; diuretics and dietary salt restriction can decrease solute load to the kidney and keep a mild sodium depletion so there is increased proximal tubular resorption; polydipsia and increased urine output is generally mild in the elderly and patients with chronic renal failure
- Primary polydipsia: Limit water intake; this can be difficult especially if the cause is psychogenic
- Diabetes mellitus: Control sugar levels with oral medications or insulin
- Hypercalcemia and hypokalemia must be corrected and the underlying cause should be sought and treated
- Eliminate causative medications if possible

135. Priapism

Priapism is an undesired, prolonged, sustained erection of the penis that may last hours to days, with or without pain. Priapism, particularly low-flow, must be considered a urologic emergency, and consultation should be sought immediately. Initial medical therapies can be attempted; however, if they are ineffective, emergency surgical intervention should be undertaken within 36 hours of onset to preserve potency and prevent corporal fibrosis.

Differential Diagnosis

- Low-flow, or "ischemic"-type: Corpora cavernosa are rigid; corpora spongiosum and glands are spared; there is decreased venous outflow, sludging, and stasis; painful
  - Intracorporeal injection for impotence (most common cause in adults): Papaverine, prostaglandin E1, phentolamine, phenoxybenzamine
  - Sickle cell disease (most common cause in children)
  - Leukemia
  - Penile infiltration with solid tumors (bladder cancer, prostate cancer)
  - Prescription drugs: Trazodone, chlorpromazine, sildenafil
  - Illicit drugs: Marijuana, crack cocaine
  - Idiopathic
  - Other (e.g., total parenteral nutrition, dialysis, vasculitis)
- High-flow: Caused by increased arterial blood flow due to arterial-cavernosal shunt; whole penis is rigid; *not* usually painful
  - Groin or straddle injury
  - Cocaine
- Less common etiologies
  - Post-spinal cord trauma or injury to the medulla (clinically similar to high-flow priapism)
  - Polycythemia
  - Thalassemia
  - Fabry's disease
  - May occur in clitoris as well as penis

Workup and Diagnosis

- History should focus on time of onset (usually hours to days), medications (e.g., antidepressants; antipsychotics; sildenafil), past medical history (e.g., sickle cell disease, anticoagulation therapy, diabetes mellitus, leukemia, genitourinary malignancies, schizophrenia, depression), prior erectile dysfunction for which treatment has been sought, and activity with onset of erection (e.g., following oral or injection treatment for impotence, with sexual activity, trauma, illicit drug use)
- Physical examination including abdomen, back, genitalia (palpate penis for areas of tenderness or induration), digital rectal examination and neurologic exam
  - Penis: Is there pain? What segments of the penis are involved? Are there signs of trauma, injection or neoplasm?
  - Testicles/scrotum: Are there masses or evidence of trauma?
  - Prostate: Palpate for signs of neoplasm
- Initial laboratory studies include CBC, urinalysis and urine screen for toxic substances
- Consider also BUN/creatinine, electrolytes, peripheral smear, ESR, and PSA
- Immediate urologic consultation is imperative to prevent continuing injury and long-term sequelae

Treatment

- Immediate urologic consultation is indicated
- Local: Ice packs; ice water enemas; if not effective, use hot water enemas; pressure dressing
- Medical: Sedatives; analgesics; may require narcotics; antispasmodic/anticholinergic drugs; estrogens; anticoagulants; procaine; amyl nitrate; IV fluids
- Injection: Local or general anesthesia; ketamine (IV or IM)
- Invasive: aspiration of the corpora cavernosa followed by injection of α-adrenergic agonist (e.g., phenylephrine, which may be repeated at 5 minute intervals)
- Surgery (urology referral): Cavernospongiosum shunt; glans-cavernosum shunt; cavernosaphenous shunt; arterial embolization
- Sickle cell disease: IV fluids; alkalinization; transfusion or exchange-transfusion; supplemental O_2

136. Proptosis/Exophthalmos

Proptosis, or exophthalmos, may be caused by inflammatory, infectious, neoplastic, traumatic, or vascular etiologies. Thyroid-associated orbitopathy is by far the most common cause of proptosis. Some may have a benign course, but others follow a fulminant course that threatens sight and/or life, and requires urgent intervention. Imaging studies are essential in almost all cases for diagnosis and planning treatment.

Differential Diagnosis

- TAO
  - Major cause of unilateral and bilateral proptosis
  - Usually bilateral, although often asymmetric
  - Course is variable
  - Associated with Graves' disease; more commonly occurs in women, smokers, and in patients treated with radioactive iodine
- Orbital cellulitis
  - Most cases occur due to contiguous spread from sinusitis
- Mucormycosis
  - Occurs primarily in diabetic and immunocompromised patients
- Orbital tumors
  - Children: Dermoid, capillary hemangioma, rhabdomyosarcoma, lymphangioma, optic nerve glioma, leukemia (chloroma or granulocytic sarcoma), metastatic neuroblastoma, plexiform neurofibroma, teratoma
  - Adults: Metastatic breast, lung, or prostate cancer; cavernous hemangioma; mucocele; lymphoid tumors; optic nerve sheath meningioma; neurofibroma; neurilemoma (schwannoma); fibrous histiocytoma; hemangiopericytoma
- Trauma (e.g., intraorbital foreign body, retrobulbar hemorrhage)
- Orbital vasculitis (e.g., Wegener's granulomatosis, polyarteritis nodosa)
- Arteriovenous malformation (e.g., carotid-cavernous fistula, retina or brain)
- Cavernous sinus thrombosis
  - Orbital cellulitis signs plus cranial neuropathies (third, fourth, fifth, and/or sixth)
  - Mental status changes
  - Usually bilateral and rapidly progressive
- Neurofibromatosis
- Pseudoproptosis
  - Enlarged globe (myopia, buphthalmos)
  - Enophthalmos of the fellow eye

Workup and Diagnosis

- History and physical examination
  - History should include age, tempo of onset, pain, fever, laterality, diplopia, thyroid disease, sinusitis, or trauma; history of diabetes, immunosuppression, or cancer; and maneuvers or conditions that worsen proptosis
  - Physical exam should include ophthalmologic, head and neck, and focal neurologic examinations
  - Measure proptosis with exophthalmometer
- Initial laboratory evaluation may include thyroid function tests (TSH, free T_4 and T_3, TSH receptor antibodies), ESR, CRP, CBC
- Consider ANCA, ANA, and blood cultures
- CT and/or MRI of orbits
- Ultrasound (with color Doppler for suspected arteriovenous malformation)
- Consider ophthalmology, neurosurgical, and/or endocrine consultation
- Consider biopsy of selected solid tumors

Treatment

- Treat the underlying cause, although treatment of Graves' disease does not always improve ophthalmopathy, and radioactive iodine may make it worse; systemic steroids for acute flareups only
- Prevent eye injury and discomfort with artificial tears and sunglasses; may patch eye while sleeping
- Surgical decompression (in TAO and retrobulbar hemorrhage with acute optic neuropathy by direct compression or by increased intraocular pressure)
- If due to infectious causes, appropriate directed systemic intravenous antibiotic therapy and/or surgical debridement
- If due to noninfectious inflammation, administer systemic steroids or immunomodulating therapy, particularly if there is acute optic neuropathy
- Incisional or excisional biopsy of orbital tumors

137. Pruritis with Rash

Pruritus, or itching, is the most common dermatologic complaint. When pruritus occurs with cutaneous findings, the clinician must carefully analyze the dermatologic findings to identify the underlying cause. Severe pruritus may lead to lifestyle disturbances by causing anxiety, depression, and loss of sleep. Pruritus without a rash should result in a search for systemic causes, such as liver disease.

Differential Diagnosis

- Infectious causes
  - Fungal infections: Dermatophyte infections (tinea), candidiasis (beefy red color with satellite papules), seborrheic dermatitis (from *Pityrosporum*, common in hair-bearing areas, with scale)
  - Bacterial infections: Erythrasma (from *Corynebacterium*), frequently in axilla
  - Viral infections: Chicken pox (Varicella)
  - Insect vectors: Scabies, pediculosis or lice (also present on spouse and other family members), flea bites (typically on legs), mosquito bites (central punctum)
  - Mixed infections: Intertrigo (present at skin folds or area of friction)
- Noninfectious causes
  - Contact dermatitis (e.g. rhus dermatitis): May be revealed in contact history, linear vesicular lesions with sharp margins
  - Atopic dermatitis: Erythematous rash in flexural areas, patient with seasonal allergies and/or asthma
  - Eczematous dermatitis: Stasis dermatitis (hyperpigmented legs of patients with vascular disease), lichen simplex chronicus (anxious patient who chronically scratches), dyshidrotic eczema (on hands and feet with scaling, erythema, and minute vesicles and painful fissures), nummular eczema (round scaly lesions on dry skin, common in the winter)
  - Pityriasis rosea: Mostly on trunk in "Christmas tree" pattern, begins as single, larger "herald" patch
  - Lichen planus: Koebner reaction (lesions occur with trauma, such as linear lesions from scratching), purple, polygonal, pruritic papules
  - Psoriasis: Koebner reaction, pink, silvery scaling plaques, extensor surfaces, nail pits
- Less common etiologies ("zebras") include mycoses fungoides (referred to as Sézary syndrome if erythroderma, lymphadenopathy, and atypical circulating white blood cells are present), dermatitis herpetiformis, miliaria (heat rash)

Workup and Diagnosis

- History and physical examination
  - Past medical and family history (e.g., asthma, psoriasis) and exposure history (e.g., poison ivy, oak, or sumac) are important, including whether the lesions are occurring for the first time or are recurrent
  - Perform a total body skin exam to evaluate distribution of rash; evaluate especially for rashes on the extensor or flexor surfaces of skin folds, and interdigital spaces
  - Note the morphology of the lesion (e.g., macule, papule, pustule, plaque, crust, vesicle, bulla, wheal)
  - Note the configuration of the lesion [e.g., linear (Koebner reaction or contact), grouped, annular, geographic]
- Scrape lesions and perform KOH test if fungal infection is suspected (hyphae visible in dermatophyte infections, and pseudohyphae visible in *Candida* infections)
- Wood's lamp test: Erythrasma turns coral red
- Scrape possible burrow site to identify a mite in scabies
- Patch testing may be done if allergic contact dermatitis is suspected
- Punch biopsy may be done to establish a histologic diagnosis (e.g., mycosis fungoides)
- Anti-gliadin antibodies and/or anti-endomysial antibodies may be found in the serum of patients with dermatitis herpetiformis
- Consider referral to a dermatologist if diagnosis remains unclear

Treatment

- Symptomatic treatment is often sufficient
  - Take cool or lukewarm rather than hot baths and showers; wash with a mild soap and apply soap only to malodorous areas
  - Apply an emollient immediately after bathing; emollients with menthol provide a cooling sensation; emollients with phenol or camphor provide an anesthetic effect
  - Oral antihistamines such as hydroxyzine or diphenhydramine may be used but are sedating
  - Nonsedating antihistamines are not effective in reducing pruritus
- Fungal infections: Topical or oral antifungal agent
- Scabies: Permethrin cream or Lindane^R lotion
- Contact dermatitis: Remove offending agent
- Eczematous dermatitis, lichen planus: Topical steroids
- Psoriasis: Steroids, tars, retinoids, UVB light, immune modulator drugs

138. Pruritis without Rash

Pruritus, or itching, is the most common dermatologic complaint. When pruritus occurs without cutaneous findings, a thorough history, physical exam, and laboratory tests must be obtained to rule out a systemic disease as a cause of pruritus. The prevalence of an underlying systemic disease in a pruritic patient is 10–50%.

Differential Diagnosis

- Hepatobiliary disorders
  - Cholestasis of pregnancy: Pruritus is most severe in third trimester, ceases after delivery
  - Primary biliary cirrhosis: Increased anti-mitochondrial antibodies
  - Biliary obstruction: Pruritus not a presenting symptom
- Endocrine disorders
  - Hypo- and hyperthyroidism
- Hematopoietic disorders
  - Polycythemia vera: Pruritus classic after emerging from bath, described as severe and prickling
  - Hodgkin's lymphoma: Pruritus may present 5 years before diagnosis; pruritus portends a poor prognosis
  - Iron deficiency anemia
- Chronic renal failure: pruritus begins 6 months after start of dialysis, affects up to 75% of patients during or immediately after dialysis
- Malignancies: Adenocarcinoma, squamous cell carcinomas
- HIV: Increasing frequency with disease progression
- Psychogenic states: May have underlying personality disorder such as OCD
- Senescence: Elderly pruritus very common
- Drug reactions
- Less common etiologies ("zebras") include multiple myeloma, carcinoid syndrome, Waldenström's macroglobulinemia, parasitic infections (e.g., hookworm, onchocerciasis, ascariasis, trichinosis), hepatitis B and C, diabetes mellitus (results in perianal pruritus)

Workup and Diagnosis

- History and physical examination
  - A focused history including past medical history, social history, family history, and sexual history is important
  - A complete review of systems may identify underlying disease (e.g., change in bowel habits with colon cancer, cold intolerance with hypothyroidism, right upper quadrant pain with hepatic disease)
  - Complete physical examination is necessary including stool exam for occult blood, and Pap smear and pelvic examination
  - Include a full body skin exam to confirm that there are no cutaneous rashes or lesions
- Initial lab tests may include CBC with differential (look for eosinophilia associated with parasites), LFTs (alkaline phosphatase is the best screening test for hepatobiliary disorders), renal function tests, thyroid function tests
- Rule out internal malignancies (e.g., chest X-ray, mammogram, stool for occult blood)
- Other labs to consider: HIV test, hepatitis B and C panel, serum iron and ferritin, serum and urine protein electrophoresis, stool for ova and parasites, blind skin biopsy with or without immunofluorescence

Treatment

- Symptomatic treatment may be sufficient
  - Take short cool or lukewarm baths and showers; wash with a mild soap and apply soap only to malodorous areas
  - Apply an emollient immediately after bathing
  - Emollients with menthol provide a cooling sensation
  - Emollients with phenol or camphor provide an anesthetic effect
  - Low-dose topical corticosteroids may be used, but only over a short duration
  - Oral antihistamines, such as hydroxyzine or diphenhydramine, may be used but are sedating
  - Nonsedating antihistamines are not as effective in reducing pruritus
  - Ultraviolet light therapy may be helpful in some cases
- Ultimate treatment is aimed at the underlying etiology

139. Ptosis

Ptosis is a drooping of the upper eyelid, which may cause decreased vision by direct visual obstruction or by inducing corneal astigmatism. Ptosis may be a harbinger of a more serious medical condition, including myasthenia gravis, CPEO (due to heart block), third nerve palsy (aneurysm), and Horner's syndrome (Pancoast or other tumors).

Differential Diagnosis

- Differentiate from lid edema (e.g., post-trauma), pseudoptosis/dermatochalasis (excess skin of upper lids), enophthalmos (narrowed palpebral fissure), hypotropia, contralateral eyelid retraction causing asymmetry, small eye (phthisis bulbi, microphthalmia, anophthalmia)

Acquired
- Aponeurotic or senile ptosis
  - Most common type of ptosis
  - Caused by disinsertion or dehiscence of the levator aponeurosis
  - Normal levator function, high lid crease
  - May be exacerbated by any ocular surgery
- Mechanical
  - Caused by mass effect of tumor or edema or by tethering by scar (cicatricial)
- Myogenic
  - Poor levator or Müller's muscle function
  - Myasthenia gravis (variable ptosis)
  - CPEO
  - Myotonic dystrophy
- Neurogenic
  - Third nerve palsy [associated supraduction deficit; may also have adduction or infraduction deficit, eye may be down and out; mydriasis]
  - Horner's syndrome [associated with miosis (1–2 mm pupil), "reverse ptosis" (lower lid higher), and often anhidrosis]; due to many etiologies, including Pancoast tumor and neuroblastoma

Congenital
- Simple congenital (myopathic) ptosis
  - Poor levator function, lid lag in downgaze
  - Subset of blepharophimosis syndrome (bilateral ptosis, horizontal shortened palpebral fissures, and telecanthus with dominant inheritance)
- Congenital Horner's syndrome (associated with vertebral anomalies)
- Marcus Gunn jaw-winking syndrome (unilateral ptosis at rest; when chewing or opening mouth the ptotic lid raises up)
- Mitochondrial myopathies

Workup and Diagnosis

- History should include age of onset, previous surgeries or trauma, variability of ptosis, diplopia, associated symptoms (e.g., dysphagia), and attempt to observe old pictures of patient, if possible
- Exam should include a complete ophthalmologic examination and focused neurologic, head and neck, and chest examinations
  - In children, rule out amblyopia from induced astigmatism or occlusion
  - Note levator function, palpebral fissure width, pupils, extraocular motility (especially supraduction), corneal sensation, corneal surface, Bell's phenomenon (eyes roll up with lid closure), and Shirmer's strips (to quantify basal secretion of tears)
- Tensilon test or ice test to rule out myasthenia gravis
- Topical cocaine and hydroxyamphetamine drops to rule out Horner's syndrome
- Visual fields with and without lids taped up to document significant superior visual field defect
- Photodocumentation; compare with old photos
- Consider CT/MRI or ophthalmology consult for possible tumors or scar
- Chest X-ray if suspect Horner's syndrome to rule out pulmonary lesion
- MRA if painful ptosis to rule out carotid dissection

Treatment

- Treat underlying medical condition when possible
- Eyelid crutches attached to glasses may be used as temporizing measures, but may limit blinking and result in dry eyes
- Eyelid surgery may be necessary
- In children under age 10, if amblyopia in induced, surgical correction should be performed as soon as possible

140. Pupillary Constriction

Pupillary constriction is effected by the action of the iris constrictor muscle, which is under parasympathetic control (cranial nerve III). Cholinergic or parasympathomimetic drugs can cause miosis. If the parasympathetic action is unopposed by the sympathetic (mydriatic) action (e.g., Horner's syndrome), anisocoria results and is more pronounced in darker surroundings (the abnormal pupil being smaller). Acute Horner's syndrome should be worked up immediately to rule out life-threatening causes.

Differential Diagnosis

- Argyll Robertson pupils (bilateral but often asymmetric; accommodate but do not react)
  - Tertiary syphilis
  - Light-near dissociation
  - Diabetes mellitus
- Coma
  - Pons lesions result in pinpoint pupils
  - Metabolic lesions and hypothalamic lesions result in small, reactive pupils
- Pharmacologic
  - Systemic opioids (e.g., heroin, morphine, codeine)
  - Systemic cholinergics (e.g., organophosphate and carbamate insecticides, nerve agents, edrophonium)
  - Topical cholinergics/miotics (e.g., pilo-carpine) or indirect cholinergics (e.g., physostigmine, echothiophate)
  - Other (e.g., phencyclidine, clonidine, phenothiazines, phytostigmine)
- Anisocoria
- Horner's syndrome: Triad of ptosis (<2 mm), miosis, and anhidrosis
  - Internal carotid artery dissection
  - Headache syndromes (cluster, migraine, Raeders paratrigeminal syndrome)
  - Herpes zoster
  - Otitis media
  - Cavernous sinus lesions
  - Tolosa-Hunt syndrome
  - Cervical lymphadenopathy
  - Orbit or neck trauma
  - Brainstem/cerebral CVA
  - Tumor (head/neck, apical lung)
  - Basal meningitis
  - Cervical cord lesion
  - High thoracic or low cervical lesions: Trauma, traction on brachial plexus, surgery, internal jugular vein catheter
- Iritis: Eye pain, redness, anterior-chamber reaction
- Mechanical: Posterior iris synechiae (pupil nonreactive or irregular)
- Long-standing Adie's pupil (see "Pupillary Dilation" entry)

Workup and Diagnosis

- Complete past medical and surgical history, with specific attention to neurologic, ophthalmologic, and head and neck region
- Physical examination should include pupil size in the light and the dark, pupil response to light and convergence, and lid position (especially with upgaze)
- If tertiary syphilis is being considered, obtain RPR/VDRL and FTA-ABS, and perform lumbar puncture with evaluation of CSF for VDRL
- If Horner's syndrome is found, consider a chest CT to rule out apical lung mass (Pancoast tumor), MRI/MRA of head/neck, carotid Doppler, and/or carotid angiogram
- Consider ophthalmologic and/or neurologic consultations

Treatment

- Treat underlying disorder if possible
- Remove offending medications
- Administer high-dose intravenous penicillin for syphilis

141. Pupillary Dilation

Pupillary dilation is effected by the action of the iris dilator muscle, which is under the control of the sympathetic system. The third order neuron originates in the superior cervical ganglion and follows the branches of the internal carotid artery. Unopposed sympathetic activity (by diminished parasympathetic action, e.g., third nerve palsy) can cause anisocoria (the abnormal pupil being larger), which is more pronounced in light. Pupil-involving third nerve palsy must be worked up for an intracranial aneurysm.

Differential Diagnosis

- Pharmacologic
  - Systemic anticholinergics (e.g., atropine, antihistamines, muscle relaxants, tricyclic antidepressants, scopolamine)
  - Adrenergic agents (e.g., caffeine, cocaine, amphetamines, methylphenidate)
  - Hallucinogens (e.g., LSD, amphetamines)
  - Other (e.g., nicotine, MAO inhibitors)
  - Topical anticholinergics and adrenergic eye drops (pupil will not constrict in response to pilocarpine 1%)
  - Serotonin syndrome
  - Drug withdrawal
- Acute closed-angle glaucoma (mid-dilated pupil)
- Trauma/surgery
  - Iris sphincter tear or surgical changes
  - Iron mydriasis (intraocular iron foreign body)
  - Head trauma
- Anisocoria greater in light (the abnormal pupil is larger)
- Adie's tonic pupil
  - Irregular pupil with segmental palsy and vermiform constriction
  - Minimal reaction to light; slow/tonic near response (constriction and redilation)
  - Supersensitive to weak cholinergics (pilocarpine 0.125%)
  - Absent deep tendon reflexes (Adie's syndrome)
- Third nerve palsy
  - Associated with ptosis and extraocular muscle palsies (see "Diplopia" entry)
  - Will not constrict in response to weak cholinergics, but will to pilocarpine 1%
- Migraine
  - Benign episodic mydriasis
- Seizures
- Congenital mydriasis
- Coma (many causes)
  - Midbrain (midposition, fixed)
  - Early brain death (midposition or dilated, unreactive to light)
  - Uncal herniation (third nerve palsy)

Workup and Diagnosis

- Complete past medical and surgical history, with specific attention to neurologic, ophthalmologic, and head and neck region
- Physical examination should include measurement of pupil size in the light and the dark, pupil response to light and convergence , and lid position (especially with upgaze)
- In cases of third cranial nerve palsy, an MRI/MRA of the head is indicated to rule out an aneurysm if pupil is involved
- Consider ophthalmology or neurology consultation

Treatment

- Treat underlying disorder if possible
- Remove offending medications if possible
- Recommend eye protection (e.g., sunglasses) if photophobia occurs
- Adie's pupil: Pilocarpine 0.125% BID-QID for cosmesis and to aid in accommodation
- Treat migraines with triptans and/or pain medications for acute attacks and antidepressants, anticonvulsants, β-blockers, or calcium channel blockers to prevent further migraine episodes

142. Purpura

Because the differential diagnosis of purpura is very large, begin by determining whether the purpura is palpable or nonpalpable. Subsequent workup is dictated by the history, physical, and review of systems to determine appropriate diagnostic tests. If, after careful evaluation, the cause of purpura cannot be determined, the patient should be referred to an appropriate consultant, usually a hematologist, unless a collagen vascular disorder is likely, in which case a rheumatologist is an appropriate choice.

Differential Diagnosis

Palpable purpura (papules or nodules that are red/purple and do not blanch with pressure)
- Leukocytoclastic Vasculitis
  - A necrotizing vasculitis of small vessels
  - Fever, malaise, fatigue and arthralgias
  - Inciting factors include drugs (e.g., NSAIDs, thaizides, and phenothiazines), infection [bacterial (e.g., RMSF, meningococcemia) or viral (e.g., hepatitis)] or, blood abnormalities (e.g., cryoglobulinemia, cryofibrinogenemia)
  - Vasculitic injury to kidneys, brain, lung, heart, and GI tract may occur
- Collagen vascular diseases
  - Systemic lupus erythematosus, Sjögren's syndrome, rheumatoid arthritis
- Granulomatous vasculitis (e.g., Wegener's, Churg-Strauss syndrome)
- Polyarteritis nodosa
- Internal malignancies
  - Myeloma, lymphoma, or leukemia
- Henoch-Schönlein purpura
- Drugs
  - Aspirin, NSAIDs, warfarin, heparin

Nonpalpable purpura (flat macules, patches similar to ecchymoses; or petechiae that do not blanch with pressure)
- Trauma
- Advancing age (senile purpura)
- Actinic changes
- Chronic stasis
- Coagulopathies (affecting platelet number or function)
  - TTP (pentad of fever, microangiopathic hemolytic anemia, thrombocytopenia, renal insufficiency, and neurologic signs)
  - ITP
  - Drug-induced thrombocytopenia
  - Bacteremia and many viral diseases
- Scurvy (vitamin C deficiency) can cause hemorrhage and purpura
- TORCH infection can cause congenital purpura ("blueberry muffin baby")
- Many systemic diseases (e.g., Cushing's and diabetes have associated nonpalpable purpura)

Workup and Diagnosis

- History and physical examination
  - History of present illness, past medical history, illness exposure, medication history, and a complete review of systems including systemic symptoms (e.g., arthralgias, myalgias, fever), characteristic spread patterns (e.g., RMSF usually starts peripherally and spreads centrifugally onto the trunk), and CNS symptoms (may suggest SLE or meningococcemia)
  - Focused physical examination with complete skin exam and notation of palpable versus nonpalpable rash
- Initial laboratory evaluation includes CBC with differential and PT/PTT/INR (to rule out coagulopathy), urinalysis (evaluate for hematuria in HSP), LFTs (to evaluate for hepatitis), BUN/creatinine (evaluate renal insufficiency (which may occur in PAN, HSP, SLE, and many other palpable purpura-inducing diseases), ESR and/or C-reactive protein (to evaluate for collagen vascular disease)
- Blood cultures and consider skin cultures by a punch biopsy if the patient is febrile
- ANA and rheumatoid factor titers and a viral hepatitis screen may be indicated
- Age-appropriate malignancy screening
- Punch biopsy is diagnostic for leukocytoclastic vasculitis

Treatment

- Discontinue causative medications
- Correct coagulopathies as necessary
- Treat malignancy as necessary
- Sun protection and avoidance of trauma will prevent actinic and age-related purpura
- Treat stasis-associated lower extremity purpura with compression stockings, elevation, and diuretics if edema is present
- Infections: Prompt antimicrobial treatment (e.g., doxycycline for RMSF, ceftriaxone for meningococcemia) is imperative to prevent mortality
- Autoimmune diseases: High-dose corticosteroids followed by steroid-sparing medications (e.g., methotrexate, cyclosporine, azathioprine, mycophenolate mofetil) for long-term treatment
- Idiopathic pigmented purpuras are most common on the lower legs of men, and may resolve spontaneously or persist indefinitely; high potency topical steroids and oral vitamin C sometimes hasten their resolution

143. Rash with Fever

The etiologies of rash with fever are vast, but a systematic approach will help the clinician quickly narrow the differential. Patients who appear "toxic" with fever and prostration must be rapidly and thoroughly evaluated to rule out life-threatening infections and illnesses. Also, the type and distribution of the rash are important in identifying the etiology, as are associated symptoms and signs (e.g., cough, URI symptoms, pharyngitis, myalgias).

Differential Diagnosis

- Viral exanthems
  - Leading cause of fever and rash in childhood
  - Most children present with low-grade fevers, viral prodromal symptoms, and a secondary diffuse exanthem that is usually nonspecific and morbilliform
  - Often last only a few days and requires only supportive management
- Drug reactions
  - Account for a large portion of rashes with associated fever
  - Immune complex disease or serum sickness has been reported with many medications
- Meningococcemia
  - Most common under age 1
  - After a brief prodrome; onset is abrupt with spiking fevers, diffuse purpuric lesions, delirium, and death
  - DIC and purpura fulminans with secondary necrosis of digits and limbs can occur
- Rocky Mountain Spotted Fever
  - A fulminant and deadly rickettsial disease transmitted by a tick bite
  - Only 60% of patients are aware of tick bite
  - Characteristic rash starts acrally on wrists and ankles and spreads toward the trunk
  - Initially, pink macules evolve over 10–24 hours into red papules, then purpuric macules and violaceous patches involving most of the body surface area
  - Necrosis and DIC may occur
- Toxic shock syndrome, *Staphylococcus aureus,* and streptococcal diseases
  - Most cases due to toxin production
  - Rapid onset of fever, hypotension with generalized skin (palms and soles common) and mucous membrane erythema ("erythroderma" in case definition), and subsequent multiorgan failure
  - Palmar/solar desquamation in 1–3 weeks
  - A morbilliform rash and skin "pain" or hyperesthesia is common
  - Nonsurgical and surgical wounds are often the source of infection in the more common nonmenstrual variant of TSS
- Fifth disease
- Measles
- Rubella
- Parvovirus
- Varicella

Workup and Diagnosis

- Because of a seemingly endless list of possible etiologies for fever and rash, a focused history and physical exam are essential to a quick, accurate diagnosis
- Determine whether the patient appears toxic; age and presence of co-morbid conditions aid diagnosis
- If there is any evidence of purpura;
  - Quickly consider the diagnosis of RMSF, meningococcemia, or systemic vasculitis
  - In the cases of meningococcemia and RMSF, the diagnosis must be made empirically, then later confirmed so that therapy is immediately initiated
- Obtain bacterial cultures from any wounds, culture the pharynx if indicated, and consider skin biopsy and culture; blood cultures are indicated in toxic patients; consider immediate lumbar puncture for CSF culture and Gram stain if meningococcemia is suspected
- Acute and convalescent antibody titers can confirm RMSF; skin biopsy with immunofluorescnce may demonstrate a vasculitis with visible rickettsial organisms within the endothelium
- TSS is often diagnosed by history and examination alone; recent cutaneous injury and nonspecific morbilliform rash in a hypotensive patient in association with the presence of epidermal necrosis on skin biopsy can confirm the diagnosis; wound cultures with growth of staph or strep

Treatment

- Supportive management and thorough evaluation for multisystem disease is imperative in this patient subset.
- Doxycycline is the treatment of choice for RMSF, while ceftriaxone is commonly used for meningococcal therapy; because these two diseases can present similarly and rapidly evolve, many clinicians empirically treat with both of these antibiotics until the diagnosis is confirmed
- Unfortunately, a complete discussion of fever and rash is far beyond the scope of this brief excerpt; the importance of rapid and accurate assessment of every patient presenting with this complaint cannot be overemphasized; rule out the most serious diagnoses first, then "a watch and wait" approach may be considered

144. Raynaud's Phenomenon

Raynaud's phenomenon is paroxysmal ischemia of the digits that manifests as changing color of the fingers, and pain and/or numbness. Sharply demarcated blanching, pallor, cyanosis, and/or erythema of the fingers, toes, or nail beds may occur. The usual sequence of color changes is white-to-blue-to-red, with eventual return to normal skin color upon removal of trigger. Repeated attacks may lead to taut, atrophic skin and shortening of the terminal phalanges (sclerodactyly). Rarely, ulcers, gangrene, and clubbing of the nails occur.

Differential Diagnosis

- Primary (idiopathic) disease
- Secondary disease associated with underlying systemic conditions
    - Scleroderma or CREST
    - Systemic lupus erythematosus
    - Rheumatoid arthritis
    - Mixed connective tissue disease
    - Sjögren's syndrome
- Arteriosclerosis obliterans
- Thromboangiitis obliterans
    - Associated with male smokers
- Arterial embolism
    - Acute onset
    - Pulseless
- Cryoglobulinemia
    - Hepatitis C
- Cold agglutinins
    - *Mycoplasma* infection
- Macroglobulinemia
    - Multiple myeloma
- Polycythemia vera
- Vasculitis (e.g., Wegener's granulomatosis)
- Hepatitis B
- Hypothyroidism
- Thoracic outlet syndrome (brachial plexus)
- Carpal tunnel syndrome
- Drugs: β-blockers, methysergide, bleomycin, vinblastine, clonidine, cyclosporine, ergot preparations
- Trauma
    - Often associated with vibratory tool workers, pianists, typists, or meat cutters
- Hypothenar hammer syndrome
- Reflex sympathetic dystrophy
- Multiple sclerosis
- Syringomyelia
- Poliomyelitis
- Neoplasms
- Vinyl chloride poisoning
- Arteriovenous fistula

Workup and Diagnosis

- Thorough history and physical examination
- CBC with differential may identify various cytopenias associated with connective tissue diseases
- TSH to rule out hypothyroidism
- Hepatitis serologies
- Creatine phosphokinase to rule out polymyositis
- Complement levels are low in SLE
- ANA, ESR, and rheumatoid factor to screen for collagen vascular diseases
- Directed autoantibody testing according to presentation
    - Anti-double stranded DNA and anti-Sm (SLE)
    - Anti-SSA (Sjögren's syndrome)
    - Anti-centromere (CREST syndrome)
    - Anti-ribonucleoprotein (mixed connective tissue disease)
    - Anti-Scl 70 (scleroderma)
    - ANCA (Wegener's granulomatosis)
- Serum cryoglobulins and cold agglutinins
- Serum protein electropheresis to rule out paraproteinemia
- EMG/nerve conduction studies to rule out brachial plexus pathology and carpal tunnel syndrome
- Age-appropriate cancer screening

Treatment

- Treat any underlying disorders
- Stop offending or exacerbating medications
- Quit smoking
- Protect hands from cold or trauma with gloves
- Avoid known triggers (e.g., cold, emotional stress, vibrating tools)
- Vasodilator drugs (e.g., long-acting oral nitrates, low-dose sustained-release nifedipine)
- Surgical treatment may include sympathectomy

145. Rectal Masses

Any mass in the anal canal or rectum should be considered cancer until ruled out. Colorectal cancer must be considered, as it is the second leading cause of cancer death in the U.S., with greater than 40,000 mortalities each year. Early detection and aggressive treatment, and a multidisciplinary approach, are the keys to improving survival.

Differential Diagnosis

- Hemorrhoids
- Rectal prolapse
- Rectal cancer
- Rectal polyp
- Prostate cancer
- Prostatitis
- Endometriosis
- Presacral neurogenic tumor
- Rectal intussusception
- Anal cancer (2% of colorectal cancers)
  - Anal canal tumors (above the anal verge) include adenocarcinoma, melanoma, and epidermoid tumors
  - Anal margin tumors (below the anal verge) include squamous cell carcinoma, verrucous (from condyloma acuminatum), basal cell carcinoma, Bowen's disease, and Paget's disease of the anus
- Foreign body
- Less common diagnoses ("zebras") include rectal carcinoid, lymphoid hyperplasia, malignant lymphoma, lipoma, dermoid cyst, teratoma, rectal duplication, and leiomyosarcoma

Workup and Diagnosis

- History should include changes in bowel habits or consistency of stool, and family history of colorectal cancer
  - Bleeding is the most common symptom associated with benign and malignant lesions; melena suggests upper GI bleeding, blood on toilet paper suggests anal fissure or hemorrhoids, bright red separate from stool suggests hemorrhoids, clots in stool suggests colonic source
  - Pain is usually associated with benign pathology
- Fecal occult blood testing may be used for screening
- Digital rectal exam and anoscopy are used initially to distinguish many anorectal lesions
- Endoscopy (sigmoidoscopy and/or full colonoscopy) with biopsy of all polyps and suspicious lesions
- Barium enema is indicated if colonoscopy unavailable
- Endorectal ultrasound is necessary to evaluate for potential rectal cancer, to appropriately stage tumor invasion and lymph node status, and to direct appropriate treatment
- Manometry may be indicated in incontinent patients

Treatment

- Rectal and anal cancers are treated by surgical resection (with sphincter preservation), radiation, and/or chemotherapy
- Hemorrhoid treatment is initially conservative: High-fiber diet, appropriate anal hygiene, Sitz baths, and topical steroids
  - Surgical options include rubber band ligation of internal hemorrhoids or surgical resection for large refractory hemorrhoids
  - Acute thrombosis of a hemorrhoid may require incision and drainage

146. Rectal Pain

Rectal complaints are common and distressing for patients. Although most causes of rectal pain and bleeding are benign and treatable, carcinoma must be considered and ruled out in older patients (>40 years) and those with suggestive findings (e.g., polyps). Many of the rectal pathologies are easily diagnosed; however, nongastrointestinal diagnoses (e.g., genitourinary or gynecologic) may present with rectal complaints and should be considered.

Differential Diagnosis

- Anal fissure
  - Acute fissure presents with pain and bleeding (noticed on toilet paper) immediately following defecation
  - Chronic fissure presents with long-standing itching and mild pain, with or without bleeding
- Perianal abscess (with or without associated fistula formation
- Thrombosed hemorrhoid
- Levator ani syndrome
- Proctalgia fugax (rectal muscle spasm)
- Coccyodynia/coccygodynia
- Fecal impaction
- Neoplasm (rectal, pelvic, or cauda equina)
- Idiopathic
- Inflammatory bowel disease (ulcerative proctitis, Crohn's disease)
- Solitary rectal ulcer syndrome
  - Misnomer: May be multiple, not restricted to rectum, and lesion may be polypoid
  - Neoplasm is a concern
- Pruritus ani
- Trauma
- Anal sex
- Constipation
- Diarrhea
- Less common causes ("zebras") include familial rectal pain, endometriosis, pelvic inflammatory disease, prostatitis, myopathies, foreign bodies, and compression or inflammation of sacral nerves

Workup and Diagnosis

- A careful history and physical exam are crucial and often diagnostic for many conditions
  - Acute anal fissure presents as an anal tear (typically posterior) with a tender perineum; no further workup is necessary if the classic history and exam are found
  - Chronic anal fissure presents as an open ulcer with drainage and sentinel pile
  - Levator ani symptoms can be elicited by digital rectal examination
  - Proctalgia fugax symptoms cannot be elicited by exam
  - Coccyodynia: Palpation of coccyx reproduces symptoms
- In cases of perianal abscess, must rule out the presence of an anal fistula and inflammatory bowel disease
- Anoscopy may be indicated to rule out inflammatory bowel disease
- If an underlying disease process is suspected, consider stool cultures, viral titers, serologies, and/or biopsy

Treatment

- Acute anal fissure: 90% heal within 3–4 weeks with conservative management (increased fiber and water intake, stool softeners, Sitz bath, topical corticosteroids)
- Chronic anal fissure: Only 40% heal with conservative treatment; sphincterotomy (<5% risk of significant incontinence) is the treatment of choice
- Perianal abscess: Requires incision and drainage followed by packing and Sitz baths until healed
- Levator ani syndrome: Decrease anal canal pressure by digital massage (3–4/week), Sitz baths, muscle relaxants
- Proctalgia fugax: Self-limited, infrequent brief attacks; primary treatment is reassurance; treat any underlying psychological disorders
- Coccyodynia: Warm Sitz baths, analgesics, and corticosteroid injections; coccygectomy may be indicated in rare cases
- Thrombosed hemorrhoid: Incision and drainage or surgical excision

147. Red Eye

A red eye is a diagnostic sign of ocular inflammation, which may be caused by a multitude of conditions. Most cases are benign and can be effectively managed by the primary care physician. Misdiagnosis of the more emergent conditions can have major vision-threatening complications; therefore, the key to management is prompt recognition of serious diseases that require ophthalmologic referral.

Differential Diagnosis

- Conjunctivitis
  - Allergic (allergens, irritants)
  - Viral (adenovirus, HSV, varicella)
  - Bacterial: Adults (*Staphylococcus aureus, S. epidermidis, E. coli, Pseudomonas* spp, *Streptococcus* spp), children (*Haemophilus influenzae* can cause otitis/conjunctivitis syndrome), *Streptococcus pneumoniae, Moraxella catarrhalis, Staphylococcus* spp), newborns (gonorrhea, *Chlamydia*)
- Corneal abrasion/ulceration
- Subconjunctival hemorrhage
- Episcleritis
- Scleritis (inflammation of conjunctiva and deep layers of globe)
- Keratoconjunctivitis sicca
  - Rheumatoid arthritis
  - Sjögren's syndrome
- Acute angle closure glaucoma
- Acute iritis
- Anterior uveitis
- Pinguecula
- Pterygium
- Viral keratitis (disruption of the corneal epithelium): Herpes simplex/zoster
- Contact lens complications (e.g., infections with *Acanthamoeba, Pseudomonas*)
- Trauma
- Chemical burns (e.g., cyanoacrylate injury)
- Orbital cellulitis (especially in children)
- Acute ethmoiditis
- Eyelid abnormalities
- Trichiasis
- Entropion
- Molluscum contagiosum
- Kawasaki's disease
- Measles
- UV radiation-induced photokeratitis
- Pseudotumor cerebri

Workup and Diagnosis

- A thorough history is key to making accurate diagnosis
  - History should focus on onset, visual changes, pain, trauma, photophobia, and fever
  - Characteristics of a discharge clarity, color, and consistency should be ascertained
  - Prior episodes and history of eye surgeries can provide valuable clues
  - Co-morbid conditions (e.g., autoimmune disorders, hypertension, diabetes) can cause ocular symptoms
  - Questions about contact lens use and medications (e.g., anticholinergics) are important
- Physical examination should include testing for visual acuity, extraocular muscles, pupil reactivity, photophobia, and disc assessment
  - Eyelid inspection with eversion
- Complete eye examination and focused head/neck and neurologic examination are indicated in all cases
- Red flags include corneal opacification, deep pain, acute vision changes, photophobia, and blurred disc margins; pain suggests increased intraocular pressure above 40 mmHg, which necessitates immediate ophthalmologic referral
- Slit-lamp examination with or without fluorescein dye
- Laboratory studies may include culture and sensitivities for suspected infective causes, CBC and ESR for suspected inflammatory causes, rheumatoid factor and ANA for autoimmune causes

Treatment

- Ophthalmologic referral for HSV/herpes zoster keratitis or conjunctivitis, acute angle-closure glaucoma, scleritis, corneal ulcer, iritis, penetrating foreign bodies
- Avoid treating patients with steroid eyedrops without ophthalmologic consultation
- Conjunctivitis
  - Allergic: Avoid offending agents, cold compresses to eyes, NSAIDs, ocular decongestants, antihistamines
  - Viral: Self-limited, good hygiene to avoid spread
  - Bacterial: Antibiotic eye drops; avoid neomycin, because allergic reactions are common
- Subconjunctival hemorrhage: Reassurance, cool compresses, clears spontaneously in 1–2 weeks
- Chemical eye injury: Immediate copious irrigation with normal saline for at least 30 minutes
- Preventative measures include proper hygiene and daily cleaning of contact lenses, proper hand-washing techniques before all contact with eyes, eye protection in occupations entailing possible ocular injury

148. Restless Legs

Restless legs are a common complaint that cannot simply be diagnosed as restless legs syndrome without an appropriate evaluation to assess for other etiologies. A careful sleep and medication history, coupled with a complete neurologic exam, are often all that is needed to establish the correct diagnosis.

Differential Diagnosis

- Normal snoring with periodic limb movements
- Nocturnal leg cramps
  - Associated with painful, crampy calves
- Chronic insomnia
- Sleep disturbance due to medication/drugs
  - Commonly associated with decongestants, steroids, caffeine, and β-blockers
  - May be due to withdrawal from tobacco, alcohol, or illicit drugs
  - Akathisia (e.g., neuroleptics, dopamine antagonists, drug withdrawal)
- Restless legs syndrome
  - Feelings of creeping, crawling, burning, pulling, itching, tugging, and discomfort in the legs are relieved by involuntary leg movement
  - Most patients are >50 years old
  - Often unilateral
  - Positive family history in 1/3 of cases
  - Symptoms are exacerbated by pregnancy, end-stage renal failure (dialysis increases restless legs activity; kidney transplant improves symptoms), and some medications (e.g., lithium antidepressants, dopamine antagonists)
- Peripheral neuropathy
  - Associated with numbness, tingling, and pain
  - Leg pain not relieved by movement
  - Consider diabetes and deficiencies of vitamin B_{12} and folate
- Peripheral vascular disease
- Deep venous thrombosis, venous stasis
- Delayed deep sleep syndrome
- Hyperthyroidism
- Sleep deprivation
- Sleep anxiety
- Spinal cord/vertebral disc disease
- Extrapyramidal symptoms due to medications (e.g., dystonic reaction, pseudoparkinsonism, neuroleptic malignant syndrome from antipsychotics)

Workup and Diagnosis

- History and physical examination
  - Restless legs is one of the most common causes of insomnia
  - Inquire about sleep patterns and sleep history from patient and bed partner
  - Determine whether pain is relieved by movement
  - Include complete medication history (e.g., tricyclic antidepressants are often prescribed for insomnia, but tend to worsen restless legs)
- Initial labs may include CBC, iron studies, fasting glucose, BUN/creatinine, electrolytes, calcium, magnesium, TSH, vitamin B_{12}, and pregnancy test
  - If anemic, a workup for blood loss is indicated (e.g., colon and upper GI evaluation, urinalysis for hematuria, consider endometrial biopsy in older women)
- Sleep study to define sleep pathology

Treatment

- Withdraw medications that may cause extrapyramidal side effects (e.g., tricyclic antidepressants, reserpine, propranolol, phenothiazines, metoclopramide, methyldopa, haloperidol, oral contraceptive pills)
- Iron replacement and treatment of underlying pathology (e.g., colon cancer) for anemic patients
- Dopamine agonists (e.g., carbidopa/levodopa, pergolide, pramipexole, ropinirole) are often useful
- Carbamazepine is useful, but may result in cognitive impairment and fatigue
- Gabapentin has been very effective and has fewer side effects (especially useful in patients with concomitant neuropathy)
- Clonidine is useful in patients with hypertension
- Narcotics may be used for short-term relief
- Offer emotional support

149. Romberg's Sign

Romberg testing is used to examine proprioception and, to some extent, cerebellar function. The test is performed by having the patient stand with feet together and eyes closed, which eliminates the visual cues that help to maintain posture. Patients with diminished proprioception begin to fall or move their feet to maintain balance. Patients with vestibular dysfunction may also exhibit Romberg's sign.

Differential Diagnosis

- Myelopathy
  - Multiple sclerosis
  - Vitamin B_{12} deficiency
  - Structural spinal cord disease
    (e.g., spondolytic myelopathy, tumor)
  - Infectious myelopathy (e.g., tabes dorsalis, HIV-related vacuolar myelopathy)
- Peripheral neuropathy: Affects large diameter, myelinated fibers
  - Vitamin B_{12} deficiency
  - CIDP
  - MGUS
  - Inherited demyelinating neuropathies
    (e.g., Charcot-Marie-Tooth disease)
- Cerebellar dysfunction
  - Multiple causes (e.g., CVA, brain tumor)
  - Most patients with midline cerebellar dysfunction have difficulty standing on a narrow base; this effect will not appreciably worsen with eye closure
- Vestibular dysfunction (peripheral)
- Drug intoxication
  - Alcohol
  - Cisplatin
  - Pyridoxine (vitamin B_6) overdose
  - Anticonvulsant toxicity (especially phenytoin) may cause difficulty standing on a narrow base, but this may not necessarily worsen with eye closure
- Friedreich's ataxia
- Miller-Fisher variant of Guillain-Barré syndrome
- Paraneoplastic sensory neuropathy
- Vitamin E deficiency

Workup and Diagnosis

- History and physical examination with comprehensive neurologic examination
  - Elicit Romberg test
  - Be sure to focus on other tests of proprioception, cerebellar function, and strength (e.g., finger-to-nose testing)
  - Most patients with a positive Romberg's sign will also exhibit abnormal proprioception and vibratory testing
- Labs may include CBC, electrolytes, glucose, calcium, BUN/creatinine, ESR, vitamin B_{12} and folate levels, RPR, drug screen, and serum/urine protein electrophoresis
- EMG/nerve conduction studies testing is the best way to objectively document or exclude a large-fiber, sensory neuropathy
- MRI is the most effective imaging option if structural spinal cord or cerebellar disease is suspected
- CSF examination may reveal elevated protein in CIDP or Miller-Fisher variant of GBS; multiple sclerosis patients may have oligoclonal bands or an elevated IgG index

Treatment

- Tell patients to be cautious when standing with eyes closed (such as when standing under the shower) or in poor lighting (such as when going to the restroom at night) to prevent falls
- Assistive devices (e.g., cane, walker) may be useful
- Surgical therapy may be necessary for compressive myelopathy, such as spondolytic myelopathy
- Supplementation for deficiency states
  - Patients with B_{12} deficiency require further evaluation to determine the cause of the underlying deficiency and if parenteral supplementation is necessary
- Eliminate exposure to offending toxic substances
- Inflammatory demyelinating neuropathies (e.g., CIDP) may improve with steroids or other immunosuppressive drugs, periodic infusion of IVIG, or plasmapheresis
- Infectious causes may be treated with the appropriate anti-infective agent (e.g., penicillin for tabes dorsalis)
- Multiple sclerosis is treated with steroids, interferons, glatiramer acetate, mitoxantrone

150. Scalp Rash

Scalp dermatitis or infection is easy to diagnose, but it can be challenging to treat. Topical therapy or topical plus systemic therapy for prolonged periods are often necessary to successfully control these disorders. Seborrheic dermatitis is a chronic condition that can be managed successfully, but is rarely "cured," whereas tinea capitis is usually treated successfully and resolves completely. Scalp lesions due to psoriasis and discoid lupus must be treated as aspects of systemic disease.

Differential Diagnosis

- Seborrheic dermatitis ("cradle cap," "dandruff")
    - The most common scalp condition, it occurs across all age ranges
    - May be caused by *Pityrosporum ovale*
    - An inflammatory condition that causes itching and loose, silvery-white scale on scalp, and occasionally blepharitis
    - May also affect the eyebrows, nasolabial folds, external auditory canals, chin, anterior chest, upper back, and groin
    - Does not cause hair loss
    - The scalp is not usually erythematous, but other affected skin areas may be red, greasy, or oily
- Tinea capitis
    - Most commonly caused by *Trichophyton tonsurans* or rarely *Microsporum canis*
    - Presents as patches of scale and/or pruritus with broken hairs, patchy hair loss (i.e., "black dot alopecia")
    - May progress to a kerion (see below)
- Kerion
    - A boggy, tender, subcutaneous fungal infection (dermatophyte)
    - Often has associated drainage and hair loss
- Scalp folliculitis
    - Presents as recurrent, itchy, crusted papules or pustules
    - An overgrowth of *Staphylococcus aureus*
- Psoriasis
    - Usually presents with plaques of thick, silvery, adherent scalp scale that overlies well-demarcated patches of erythema
    - Often occurs at the ears and occipital area
    - May be limited to the scalp, but often has skin disease, nail pitting, or nail dystrophy
- Dissecting cellulitis of the scalp
    - Chronic, tender, boggy, often suppurative subcutaneous fluctuant masses
    - Occurs in black patients
    - May be associated with acne keloidalis, which can cause a scarring hair loss at the occiput
- Discoid lupus
    - Presents initially as well-demarcated erythematous plaques of patchy, scarring scalp hair loss, then spreads centrifugally
- Contact dermatitis

Workup and Diagnosis

- History and physical examination
    - If the scalp scale is diffuse, white, and nonadherent, seborrheic dermatitis is the likely diagnosis
- Bacterial culture from any intact scalp pustule or suppurating area may be helpful to confirm bacterial folliculitis or dissecting cellulitis
- KOH prep of scalp scale or scalp hair can be assessed under a microscope in the office to confirm the presence of endothrix (spores within the hair shaft) in the hair or branching hyphae in the scalp scale
- Fungal cultures can be obtained from the drainage of a kerion or from scalp scale scraped by a tongue depressor or sterile toothbrush
    - Hairs from the affected area can also be sent for fungal culture to rule out tinea capitus; the hairs must be plucked so that the root of the hair is available
    - Cultures may take several weeks and sensitivity varies widely based on clinician technique and lab handling
- A punch or shave biopsy is usually unnecessary, but can aid in the diagnosis of seborrheic dermatitis
- In cases of tinea capitis, only *M. canis,* which is uncommon in the U.S., fluoresces with a Wood's lamp

Treatment

- Seborrheic dermatitis: Zinc pyrithione, ketoconazole, tar, and salicylic acid shampoos
    - If monotherapy fails, the addition of a topical steroid solution or ointment (e.g., betamethasone, fluocinonide) during flareups may be useful
- Tinea capitis and kerion: Systemic antifungal therapy (e.g., griseofulvin, diflucan, terbenafine, ketoconazole, itraconazole) for 4–8 weeks; steroids
- Scalp folliculitis: Treat with 2–4 weeks of a first-generation cephalosporin or tetracycline derivative
    - Topical clindamycin or erythromycin solutions may also be used
- Discoid lupus and psoriasis: Intralesional steroid injection and/or systemic treatments
- Dissecting cellulitis: Incision and drainage of suppurative lesions, intralesional steroids, and systemic retinoids or antibiotic therapy

151. Scoliosis & Kyphosis

Scoliosis is a curve of the spine in the coronal plane (i.e., lateral curve) that is often associated with a rotational deformity as well. Kyphosis is an alteration in normal spinal curvature in the sagittal plane, and it refers to a curve with an anterior concavity. Normally, some degree of thoracic and sacral kyphosis exists. Lordosis (convex anterior) is normal in the cervical and lumbar spines.

Differential Diagnosis

Scoliosis
- Idiopathic (75–80% of cases) scoliosis usually occurs in otherwise healthy patients; pain and neurologic deficits are rare; right thoracic curve is most common, then double curve (right thoracic and left lumbar); named by convex side
  - Infantile (birth to 3 years): Rare in the U.S.
  - Juvenile (4–10 years): Uncommon
  - Adolescent (11 years to skeletal maturity): Occurs mostly in females
- Neuromuscular scoliosis
  - Common with paralytic disorders
  - More severe, almost always progressive
- Congenital scoliosis
  - Failure of formation or segmentation

Kyphosis
- Postural roundback
- Scheuermann's disease
  - Second most common pediatric spinal deformity
  - Cannot voluntarily correct
  - Angulation in mid- to low-thoracic spine
- Congenital kyphosis

Less common etiologies ("zebras")
- Post-thoracotomy
- Marfan's syndrome
- Neurofibromatosis
- Achondroplasia
- Diastrophic dwarfism
- Specific neuromuscular disorders (e.g., cerebral palsy, syringomyelia, polio, muscular dystrophy, cord tumor/trauma)

Workup and Diagnosis

- History and physical examination, including peripheral neurologic exam
  - Scoliosis: Inspect the back, shoulders, and pelvis for scapular prominence; rib prominence (especially with Adams forward bend test), shoulders, or pelvis not level; "rib hump" measured with scoliometer on bending; assess decompensation by using plumb bob to measure location of C7 with respect to gluteal cleft
  - Kyphosis: Inspect the spine for curve greater than normal of 25–45° in the thoracic spine; assess patient's ability to extend to correct curvature
- A/P and lateral X-rays of entire spine with extra long cassette (scoliosis series)
- Scoliosis: Curve is measured by Cobb method (angle between the axes of the inferior and superior vertebrae with maximal tilt)
  - Stagnara view for severe curves: A/P X-ray of vertebral bodies
  - Bending versus traction views if surgery is contemplated
  - MRI or CT if abnormal neurologic exam, unusual curves, rapid progression, or congenital
  - Pulmonary function tests are indicated in severe disease to evaluate for pulmonary dysfunction due to decreased rib cage space
- Kyphosis: Supine hyperextension films

Treatment

- Scoliosis
  - Treat underlying cause if applicable (e.g., tumor)
  - <20–25° of deformity: Observation
  - 20–40° of deformity: Bracing (preferably to be worn 23 hours/day); bracing stops progression only; Milwaukee brace (includes neck ring) gives best results but poor compliance; lumbosacral orthosis (Boston brace) has poorer results but better compliance
  - >40° of deformity: Surgery (posterior spinal fusion with rods) is usually indicated; progression is very likely
  - More aggressive treatment is usually indicated if progression >5°, female, younger, or if secondary, treatment generally more aggressive
- Kyphosis: Bracing or surgery, similar to scoliosis

152. Scrotal Masses

Scrotal masses and swelling can involve the contents of the scrotum, the wall of the scrotum, and the scrotum itself. Ultrasonography should be used liberally in evaluating scrotal masses. All solid masses must be evaluated by surgical exploration. Torsion of the testis should be reduced as quickly as possible; however, surgical intervention will still be needed to prevent future torsion in the affected or contralateral testis. Swelling of the scrotum without a mass is usually associated with a separate medical condition, such as heart failure or anasarca.

Differential Diagnosis

Painful masses
- Torsion of the spermatic cord
  - Testicle rides higher on affected side
  - Neonate to early 20s
  - Sudden pain in one testicle, followed by swelling and erythema of scrotum
- Epididymitis
  - Testicle position is normal; tenderness at top and posterior of testicle
  - Childhood to old age
  - <35 years: *Chlamydia,* gonorrhea
  - >35 years: *Enterobacteriaceae*
- Orchitis
  - Testicle position normal
  - Usually with epididymitis due to *E. coli, Klebsiella, Pseudomonas;* mumps
- Strangulated hernia (vascular compromise)
- Trauma

Nonpainful masses
- Hernia
- Varicocele
  - A collection of dilated tortuous veins posterior to and above testis
- Testicular cancer
  - Most common at ages 15–35
  - Gradual onset, though may only be noticed incidentally following trauma
- Spermatocele
  - Firm, cystic mass containing sperm above and posterior to testis
- Hydrocele
  - Covers anterior surface of the testicle
  - Seen in infants but usually closes before 1 year of age, then reappears in men over 40
- Scrotal swelling
  - Edema from cardiac, hepatic, or renal failure
- Epididymal cyst
  - More common in males with in utero DES exposure
- Sperm granuloma
  - Usually at the site of a prior vasectomy
- Less common etiologies include torsion of the appendices of the testis and epididymis, urinary extravasation, lipoma of spermatic cord, and pyogenic or granulomatous orchitis

Workup and Diagnosis

- History and physical examination including abdomen, back, genitalia, and digital rectal examination
  - Onset/duration of symptoms, evidence of trauma, past medical history (e.g., cryptorchidism, testicular atrophy or dysgenesis), family history (e.g. testicular cancer significantly increases risk), sexual activity, and history of GU instrumentation
  - Constitutional: Fever, weight loss, pain, face (e.g., parotid glands are enlarged in mumps), breast (e.g., gynecomastia), penis (e.g., ulcers, plaques, induration, urethral discharge), scrotum, and testicles
  - Compare size, position, and tenderness of testicles; transilluminate all masses; palpate spermatic cord and inguinal canals (explore for hernias, hidden testicles, cord tenderness); and digital rectal exam
  - Lift testicle up over symphysis pubis: Pain relieved in epididymitis (Prehn's sign); no change with torsion
- Initial laboratory testing may include CBC, urinalysis, urethral gram stain and culture
- Ultrasound is indicated in all patients; include Doppler flow study if torsion is suspected
  - Intratesticular masses are considered to be cancer until proven otherwise
- If solid mass is found, consider chest X-ray, CT of abdomen, serum tumor markers (AFP, β-hCG), LDH, electrolytes, BUN/creatinine, calcium, PT/PTT, and obtain urology consult and consider hematology-oncology consult

Treatment

- Torsion
  - Detorsion maneuver: Infiltrate spermatic cord with 10–20 mL of 1% lidocaine, then twist testes counterclockwise on left or clockwise on right; successful detorsion is indicated by immediate relief
  - Urologic referral: Emergent if unsuccessful; for orchiopexy if successful
- Epididymitis and orchitis: Treat with antibiotics
  - <35 years: (presumed to be sexually acquired): Treat with ceftriaxone or fluoroquinolone; plus doxycycline or azithromycin or tetracycline
  - >35 years: Trimethoprim-sulfamethoxazole or fluoroquinolone, unless history reveals that infection is sexually acquired
  - Analgesics
  - Scrotal support
  - Hospitalize if septic
- If a mass is found that does not have a clear etiology after appropriate evaluation, consult urology

153. Seizures/Convulsions

Seizures are a symptom of some identifiable underlying cause or are idiopathic. Epilepsy is recurrent unprovoked seizures. Seizures may or may not be associated with convulsive activity. Correct classification of the seizure type helps to suggest etiology and treatment.

Differential Diagnosis

- Partial seizure (involve only part of the brain)
  - Simple (no altered consciousness)
  - Complex (with altered consciousness)
- Generalized seizure (involve both hemispheres)
  - Tonic-clonic
  - Atonic
  - Tonic
  - Myoclonic
  - Absence
- Epilepsy
  - Recurrent unprovoked seizures of any or multiple types, which may be idiopathic or symptomatic
- Secondary seizure
  - Metabolic abnormalities (e.g., electrolyte disturbances, hypoglycemia)
  - Drug effects, intoxication, or withdrawal
  - Head injury/trauma
  - Febrile seizures in children
  - Structural lesions (e.g., tumor, subdural hematoma)
  - Cerebrovascular etiologies (e.g., cerebral infarct, intracerebral hemorrhage, subarachnoid hemorrhage)
  - Hypoxic-ischemic encephalopathy
  - Infection (e.g., meningitis, encephalitis)
  - Hypoxia
- Nonepileptic seizure
  - Not associated with abnormal electrical activity in the brain
  - Patients with loss of consciousness secondary to cerebral hypoperfusion (fainting, syncope) may occasionally exhibit brief periods of twitching or convulsive movements resembling seizure activity
  - Psychological disturbances (pseudoseizure)
- Inborn errors of metabolism
  - Disorders of amino acid metabolism
  - Organic acidemias
  - Urea cycle disorders
  - Mitochondrial disorders
  - Peroxisomal disorders
  - Glycogen storage disorders
  - Disorders of sugar metabolism
- Rasmussen's encephalitis
  - Causes seizures and progressive hemispheric dysfunction in infants

Workup and Diagnosis

- History and physical examination
  - In many instances, the most useful history is obtained from a witness of the seizure rather than the patient him- or herself, because seizures commonly cause altered consciousness and may result in postictal confusion
  - Appropriate classification of seizure type may help to suggest etiology and treatment (e.g., a partial seizure resulting in isolated clonic jerking of the right arm is suggestive of pathology in the left frontal lobe)
  - Evidence of postictal paralysis on examination may also help to suggest the part of the brain involved
- Initial labs should include CBC, electrolytes, glucose, O_2 saturation, calcium, magnesium, glucose, and BUN/creatinine
- CT is suitable for emergent evaluation, but MRI is more sensitive
- CSF examination if CNS infection (e.g., meningitis) or subarachnoid hemorrhage is suspected
- Drug screen and ethanol level
- EEG
- Video EEG monitoring may be useful in cases of refractory epilepsy as part of evaluation for epilepsy surgery or suspected nonepileptic seizures

Treatment

- Generalized status epilepticus (continuous or recurrent seizure activity without a return to baseline for >30 minutes) is a medical emergency and should be treated aggressively with IV antiepileptic medications
- Remove offending intoxicants or medications
- Correct metabolic abnormalities as necessary
- Numerous anticonvulsant medications are available for acute and chronic use
  - Select the most appropriate agent on the basis of the clinical situation, seizure type, and side effect profile
  - Combination anticonvulsant therapy may be effective for patients refractory to a single agent
- Vagus nerve stimulators are effective in patients refractory to anticonvulsant therapy
- Epilepsy surgery also may be effective in controlling seizures in carefully selected surgical candidates who are refractory to chronic anticonvulsant medication
- Lifestyle modification and avoidance of triggers (e.g., sleep deprivation, alcohol)

154. Shoulder Pain/Swelling

The shoulder is a complex arrangement of the humerus held loosely in place by ten muscles acting on the scapula, clavicle, and humerus, which form three articulations (acromioclavicular, glenohumeral, and sternoclavicular). Acute injuries are generally due to trauma (e.g., forced hyperabduction) or excessive demands; most chronic cases are due to overuse. The glenohumeral joint is the most frequently dislocated joint in the body (anterior in 95% of cases).

Differential Diagnosis

- Trauma and sports related injuries
  - Acromioclavicular dislocation ("separated shoulder")
  - Sternoclavicular dislocation
  - Glenohumeral dislocation
  - Proximal humeral fractures
- "Impingement syndrome"
  - Progressive degeneration and inflammation of the subacromial contents (rotator cuff and subacromial bursa) in part due to compression between the acromion and the head of the humerus
  - May result in rotator cuff tear
- Rotator cuff strain, tear, or rupture
  - May occur acutely (secondary to trauma) or, more commonly, due to a relatively mild (e.g., reaching overhead) insult to a chronically degenerative cuff
- Degenerative joint disease
- Tendonitis
- Subacromion and/or subcapsular bursitis
- AC joint inflammation
- Calcific tendonitis
  - Deposition of calcium crystals in the rotator cuff with resulting inflammation and severe pain
- Suprascapular nerve entrapment
- Bicipital tendonitis
- Adhesive capsulitis
  - Thickened, scarred joint capsule and "frozen shoulder" due to prolonged postinjury or postsurgery immobilization
- Cervical disc disease and radiculopathy
- Gout
- Pseudogout
- Connective tissue disease (e.g., rheumatoid arthritis, SLE)
- Brachial plexus injury
- Septic arthritis
- Referred pain from MI, cholecystitis, splenic injury
- Malignancy (e.g., apical lung)
- Lyme disease
- Fibromyalgia
- Thoracic outlet syndrome
- Reflex sympathetic dystrophy
- Rib dislocation/rib pain
- Acute axillary vein thrombosis

Workup and Diagnosis

- History and physical examination
  - Inspection for asymmetry, dislocation, or atrophy
  - Note range of motion, strength, sensory, crepitus, pain with passive and/or active motion
  - Perform a complete neurovascular exam
- Plain X-rays of shoulder; cervical spine films and chest X-ray may also be useful
- X-ray or CT scan may identify chronic, degenerative arthritis
- Shoulder MRI evaluates the anatomy of the rotator cuff and associated soft tissue; may differentiate partial from complete tears
- EMG can help discern nerve entrapments, cervical disc disease, or brachial plexus injury
- Diffuse shoulder or acromioclavicular pain may require workup for medical etiologies, including ESR, ANA, rheumatoid factor, and TSH

Treatment

- Slings may be used for comfort but early range of motion (24–48 hours) is necessary to prevent adhesive capsulitis
- Conservative therapy is beneficial for most cases of shoulder pain: Rest, ice, NSAIDs, and opioid narcotics
- Subacromial cortisone injection if other anti-inflammatory methods fail; however, multiple injections are discouraged because of possible tissue atrophy
- Physical therapy is generally the mainstay of treatment
  - Conditioning and strengthening
  - Progressive range of motion exercises for adhesive capsulitis
- Full thickness rotator cuff tears may require surgical repair
- Adhesive capsulitis may require surgical lysis of adhesions
- Prevent future injuries by promoting strength and flexibility

155. Skin Pigmentation (Decreased)

Distinguishing between hypopigmentation and depigmentation is crucial to narrowing the differential diagnosis. Hypopigmentation is a decrease in the level of pigmentation of the skin, whereas depigmentation is a total loss of skin pigment. Both can be either localized or generalized, which also helps narrow the differential. Skin biopsies are rarely helpful in this scenario.

Differential Diagnosis

- Vitiligo
  - Affects 1% of the population
  - Begins as a focal or diffuse (more common) hypopigmented patch that progresses to total loss of pigmentation of the affected skin (chalk white)
  - Usually symmetric; often tops of hands, perioral, periorbital skin, knees, elbows
- Pityriasis alba
  - Very common, especially in black children
  - Less distinct borders than in vitiligo, does *not* result in complete depigmentation
  - Plaques may appear lighter than surrounding skin and may be scaly
  - Often secondary to mild inflammation, such as tinea versicolor or atopic eczema
  - Completely reversible and does not cause permanent hypopigmentation
- Piebaldism
  - Congenital, permanent, and irreversible
  - Newborns often have a patch of white scalp hair and depigmented patches on the trunk with normally pigmented patches within these larger depigmented areas
- Chemical leukoderma (depigmentation)
  - May be caused by phenols, germicides, and many other caustic chemicals
  - Results in confetti-like macules of depigmentation in exposed skin
- Albinism
  - Congenital
  - Disorder of melanin synthesis with several phenotypes, ranging from complete lack of pigmentation (white hair and translucent or "red" iris) to the more common diffuse hypopigmentation or "yellow" albinism that is prevalent in the black population
  - Affects the skin, hair, and eyes
  - Photophobia, decreased visual acuity, strabismus, and risk of skin cancer are the main problems faced by these patients
- Congenital birthmarks (e.g., nevus anemicus, nevus depigmentosis) are isolated patches of hypo- or depigmentation that remain unchanged over time
- Tuberous sclerosis is an inherited systemic disorder that results in hypopigmented macules in the shape of an "ash leaf" on the trunk, and confetti-type depigmented macules on the arms/legs

Workup and Diagnosis

- History and physical examination
  - Determine whether the skin is completely depigmented (chalk white) or merely hypopigmented (lighter than surrounding skin but with residual pigmentation)
  - Vitiligo is easily diagnosed on clinical exam alone
  - Family or personal history of thyroid disease, other endocrine disorders, diabetes, or exposure to chemicals
  - History of allergies, hay fever, or asthma, which may support the diagnosis of postinflammatory hypopigmentation from atopic dermatitis
  - History of erythema or rash at the hypopigmented spot suggests pityriasis alba or postinflammatory hypopigmentation
  - Perform an eye exam to rule out strabismus or iris translucency that can be present in albinism
- Wood's lamp examination can be used to highlight the borders of hypo- and depigmented patches
- Skin biopsy can support the diagnosis of vitiligo but is not specific
- Check thyroid function tests in patients with recent-onset vitiligo, and consider fasting glucose or ACTH stimulation test to rule out diabetes and Addison's
- CBC (anemia, macrocytosis) may be indicated to screen for pernicious anemia, if suspected in patients with vitiligo

Treatment

- Topical steroids may stimulate repigmentation of vitiligo and pityriasis alba
- Sunscreens are crucial to protect vulnerable skin
- Since some patients develop vitiligo in areas of trauma (i.e., Koebner effect), trauma should be avoided
- Repigmentation may be facilitated by systemic or topical photochemotherapy with psoralens plus UVA
- Punch minigrafting from normal donor skin areas to vitiligo areas stimulates melanocyte repopulation
- Patients with diffuse or unresponsive vitiligo may diffusely and irreversibly depigment their skin by applying monobenzylether or hydroquinone.
- Treatment of any associated thyroid disorder or diabetes, pernicious anemia, etc., does *not* alter or improve the course of the associated vitiligo
- Oral β-carotene can be taken long term by patients with diffuse vitiligo or albinism and may impart a more "normal" skin color

156. Sore Throat

Sore throat is a common symptom. Many patients incorrectly believe that antibiotics improve the clinical course in all sore throats. Although the vast majority of sore throats are of viral origin and should be managed conservatively, an appropriate history and physical exam usually identify other causes of sore throat. Use of the clinical criteria listed below to determine the likelihood of strep pharyngitis will assist in making the work up more cost effective.

Differential Diagnosis

- Viral pharyngitis/laryngitis
  - Most common cause of sore throat
  - Associated with cough, low-grade fever, nasal congestion, and sneezing
  - Influenza occasionally causes sore throat with high fever, cough, severe myalgias
  - Rhino-, adeno-, coxsackie-, and herpesvirus
  - Acute HIV infection
- Mononucleosis
  - Associated with fever, headache, and excessive fatigue
  - Most common in teen and college ages
  - May have associated lymphadenopathy, splenomegaly, hepatitis, or encephalitis
- Streptococcal pharyngitis
  - May be associated with scarlatiniform rash, fever >101°F (>38.3°C), exudative pharyngitis, tender cervical lymphadenopathy, and *absence* of cough
  - More common in winter months, ages 5–10, and with history of group A *Streptococcus* exposure
- Allergic pharyngitis
- Gonococcal pharyngitis
- Fungal pharyngitis (e.g., *Candida*)
- Foreign body in throat
  - Most often occurs in smaller children
  - Associated with sudden onset of audible wheezing, stridor, drooling
- GERD
- Sore throat secondary to postnasal drip
- Irritation secondary to inhalants (e.g., cigarette smoke), chemicals (e.g., alcohol), hot foods
- Voice abuse (e.g., excessive screaming)
- Deep neck space infections (e.g., retropharyngeal abscess, peritonsillar abscess, Ludwig's angina)
- Epiglottitis/bacterial tracheitis
  - Occurs in children ages 2–7 and increasingly in adults
- Diphtheria
- Trauma
- Lymphadenitis (cervical)
- Cancer (e.g., tonsillar, tongue, laryngeal, esophageal)
- Caustic ingestions .
- Thyroiditis
- Angina/acute coronary syndrome

Workup and Diagnosis

- History and physical exam often make the diagnosis
  - Consider exposure history, age, associated symptoms, past medical history (e.g. immunocompromise), use of inhaled steroids (e.g. with *Candida* pharyngitis), allergy history)
  - Focus on head and neck, lung, and abdominal examinations
- Streptococcal pharyngitis is often a clinical diagnosis
  - Presence of three out of four of the following criteria suggests the diagnosis: Exudative pharyngitis (not just a red throat); tender anterior lymphadenopathy; presence or history of fever; and *absence* of a cough; whereas if none or one of the criteria exists, group A β-hemolytic streptococcus is unlikely
  - Streptococcal culture is the gold standard (inexpensive; identifies group A and others; 1–2 days for results)
  - Rapid strep testing is more expensive and identifies only group A strep, but gives immediate results; very specific (95%) but less sensitive (60–70%), so consider culture if negative
- Monospot or CBC showing atypical lymphocytes is diagnostic for mononucleosis
- X-ray for foreign body; laryngoscopy if unable to verify
- Lateral neck X-ray may diagnose epiglottitis and retropharyngeal abscess
- Gonococcal and diphtheria cultures if necessary
- Barium swallow, upper GI series, or EGD for GERD

Treatment

- Viral pharyngitis: Treat symptomatically with hydration, decongestants, saline nasal spray, analgesics, and rest
- Strep pharyngitis: Appropriate antibiotics (e.g., penicillin, erythromycin) and symptomatic treatment with analgesics
- Mononucleosis: Symptomatic treatment with analgesics; limit contact sports if splenomegaly is present
  - Hospitalization in patients with encephalitis, airway compromise, or dehydration due to nausea/vomiting secondary to hepatitis
- Allergic pharyngitis: Antihistamines, nasal steroids
- Foreign body: Protect airway; removal by ENT doctor
- GERD: H2 blockers (e.g., ranitidine) or proton pump inhibitors (e.g., omeprazole), elevate head of bed, weight loss, small meals

157. Splenomegaly

The spleen is the largest lymphatic organ of the body. Splenomegaly, or enlargement of the spleen, occurs when the spleen exceeds 12 cm in length, 7 cm in width, or 150 g in mass. Although a normal spleen is not usually palpable, dullness can be percussed between the ninth and eleventh ribs (Traube's space) with the patient lying on the right side. Palpation is best performed with the patient supine with knees flexed. The spleen is best felt as it descends during inspiration. However, physical diagnosis is not sensitive.

Differential Diagnosis

- Mononucleosis
- Congestive heart failure
- Portal hypertension
  –Most often secondary to cirrhosis
- Hepatitis
- Hereditary spherocytosis
- Sickle cell disease
- Thalassemia major
- Polycythemia vera
- Malaria
- Tuberculosis
- Other infections: *Mycobacterium avium* complex, HIV, CMV, RMSF
- Endocarditis
- Malignancy (e.g., leukemia, lymphoma, metastases)
  –Massive enlargement of the spleen usually signifies a lymphoproliferative or myeloproliferative disorder
- Systemic lupus erythematosus
- Felty's syndrome (rheumatoid arthritus, splenomegaly, and granulocytopenia)
- Splenic hemangioma, hamartoma, or cyst
- Trauma
- Splenic vein thrombosis
- Less common causes ("zebras") include Gaucher's disease, amyloidosis, kala-azar (visceral leishmaniasis), schistosomiasis, rickets, syphilis, babesiosis, typhoid fever, histoplasmosis, and toxoplasmosis

Workup and Diagnosis

- History and physical examination
- CBC with differential cell counts
  –Decreases in one or more cell lineages may indicate hypersplenism
  –Neutrophilia suggests infection
- Examination of the peripheral smear
  –Atypical lymphocytes suggest mononucleosis
  –Spherocytes suggest hereditary spherocytosis
  –Teardrop-shaped RBCs suggest bone marrow invasion
- Further laboratory studies may include electrolytes, BUN/creatinine, urinalysis, chest X-ray, ANA, rheumatoid factor, HIV testing, and sickle cell prep
- Abdominal CT or ultrasound better delineate the splenomegaly and may reveal associated abdominal pathology
- Bone marrow biopsy may be indicated to evaluate for leukemia, myelofibrosis, and/or infection
- Biopsy, fine needle aspirate, and/or splenectomy may be necessary

Treatment

- Infectious etiologies require appropriate antibiotic regimens
- Leukemia and lymphoma are treated with combination chemotherapy
- Systemic lupus erythematosus and rheumatoid arthritis are treated with steroids and/or cytotoxic agents
- Hemolytic anemia is treated with steroids
- Splenectomy may be required for patients with traumatic spleen injury with persistent bleeding; patients without a spleen are at increased risk of sepsis and should receive regular pneumococcal and *Haemophilus influenzae* vaccinations

158. Stomatitis

Stomatitis refers to inflammation of the oral mucous membranes. It represents a heterogeneous group of underlying conditions, many of which are infectious in etiology. A careful history and physical examination are often sufficient to effectively narrow the differential diagnosis. In uncertain cases, a biopsy of the lesions and/or referral to an otolaryngologist, dermatologist, or oral surgeon is appropriate.

Differential Diagnosis

- Aphthous stomatitis is the most common cause of recurrent oral lesions
  - Presents as gray-yellow tender ulcer in anterior part of oral cavity
  - Major, minor, and herpetiform subtypes
  - Herpetiform ulcers: Multiple vesicles on tip or sides of tongue
- Infectious stomatitis
  - Herpes simplex virus may present as a primary infection (herpetic gingivostomatitis) with ulcers/vesicles in anterior oropharynx or as a secondary infection with "fever blisters" on lips
  - Herpangina: Caused by coxsackievirus; results in 1–2 mm vesicles on soft palate that rupture to become white ulcers; seen primarily in children, may be associated with palmar and plantar lesions in hand-foot-and-mouth disease
  - Syphilis (condyloma lata) results in *painless* oral chancres on lips, buccal mucosa, gingival
  - Varicella or chicken pox
  - Condylomata acuminata (warts) and molluscum contagiosum lesions resemble their characteristic genital lesions
  - Primary HIV infection
  - Candidiasis
- Stomatitis in immunocompromised patients
  - Breakdown in epithelium results in superinfection by *Candida,* HSV, VZV, or CMV
  - May occur secondary to chemotherapy
- Stevens-Johnson syndrome
- Gangrenous stomatitis (acute necrotizing ulcerative gingivitis)
  - Also known as "trench mouth"
  - Primarily affects children with severe malnourishment or debilitation
  - Causative agent is most commonly a spirochete (e.g., *Borrelia vincentii*)
  - Presents as painful, red vesicle on gingiva; progresses to necrotic ulcer, then cellulitis
- Chronic granulomatous disease
- Behçet syndrome (presents as recurrent oral and genital ulcers)
- Lichen planus
- Vitamin C deficiency
- Cancers (e.g., mouth cancer, leukemia, mucositis following chemotherapy)

Workup and Diagnosis

- Diagnosis usually evident by history and clinical observation
  - Focus on onset, duration, pain, associated symptoms (e.g., hand or foot lesions, dermatologic complaints, fever, past medical history, and exposure/sexual history)
  - Physical examination should focus on the eyes, ears, nose, throat, neck, and skin, with a cursory systemic evaluation
- For infectious causes, specific microbe identification by culture, antigen detection assays, and histologic studies is necessary, especially in immunocompromised patients
- Laboratory evaluation may include CBC, RPR, viral titers, ESR, HIV and others
- Chronic granulomatous disease: Lab studies may show anemia of chronic disease, leukocytosis, and elevated ESR
  - Diagnosis by NBT slide test: In absence of oxidase activity, neutrophils from CGD patients do not stain with NBT dye
- A biopsy may be necessary for definitive diagnosis; if an infectious etiology is being considered, send one part of the specimen for biopsy in formalin and a second piece in nonbacteriostatic saline for cultures
- Consider a referral to a dermatologist, otolaryngologist, or oral surgeon in uncertain cases

Treatment

- Aphthous stomatitis: Symptomatic treatment only; lesions spontaneously resolve within 2 weeks
  - Strict oral hygiene (e.g., antiseptic mouthwash)
  - Topical anesthetics may relieve pain
  - Judicious use of topical and oral steroids in severe disease
  - Oral thalidomide reportedly helpful in severe disease (e.g., AIDS patients)
- Infectious stomatitis: Target specific organism with appropriate antimicrobial treatment
  - Topical antiseptic/anesthetic
  - Coating agents (e.g., milk of magnesia, aluminum hydroxide) may be helpful
- Gangrenous stomatitis
  - High-dose IV penicillin
  - Correct underlying malnutrition or debility
  - Surgery may be necessary
- Chronic granulomatous disease: Early recognition and aggressive management of infections

159. Stridor & Wheezing

Stridor is characterized by a high-pitched grating sound on inhalation or exhalation, but it is caused by narrowing or obstruction of the upper airway. Wheezing is a high-pitched musical sound on inhalation or exhalation that is due to oscillations of narrowed lower airway walls. The age of the patient is important in determining the specific etiology: Younger patients are much more likely than older patients to have symptoms of respiratory infections or a foreign body; older patients are more likely to suffer from pulmonary edema, COPD, and cancers.

Differential Diagnosis

Stridor (inspiratory)
- Croup (laryngotracheobronchitis)
  - Viral infection with tracheal narrowing due to airway edema
  - "Bark-like" cough, hoarseness
- Epiglottitis
  - Airway emergency most commonly due to *Haemophilus influenzae* or group A streptococcus infection
  - Abrupt onset of high fevers, sore throat, hoarseness, dysphagia, respiratory distress
- Foreign body lodged in the upper airway
- Allergic reaction/anaphylaxis
  - May have urticaria and angioedema (subcutaneous or mucosal swelling, often of the lips)
- Trauma
- Postendotracheal intubation
- Psychogenic (e.g., paroxysmal vocal cord dyskinesia)

Stridor (expiratory)
- COPD (expiratory vocalization to prolong time to airway closure and avoid air trapping)
- Cardiac failure (expiratory vocalization to prolong increased intrathoracic pressure and unload left ventricle)

Wheezing
- Asthma
  - Triad of chronic cough, dyspnea, wheezing
  - Wheezing may be absent in cases of severe obstruction (insufficient air movement)
- Pulmonary edema
  - Leakage of fluid into the interstitium and alveoli due to elevated capillary pressure (cardiogenic) or abnormal capillary permeability (noncardiogenic)
- COPD
- GERD
- Respiratory infection
  - Upper respiratory infection
  - Bronchiolitis
  - "Atypical" pneumonia
- Aspirated foreign body
  - Abrupt onset of unilateral wheezing or stridor (if lodged in the upper airway), cough, and decreased breath sounds
- Allergic reaction/anaphylaxis
  - Urticaria, throat swelling (angioedema), and lip/tongue edema may be present

Workup and Diagnosis

- History and physical examination
- Initial labs may include CBC with differential, pulse oximetry, electrolytes, BUN/creatinine, calcium, and glucose
- Consider blood and/or sputum cultures if infectious cause is suspected
- Chest X-ray helps to differentiate respiratory infection from pulmonary edema, diagnose radiopaque foreign bodies, and shows "steeple sign" in cases of croup
- Lateral neck X-ray may reveal swelling of the epiglottis in cases of epiglottitis or abscess
- Chest CT with contrast provides excellent views of the lung parenchyma and helps to identify tumors and bronchiectasis
- Bronchoscopy may be diagnostic and therapeutic in cases of obstruction due to foreign body
- Lung biopsy or bronchoalveolar lavage can be performed in cases of suspected malignancy
- Echocardiogram may be indicated to evaluate for structural heart disease, valve disease, and left ventricular function

Treatment

- Attention to airway, breathing, and circulation
- Administer supplemental O_2
- Asthma: Avoid triggers; bronchodilation with inhaled β_2 agonists (e.g., albuterol) and anticholinergics (e.g., ipratropium); inhaled, oral and/or IV steroids
- Epiglottitis: Emergent airway intervention (endotracheal intubation or tracheostomy); cephalosporin antibiotics
- Respiratory infection: Appropriate antibiotics if bacterial cause is suspected; β agonists
- Anaphylaxis: Patients in extremis require immediate subcutaneous epinephrine injection; antihistamines (e.g., diphenhydramine); inhaled β_2 agonists (e.g., albuterol); steroids
- Croup: Supportive care; nebulized steroids; epinephrine

160. Syncope

Syncope is often referred to by patients as "fainting" and is defined as a loss of postural tone and consciousness. Syncope usually lasts for brief periods of a few minutes. Longer periods are of more concern, because of the possibility of major cardiac or neurologic problems. The patient's and other observer's descriptions of symptoms immediately before and after the episode are key to determining the etiology of the syncopal episode. Particularly in healthy children and adults, vasovagal syncope from decreased cerebral blood flow is the most common type of brief syncopal episode.

Differential Diagnosis

- Vasovagal episode
  - Most common cause of syncope
  - May be triggered by heat, fatigue, stress, hunger, alcohol, and severe pain
  - Associated with diaphoresis, weakness, blurry vision, lightheadedness
  - Almost always benign
- Orthostatic hypotension
  - Fall in blood pressure upon standing, due to failure of vasoconstrictor reflexes
  - Precipitated by sudden standing from recumbent position
  - Often associated with antihypertensive medications (diuretics, vasodilators, α- or β-blockers) and dehydration/hypovolemia
  - May occur with autonomic disorders (e.g., Shy-Drager syndrome)
- Situational syncope
  - Increased intrathoracic pressure (e.g., cough, micturition, defecation) leads to decreased venous return and resulting diminished blood flow to the brain
- Cardiac arrhythmias
  - Very slow (<30 bpm) or fast (>180 bpm) heart rates may result in decreased cardiac output and resulting diminished blood flow to the brain
- Valvular disease
  - Most commonly due to aortic stenosis
- Myocardial disease
- Cerebrovascular disease
  - Usually due to carotid or vertebrobasilar atherosclerosis
- Hypoglycemia
- Anemia
- Seizure
- Anxiety attack
- Migraine
- Medications (e.g., anticholinergics)
- CVA
- Hemorrhage
- Trauma

Workup and Diagnosis

- History and physical exam will often suggest the underlying etiology
  - Note pre- and postsyncopal symptoms (e.g., chest pain, dizziness, lightheadedness, nausea/vomiting, headache, diaphoresis, blurry vision, blindness)
  - Full HEENT, neurologic, and cardiovascular exam
  - Examine for trauma following syncope
  - Record BP in supine, sitting, standing, and in both arms
  - Strategically attempt to reproduce syncope by Valsalva maneuver (e.g., coughing, deep breathing for 2–3 min)
- Initial labs should include CBC, electrolytes, calcium, magnesium, glucose, toxicology screens, and ECG
- Further cardiovascular testing may include cardiac enzymes if ischemia is suspected, 24-hour Holter monitor, echocardiogram, stress testing, and/or invasive cardiac monitoring
- Head CT to rule out cerebral disease
- Doppler ultrasound of carotids if bruit is heard
- EEG may be useful if seizure disorder is suspected
- Tilt table test may induce vasovagal episode
- Plasma aldosterone/mineralocorticoid levels to evaluate for hypovolemia due to adrenocortical insufficiency

Treatment

- Identify, treat, and/or refer on the basis of underlying cardiac, neurologic, autonomic or other causes
- Vasovagal episode: Rehydrate, treat possible triggers (e.g., relieve pain)
- Orthostatic hypotension: Adjust medications, make lifestyle changes (e.g., rise slowly from sitting)
- Cardiac arrhythmias: Medical management and/or pacemaker placement
- Myocardial disease/valvular disease: Assess severity, consider medical versus surgical treatment
- Cerebrovascular disease: Reduce risk factors; consider medical versus surgical treatment
- Hypoglycemia: Identify underlying cause; adjust medications and diet to prevent further episodes
- Seizures: Adjust medications to prevent seizures; no driving

161. Tachycardia

Tachycardia is defined by a heart rate ≥100 beats per minute. Most tachyarrhythmias occur as a result of triggered activity, increased automaticity, or re-entry circuits. A 12-lead ECG is essential to determining the type of tachyarrhythmia present. Wide complex tachycardia must be worked up and treated as ventricular tachycardia until proven otherwise.

Differential Diagnosis

- Sinus tachycardia
  - Regular rhythm, narrow QRS complex
  - Originates at sinus node (normal P waves)
  - Occurs in response to physiologic stimuli (e.g., volume depletion, fever, pain, thyrotoxicosis)
- Ectopic atrial tachycardia
  - Regular rhythm, narrow QRS complex
  - Atrial focus other than sinus node
  - P waves are often inverted in inferior leads
- Atrial flutter
  - Narrow QRS complex
  - Usually regular, but may be irregular
  - Caused by a re-entrant circuit in atrium
  - Characteristic "sawtooth" pattern on ECG
  - Atrial rate typically 250–350 bpm
  - Ventricular rate usually 1/2 atrial rate (2:1 block), but may be 3:1, 4:1, etc.
- Junctional tachycardia
  - Regular rhythm, narrow QRS complex
  - Originates in AV node
  - P waves may be absent or retrograde
- AVNRT
  - Regular rhythm, narrow QRS complex
  - Due to reentrant circuit in or near AV node
  - Rate typically 170–220 bpm
  - P waves may be absent or retrograde
- Orthodromic AV reentrant tachycardia
  - Regular rhythm, narrow QRS complex
  - Caused by reentrant circuit at AV node
  - Abrupt onset/offset
  - WPW syndrome is most common example
  - ECG reveals delta waves
- Ventricular tachycardia
  - Regular rhythm, wide QRS complex
  - AV dissociation on ECG
  - May cause sudden cardiac death
  - Typically occurs in setting of acute coronary ischemia; other causes include cardiomyopathy, electrolyte disturbances (e.g., hypokalemia, hypomagnesemia), drug toxicity, or congenital abnormalities
  - Torsade de pointes is a specific form of VT associated with electrolyte abnormalities and drug toxicity
- Antidromic AVRT
  - Wide QRS complex
  - Conduction occurs down bypass tract and up AV node
  - Less common than orthodromic AVRT

Workup and Diagnosis

- History and physical examination
  - Associated symptoms may include lightheadedness, palpitations, dyspnea, chest pain, and syncope
  - Assess for hemodynamic instability (blood pressure, level of consciousness) and jugular venous pulsations (cannon A waves are highly suggestive of AV dissociation)
- ECG is the key tool for establishing diagnosis
  - Determining supraventricular versus ventricular origin is the most critical distinction
  - Adenosine IV push may be used to transiently block the AV node to identify underlying rhythms
- Any wide-QRS complex tachycardia (QRS >0.12 seconds) is considered ventricular tachycardia until proven otherwise
  - Nonsustained VT lasts <30 seconds and is asymptomatic
  - Sustained VT lasts >30 seconds or results in hemodynamic compromise
  - Monomorphic VT is a single stable QRS complex
  - Polymorphic VT is a changing QRS morphology and axis—may have normal or prolonged QT interval (e.g., torsade de pointes) on baseline ECG

Treatment

- Ventricular tachycardia must be treated emergently
  - Unstable VT with hypotension or cardiac ischemia requires immediate cardioversion
  - IV amiodarone or lidocaine if cardioversion fails
  - Stable VT should be treated initially with antiarrhythmic medications (e.g., IV amiodarone, lidocaine, procainamide), correction of electrolyte abnormalities, and/or IV magnesium; cardiovert if there is no response
- Supraventricular tachycardias
  - Control rate, terminate rhythm, prevent recurrence
  - Vagal maneuvers (e.g., carotid sinus massage) to transiently block AV node may be useful (avoid in elderly, carotid bruits, or known carotid artery stenosis)
  - Medications include AV nodal blocking drugs (e.g., β-blockers): Slow conduction to ventricles; antiarrhythmics terminate rhythm, prevent recurrence
  - Cardioversion is reserved for symptomatic patients
  - Radiofrequency ablation is more definitive means of terminating arrhythmias and preventing recurrences

162. Tachypnea

Tachypnea is defined as an increase in the normal respiratory rate. The normal respiratory rate varies with age (24–38 respirations per minute for children <1 year of age; 12–19 rpm for adults). Tachypnea is typically associated with dyspnea (the feeling of inadequate respiration); however, processes that cause metabolic acidosis will result in a Kussmaul breathing pattern, characterized by "comfortable" tachypnea.

Differential Diagnosis

- Cardiovascular etiologies
  - Pulmonary embolism: Associated with pleuritic chest pain, tachycardia, hypoxia, possible cyanosis, hypercoagulable states
  - CHF: Associated with history of ischemic heart disease, pitting peripheral edema, elevated jugular venous pressure, third heart sound, dyspnea
  - Acute MI/angina: Associated with chest pain, diaphoresis, dyspnea, nausea
  - Hypotension (e.g., cardiomyopathy): Low BP, tachycardia if acute, may be due to medications
- Pulmonary etiologies
  - COPD/asthma: Associated with a history of wheezing, cigarette use
  - Pneumonia: Associated with fever, cough, sputum production, dyspnea
  - Pneumothorax: Associated with pleuritic chest pain, history of rib trauma, COPD, hyperresonance to percussion
  - Restrictive lung diseases: Interstitial lung disease, thoracic abnormalities (e.g., kyphosis, pneumonectomy), neuromuscular diseases (e.g., ALS, Guillain-Barré, diaphragmatic paralysis)
- Metabolic and toxicologic etiologies
  - Diabetic ketoacidosis: Associated with dehydration, Kussmaul respirations, acetone breath
  - Severe dehydration: May occur in the setting of vomiting, diarrhea, burns, inadequate fluid intake
  - Salicylate toxicity: Associated with nausea, vomiting, tinnitus, altered mental status, convulsions
  - Metabolic acidosis
- Neurologic etiologies
  - CVA
  - Head trauma
- Anxiety/hyperventilation
- Sepsis
- Hyperthyroidism
- Medications/drugs
  - Sympathomimetics (e.g., cocaine)
  - Aspirin
  - β-agonists
  - Methylxanthines
- Less common etiologies ("zebras") include pericardial effusion, malignancy, tuberculosis, pheochromocytoma

Workup and Diagnosis

- History and physical examination focusing on precipitants, time course, associated symptoms, and past medical history
- Initial laboratory studies may include pulse oximetry, CBC, electrolytes, renal function, glucose, urinalysis, blood culture, urine culture, pulmonary function tests, serum aspirin level, and urine toxicology screen
- Electrocardiography and cardiac enzymes to rule out myocardial ischemia/infarction
- Chest X-ray
- Arterial blood gas
  - Determine whether cause is primary respiratory alkalosis or secondary to primary metabolic acidosis
  - Increased A-a gradient suggests pulmonary disease or pulmonary embolism
- V/Q scan may be used to evaluate for pulmonary embolism and infarction
- CT scan of the chest may be used to better visualize the lung parenchyma and can also be used to evaluate for pulmonary embolism
- Echocardiography is useful in cases of suspected congenital heart disease, pericardial effusion, and can also be used to evaluate left ventricular function in patients with congestive heart failure or myocardial infarction

Treatment

- Immediate assessment of ABCs (airway, breathing, circulation)
- Administer supplemental O_2
- Treat pain if appropriate
- Evaluate for toxic ingestions and treat immediately as per toxicology protocols
- Treat underlying etiologies as appropriate

163. Tactile Fremitus

Tactile fremitus is performed by placing your hands firmly on the patient's chest and having them repeat "99" several times to feel the vibration of the conducted sound. Then, examine the rest of the chest in the same fashion. An increase in fremitus indicates a direct solid communication from the bronchus to the chest wall or a consolidation. A decrease in fremitus indicates the presence of air, fluid, or solid material in the pleural space or obstruction of the bronchi.

Differential Diagnosis

- Increased fremitus (increased transmission of sound through the chest)
  - Consolidative pneumonia (e.g., *Streptococcus pneumoniae*, lobar pneumonias)
  - Diffuse alveolitis
  - Diffuse fibrosis (e.g., cystic fibrosis)
- Decreased fremitus (decreased transmission of sound through the chest)
  - Pleural effusion: Due to CHF, pneumonia, cancer, pulmonary embolus, connective tissue disease (e.g., SLE, RA), pancreatitis, and renal and liver disease
  - Hemothorax: Due to chest trauma or instrumentation
  - Chylothorax: Due to traumatic disruption of the thoracic duct or malignancy
  - Pneumothorax: May occur spontaneously or following trauma or instrumentation
  - Asthma
  - Bronchitis
  - Emphysema
  - Atelectasis: May be acute (e.g., postoperative) or chronic (airlessness, infection, bronchiectasis, destruction, fibrosis)
  - Foreign body aspiration
  - Pleural thickening
- Rhonchal fremitus
  - Due to airway secretions
- Friction fremitus
  - Due to pleural friction rub

Workup and Diagnosis

- Complete history and physical exam
  - Note egophany ("E" to "A" changes), symmetry of chest movement, auscultation, percussion
- Initial labs may include CBC, pulse oximetry, electrolytes, BUN/creatinine, calcium, and glucose
- Consider blood and/or sputum cultures if suspect an infectious cause
- Chest X-ray may reveal pneumothorax, pneumonia, effusion, atelectasis, and other diagnoses
- Consider chest CT scan if unexplained abnormal chest X-ray or to better delineate fibrosis or cause of effusions
- Arterial blood gas may be indicated
- Pulmonary function tests may be indicated to identify restrictive or obstructive disease and barriers to diffusion

Treatment

- Attention to airway, breathing, and circulation
- Administer supplemental O_2
- Chest tube insertion may be indicated for pneumothorax, hemothorax, or chylothorax
- Treat the underlying cause

164. Testicular Pain

Testicular pain must be considered a testicle-threatening emergency because of the possibility of testicular torsion or Fournier's gangrene, although the most common etiologies are neither serious nor emergent. Testicular pain often is accompanied by significant concern on the part of the patient who worries that this might be cancer.

Differential Diagnosis

- Epididymitis
  - Insidious onset of symptoms seen in adolescent (postpuberty) boys
  - Bacterial (e.g., *Chlamydia, Enterobacter*) versus viral (mumps, mononucleosis, adenovirus)
- Testicular torsion
  - Twisting of the spermatic cord results in testicular ischemia
  - Acute onset of severe pain, diffuse tenderness
  - Negative urinalysis; absent cremasteric reflex
  - Testes on affected side are tender, shortened, and lie transversely
  - Duration of ischemia (time until detorsion is completed) determines the viability of the affected testicle
- Hydrocele
  - A collection of fluid between the layers of the tunica vaginalis; usually nontender
- Varicocele
  - Palpated as a "bag of worms" above testes
  - Dull ache exacerbated by strenuous exercise; left > right
- Epididymal or testicular appendage torsion
  - Subacute onset seen in prepubertal boys
  - Localized to the upper pole of testicle
  - Negative U/A; normal cremasteric reflex
- Ruptured abdominal aortic aneurysm
- Peritonitis
- Referred pain due to an incarcerated hernia, constipation, or kidney stone
- Scrotal trauma
  - Results from a direct blow or saddle injury
  - May result in traumatic epididymitis, hematocele, or laceration of the tunica albuginae (testicular rupture)
- Fournier's gangrene
  - Necrotizing fasciitis of the perineum
  - Seen primarily in older men
- Henoch-Schönlein purpura
  - Systemic vasculitis resulting in scrotal pain, abdominal pain, arthralgias, nonthrombocy-topenic purpura, and renal disease
  - Occurs in prepubertal boys
- Tumor
  - Painless scrotal mass is a testicular neoplasm until proven otherwise

Workup and Diagnosis

- History and physical examination including abdomen, back, genitalia, and digital rectal examination
  - Note character of onset (sudden or subacute), duration (minutes, hours, or days), location (generalized or localized), quality (sharp or dull, moderate or severe, constant or intermittent), and previous episodes
  - Palpate testicle and spermatic cord to assess for tenderness, effusion, subcutaneous emphysema, size, and lie of testicle, and assess for hernias
  - Transilluminate for presence of fluid
  - "Blue dot sign": Bluish discoloration along upper pole seen in about 20% of cases of torsion of the testicular appendix and due to infarction and necrosis
  - "Prehn's sign": Relief of pain with elevation of the testis in testicular torsion
- If testicular torsion is suspected, emergent detorsion is necessary, generally by a urologic specialist
- Culture for *Neisseria gonorrhoeae* and *Chlamydia trachomatis* in sexually active males before urinalysis
- Urinalysis in all patients: Elevated WBC or RBC levels suggest infection (e.g., epididymitis)
- Ultrasound of the testicles using color Doppler measures blood flow and evaluates for masses
- Radionucleotide scintigraphy may also be used to assess blood flow
- Recent studies have advocated the use of MRI

Treatment

- Testicular torsion is a surgical emergency
  - Immediate detorsion is necessary to salvage the testicle
  - If surgery unavailable, attempt manual detorsion
  - Detorsion maneuver: Infiltrate spermatic cord with 10–20 mL of 1% lidocaine, then twist testes counterclockwise on left or clockwise on right; successful detorsion is indicated by immediate relief
  - Urologic referral is indicated emergently if detorsion is unsuccessful; also refer for orchiopexy
- Incarcerated inguinal hernias and testicular rupture require surgical repair
- Epididymitis
  - Appropriate antibiotic therapy (empiric treatment)
  - NSAIDs and scrotal elevation for pain control
  - Viral causes require only supportive care
- Varicocele requires urology referral to optimize fertility
- Henoch-Schönlein purpura: Medical management
- Tumor: Resection
- UTI/pyelonephritis: Appropriate antibiotic therapy

165. Tinnitus

Tinnitus is a perception of noise (usually ringing, buzzing, or hissing) in the ears, which may be constant or intermittent, temporary or permanent. The pitch and other characteristics of tinnitus should be identified, if possible, to more effectively narrow the differential diagnosis. Additionally, the presence or absence of associated symptoms, including hearing deficits, further narrow the differential, and a hearing test is indicated in most cases of tinnitus when the diagnosis is unclear. The degree of distress caused by tinnitus varies widely.

Differential Diagnosis

- Acute or chronic otitis media
- Impacted cerumen
- Eustachian tube dysfunction
  - "Ocean roar" that may wax and wane with respiration
- Dysfunctional hearing aid
- Presbycusis (high pitch)
- Idiopathic (low pitch)
- Noise-induced hearing loss (high pitch)
- Meniere's disease
  - Triad of tinnitus, hearing loss, and vertigo
- Ototoxicity secondary to drugs
  - High pitch
  - May persist after medication (e.g., aminoglycosides)
  - May be dose-related (e.g., aspirin)
- Trauma
  - Commonly associated with airbag, whiplash, barotrauma
  - May have ruptured tympanic membrane
- TMJ syndrome
  - Nonpulsatile tinnitus (Costen's syndrome)
  - Associated jaw symptoms (e.g., pain, clicking)
- Migraine headache
- Vascular disease (e.g., atherosclerosis, diabetic vasculopathy, arteriovenous malformation, small vessel disease, hypertension)
- Stroke
- Otosclerosis
  - Associated with chronic otitis media or tympanic membrane trauma
- Pseudotumor cerebri
- Tumor
  - Glomus tympanicum or jugulare: Pulsatile tinnitus with hearing loss
  - Acoustic neuroma: Unilateral hearing loss and tinnitus, headache
- Infections (e.g., meningitis, Lyme disease, rubella)
- Less common etiologies ("zebras") include thyroid disease, Paget's disease, myoclonus of palatal muscles, fetal insults (infections, toxins), sickle cell disease, osteogenesis imperfecta, neurosyphilis, symptomatic Chiari malformation, late onset congenital hearing loss, dissecting aneurysm, carotid cancer, and multiple sclerosis

Workup and Diagnosis

- History and physical exam, including medication history and complete head and neck examination
  - Include neurologic and/or systemic exam if indicated by history
  - Evaluate temporomandibular joint for clicking, popping, and dislocation
- Tympanometry to diagnose otitis media and eustachian tube dysfunction
- Full audiology evaluation if possible sensorineural etiology
- Consider CBC (anemia) and glucose tolerance test (occult diabetes mellitus)
- Head CT scan is indicated if glomus tumor is suspected (delineates base of skull involvement)
- MRI (with enhancement) if possible Chiari malformation, multiple sclerosis, pseudotumor cerebri, or acoustic neuroma
- Angiography
- MRA if CT and MRI are negative but vascular etiology is suspected
- Consider referral to otolaryngologist or neurologist
- Consider screening for secondary depression or insomnia, because this is common in patients with tinnitus

Treatment

- Treat underlying cause if possible
- Discontinue ototoxic medications
- Presbycusis: Hearing aids
- Tinnitus retraining therapy may reduce tinnitus by habituation training
- Masking devices may be used to create a low level sound to decrease or eliminate perceived tinnitus
- Biofeedback or stress reduction may be useful, because tolerance to tinnitus decreases with stress and fatigue
- Surgery to correct conductive defect with outer or middle ear disease or to remove tumors
- Cochlear implants are indicated for severe hearing loss in patients that do not benefit from hearing aids
- Botulinum toxin injection is used for myoclonus of palatal muscles
- Treat underlying depression and insomnia if present

166. Toe Pain/Swelling

Toe pain and swelling can be caused by local processes such as infection or trauma, or it may be a symptom of a systemic disorder, such as rheumatoid arthritis, endocarditis, or atherosclerotic vascular disease. Gout, or podagra, is the most common cause of pain, redness, and swelling of the great toe (first metatarsophalangeal joint). It is often so severe that the weight of a bed sheet can be excruciating.

Differential Diagnosis

- Gout
  - Monosodium urate crystal deposition occurs secondary to hyperuricemia
  - Severe pain, redness, and swelling occurring in one joint (80% of cases), usually of the lower extremity, and most classically at the metatarsophalangeal joint of the great toe (podagra)
  - Tophi: Collections of solid urate in connective tissue
- Ingrown toenail
  - Causes severe pain in the distal nail folds with associated erythema, edema, and tenderness
- Trauma
  - Contusion
  - Fracture
- Pseudogout
  - Calcium pyrophosphate deposition disease
  - Can affect the toe, but the knee is most common
- Seronegative spondyloarthropathy
  - Psoriatic arthritis: Spondyloarthropathy involving middle-aged patients at multiple joints associated with classic skin lesions
  - Reiter's syndrome: Arthritis, uveitis, urethritis
- Septic arthritis
  - Fever, joint redness, pain with passive and active range of motion
  - Most often due to skin flora such as *Staphylococcus aureus* and various streptococci
  - *Neisseria gonorrhoeae* in young sexually active adults
  - Often associated with previous penetrating trauma to the toe
- Less common etiologies ("zebras") include cholesterol emboli, infective endocarditis, Lyme disease (presents as monoarticular arthritis in 10% of cases), and paronychia (bacterial infection of the posterior nail folds)

Workup and Diagnosis

- History and physical examination
- Initial laboratory studies may include CBC, electrolytes, BUN/creatinine, calcium, magnesium, phosphorus, ESR
  - Blood cultures and Lyme titers may be indicated
  - Iron studies (ferritin, iron, TIBC) may be useful if suspect pseudogout, as many patients have underlying hemochromatosis)
- Aspiration of the affected joint and synovial fluid analysis
  - Look for infection, inflammation, blood (hemarthrosis of trauma), and crystals
  - Gram stain, culture, and polarized light microscopy
  - Fluid cell counts typically reveal <50,000 white blood cells/mL in inflammatory processes, and >50,000 white blood cells in infectious arthritis
  - Gout: Needle-shaped, negatively birefringent crystals
  - Pseudogout: Linear-shaped weakly positively birefringent crystals
- Radiographs may reveal fractures, chondrocalcinosis (pseudogout), signs of osteomyelitis (septic arthritis), or erosive distal bone changes (psoriatic arthritis)

Treatment

- Gout: NSAIDs, corticosteroids, colchicines for acute attacks; colchicine, urate-lowering agents (e.g., allopurinol, probenecid) for chronic management
- Ingrown toenails: Warm soaks, removal of toenail if persistent
- Pseudogout: NSAIDs, corticosteroids, colchicines for acute attacks; NSAIDs, colchicine, urate for chronic management
- Trauma: Most closed toe fractures can be treated with stiff-soled shoes (to unload the metatarsal heads); "buddy-tape" immobilization may help relieve pain; rest, ice, NSAIDs, elevation
- Reiter's syndrome: Prednisone, indomethacin, sulfasalazine, methotrexate; local injection of steroid
- Septic arthritis: Treatment is based on clinical scenario and initial Gram stain; ceftriaxone for gram-negative infections, cefazolin for gram positives, add gentamicin for pseudomonal infections

167. Toothache

Toothache or tooth pain is caused when the nerve root of a tooth becomes irritated. Tooth infection, decay, injury, or loss of a tooth are the most common causes of dental pain. Pain may also occur after an extraction (removal of a tooth). Pain sometimes originates from other areas and radiates to the jaw, thus being perceived as tooth pain, most commonly from the temporomandibular joint, ear, and even occasionally cardiac problems.

Differential Diagnosis

- Pulp pain (pulpalgia) secondary to dental caries
- Traumatic tooth injury (e.g., tooth fracture, restoration fracture, avulsion)
- Traumatic occlusion
  - Secondary to a new restoration or bruxing
  - Galvanic "shock" due to contact by two dissimilar metals (e.g., gold crown with amalgam filling)
- Periradicular or periapical pain due to infection of the tooth root or abscess formation
- Referred pain from a tooth in the opposing arch
- Sinusitis
  - Maxillary sinusitis is the most common extraoral source of tooth pain
  - All or most teeth in the upper arch may become sensitive secondary to sinusitis
- Headache
- Temporomandibular joint pain (TMJ)
- Trigeminal neuralgia
- Barodontalgia from high altitudes
- "Dental migraine"
  - Associated with patients with depression
- Salivary gland disorders (e.g., Sjögren's syndrome, systemic lupus erythematosus)
- Otitis media and/or mastoiditis
- Angina pectoris
- Dry socket (osteitis)

Workup and Diagnosis

- History and ear, nose, throat, neck, and cardiac exam and intraoral exam should include mobility tests, percussion, electric pulp test, and thermal tests (ice)
  - Tooth mobility is tested by using the back ends of two mouth mirrors on both sides of the tooth
  - Reversible pulpitis pain is sharp, intermittent pain of short duration that is provoked by hot, cold, sweets, or biting; the pain does not linger more than a few seconds when the stimulus is removed
  - Irreversible pulpitis pain lasts more than 30 seconds upon withdrawal of the stimulus and may occur spontaneously, such as when sleeping
  - If an abscess is present, the tooth may be slightly elevated in its socket and mobile
  - Periapical abscesses may have systemic findings such as lymphadenopathy or fever
  - Toothache or TMJ pain in the morning may occur due to bruxing at night
- Transillumination may show fracture lines in teeth
- Pulp necrosis will not have any response to stimulation or via the electrical pulp tester
- Dental radiographs
- Consider sinus X-rays or CT scan if sinusitis likely
- Consider referral to dentist (e.g., tooth decay, abscess) or otolaryngologist (e.g., mastoiditis)

Treatment

- Reversible pulpitis from tooth decay can be treated with a restoration (e.g., filling or crown)
- Irreversible pulpitis requires root canal or tooth extraction if the tooth is not salvageable
- Incision and drainage of an abscess will often result in instant relief of pain
- Penicillin for oral infections (clindamycin if severe)
- Appropriate oral antibiotics (e.g. amoxicillin, trimethoprim-sulfamethoxazole) for sinusitis or otitis
- TMJ: avoidance of gum chewing and bruxing, bite block, NSAIDs, topical ice massage
- Migraine: pain relievers (e.g., acetaminophen, NSAIDs) migraine specific medications (e.g., triptans) and preventative therapy (e.g., gabapentin, riboflavin)

168. Tremor

Tremors are abnormal, rhythmic, involuntary movements. They are classified as resting and intention or action tremors, the former occurring at rest (resting tremor) or in a static position (postural tremor), such as when holding the arms outstretched, and the latter occurring or increasing with purposeful activity, such as reaching for an object. A very common type of resting tremor is the physiologic tremor, which is not usually visible, but can be enhanced by anxiety, medications (e.g., caffeine), and other circumstances.

Differential Diagnosis

Resting tremors
• Parkinson's disease
  –"Pill-rolling" appearance
  –Associated cog-wheel rigidity, shuffling gait, akinesis, and/or depression
• Benign familial or essential tremor
  –Especially common with head tremor (e.g., actress Katherine Hepburn)
  –Positive family history
  –No other neurologic findings
• Drug or toxin-induced tremors (e.g., MPTP)
• Postural tremors: Elicited when a limb is held up against gravity; caused by metabolic conditions (e.g., thyrotoxicosis)
• Voluntary movement (hyperkinetic) tremors
• Wilson's disease
• Stroke
• Cerebellar disease

Movement tremors
• Intentional tremor: Occurs with movement toward a target; associated with a cerebellar deficit which would inhibit (e.g., multiple sclerosis, midbrain injury or stroke)

Workup and Diagnosis

• Evaluation of tremors includes a complete history and physical examination with attention to the onset and other characteristics of the tremor; medication history; a limited general physical examination and a comprehensive neurologic examination
• CT or MRI of head to rule out mass lesions, CVA, and normal pressure hydrocephalus
• Initial labs may include TSH, T_4, CBC, vitamin B_{12} and folate, RPR, and a comprehensive metabolic panel (electrolytes, calcium, glucose, BUN/creatinine, liver function tests, and albumin)
• Essential or familial tremor is diagnosed by excluding other etiologies and by a positive response to propranolol
• Parkinson's disease is diagnosed by the characteristic constellation of symptoms and response to treatment (Parkinson's is often diagnosed and treated before tremor develops)
• Toxicology screen to rule out drug ingestion
• The following types of movement may be confused with tremor, but are actually separate entities
  –Tics are usually unifocal and slower and are not tremors
  –Chorea causes jerky irregular movements
  –Myoclonus is rapid and irregular
  –Athetosis and dystonia are slow movements
  –Asterixis results from inhibition of muscle contractions due to hepatic encephalopathy

Treatment

• Parkinson's disease
  –Anticholinergic medications (e.g., benztropine)
  –Amantidine
  –Levodopa-carbidopa
  –Dopamine agonists (e.g., bromocriptine)
  –Selegiline treats symptoms, but may also have a neuroprotective effect that slows disease progression
  –Surgical intervention had been the used in the past
  –Transplantation of fetal nigral cells into the putamen is under investigation
• Essential or familial tremor responds well to propranolol (10–80 mg BID), primidone, mysoline, or low-dose valium; however, treatment is only symptomatic
• Thyrotoxicosis is treated by surgery or nuclear ablation, propranolol, and/or antithyroid medications (tapazole or propylthiouracil)
• Drug and alcohol withdrawal is treated with detoxification
• Wilson's disease is treated with chelation

169. Unequal Pulses

Unequal pulses is a difference in blood pressure measurements between both arms or between the arms and the legs. The presence of unequal pulses can help diagnose significant underlying disease. A thorough vascular examination is an integral part of every cardiac exam.

Differential Diagnosis

- Atherosclerosis
  - Most common cause of unequal pulses
  - Manifestations include claudication, rest pain, ischemic ulcers, and gangrene
- Aortic dissection
  - Sharp, "tearing" chest or back pain
  - Etiologies include hypertension, Marfan's syndrome, bicuspid aortic valve, cocaine, trauma
- Aortic aneurysm
  - Focal or diffuse dilation 50% larger than normal diameter of vessel
  - Etiologies include atherosclerosis (most common for abdominal, descending thoracic aneurysms), cystic medial necrosis (most common for ascending aneurysms), connective tissue disorders (Marfan's, Ehlers-Danlos), congenital abnormalities (bicuspid aortic valve), syphilitic aortitis, spondyloarthropathies, vasculitis
- Takayasu's disease ("pulseless disease")
  - Idiopathic inflammatory disorder of aorta
  - Most common in women aged 10–40 years
  - Often presents with systemic complaints (fever, malaise, weight loss, fatigue)
  - Aortic inflammation causes narrowing of aortic branches, ultimately resulting in vascular insufficiency
- Coarctation of aorta
  - 6–8% of all congenital heart disease
  - More common in males
  - May rarely result in diminished left brachial pulse when origin of left subclavian artery is distal to coarctation
  - Narrowing of section of aortic arch resulting in decreased BP in lower extremities, may present as HTN in upper extremities
  - May also have bicuspid aortic valve, ventricular septal defect, patent ductus arteriosus, left ventricular outflow obstruction
- Subclavian steal syndrome
  - Syncope or dizziness following exercise of the arms
- Compartment syndrome
  - Increased pressure in a closed compartment may decrease the blood pressure to tissues
  - Look for the "five P's" (pain, pallor, pulselessness, paresthesia, paralysis)

Workup and Diagnosis

- History and physical examination
  - Elicit risk factors and identify predisposing conditions
  - Atrophic changes and dependent rubor suggest atherosclerosis
  - Pulsatile abdominal mass and abdominal bruit suggest aortic aneurysm
  - Hypertension, diastolic murmur of aortic insufficiency, and left pleural effusion suggest aortic dissection
  - Continuous murmur suggests coarctation of the aorta
  - Asymmetric blood pressure suggests aortic dissection, coarctation of the aorta, or Takayasu's disease
- ABI of systolic pressure <0.9 is consistent with peripheral arterial disease; values <0.5 are consistent with severe ischemia
- Chest X-ray may reveal widened mediastinum, pleural effusion, and tracheal deviation in aortic dissection; "rib notching" is due to intercostal artery collateral channels in coarctation of the aorta
- CT or MRA may be used to diagnose Takayasu's, aortic aneurysm, and peripheral arterial disease
- MRA, transesophageal echocardiogram, or CT scan are used to diagnose aortic dissection
- Angiography is the definitive test for Takayasu's arteritis, peripheral artery disease, aortic dissection, and coarctation of the aorta

Treatment

- Atherosclerosis
  - Nonpharmacologic interventions include exercise, smoking cessation, lipid-lowering therapy, aggressive blood sugar control, adequate foot care
  - Medical therapy includes antiplatelet agents (aspirin, dipyridamole, clopidogrel), pentoxifylline, cilostazol
  - Revascularization procedures may be necessary
- Aortic dissection requires prompt, aggressive therapy to lower BP and decrease left ventricular contractility
  - All patients should be treated with β-blockers
  - Surgery may be indicated
- Aortic aneurysm: Blood pressure reduction; surgical correction if symptomatic, large, or rapidly expanding
- Takayasu's disease: Corticosteroids, methotrexate, and possible revascularization procedures
- Coarctation of aorta is treated with angioplasty or surgical correction
- Compartment syndrome requires immediate decompression by fasciotomy

170. Urinary Stream (Decreased)

A perceived or observed decrease in the strength or flow of one's urine stream is a common complaint. This is often of concern to the patient because of the concern about both a serious medical problem and the slowing of urination and associated dribbling or incomplete emptying that accompanies the decreased stream intensity. Benign prostatic hypertrophy is by far the most common etiology of this complaint, and it is often accompanied by nocturia, urgency, frequency, dribbling, and incomplete emptying.

Differential Diagnosis

- Benign prostatic hyperplasia
  - Most common cause of decreased urinary stream in men >40
- Urethral stricture
  - May be congenital or acquired
- Chronic urethritis
  - May be secondary to stricture or chronic infection
- Prostate cancer
  - More frequent in men >40
- Neuropathic bladder
  - Spinal cord trauma
  - Herniated disc
  - Multiple sclerosis
  - Spina bifida
  - CVA
  - Parkinson's disease
  - Nerve injury secondary to pelvic surgery (e.g., prostatectomy)
- Bladder neck contracture
  - May be congenital or acquired (e.g., post-prostatectomy)
- Urethral or bladder foreign body
- Bladder stones
- Bladder neck cancer
- Urethral cancer
- Urethral polyp
- Posterior urethral valves
  - Frequently presents with recurrent UTIs

Workup and Diagnosis

- History and physical examination, including abdomen, back, genitalia (palpate penis for areas of tenderness or induration), digital rectal examination, neurologic exam
  - Note previous urinary tract instrumentation and STDs
  - Exploration of urethra with catheter to check for obstruction and postvoid residual (normal <100 mL)
- Initial labs include urinalysis (pyuria indicates secondary infection), urine culture and sensitivity, CBC (may reveal leukocytosis in infection, anemia in chronic disease), BUN/creatinine (elevated in acute renal failure, such as obstruction), and electrolytes
- Consider PSA, which is elevated in prostate cancer and prostatitis; may be mildly elevated in BPH
- Consider urine cytology and alkaline phosphatase (elevated in metastatic prostate cancer)
- Uroflowmetry: Calculate urine flow rate during timed void (normal 20–25 mL/second; <10 indicates obstruction)
- Consider renal ultrasound to rule out hydronephrosis and stones
- Consider abdominal/pelvic CT scan to detect stones and workup cancer
- Consider cystoscopy (to rule out cancer and anatomic problems), retrograde urethrography (to assess for strictures), voiding cystourethrogram (pressure/volume curves), transrectal ultrasound with needle biopsy (prostate CA), and/or intravenous pyelogram (stones and anatomic abnormalities)

Treatment

- Initial evaluation for urinary retention, which must be treated immediately with catheterization to prevent additional injury and relieve pain; thereafter, evaluation and treatment of infection and pain is indicated
- BPH: "Watchful waiting," α-blockers, 5α-reductase inhibitors, TURP or other transurethral procedures, and/or open prostatectomy
- Urethral stricture: Dilation, lysis, open surgical repair
- Chronic urethritis/prostatitis: Long-term antibiotics
- Prostate cancer may require prostatectomy or no intervention, depending on stage of the cancer and patient issues (e.g., age, co-morbid conditions)
- Bladder cancer: Transurethral resection, intravesical chemotherapy; radical cystectomy for late disease, external radiation, and/or systemic chemotherapy
- Neuropathic bladder: Parasympatholytic medications, intermittent or permanent catheterization, or surgical options (section of sacral nerve roots, ureteral diversion, and/or artificial sphincter)

171. Urticaria

Urticaria, also known as hives, is a very common clinical presentation characterized by transient (<12 hours), itchy dermal wheals. Angioedema is defined as subcutaneous or mucosal (often of the lips) swelling that is episodic and recurrent; it may occur alone or in association with urticaria. Chronic idiopathic urticaria and/or angioedema in children may be exacerbated during puberty.

Differential Diagnosis

- Idiopathic urticaria without angioedema
  - Most common diagnosis in patients with hives
  - Often related to food or drug allergies, bites, or stings
  - 25% of patients with one episode will progress to chronic urticaria
- Chronic urticaria
  - Idiopathic in 50% of cases
  - Chronic idiopathic urticaria spontaneously resolves within 2 years in 80% of patients
  - Criterion for chronic urticaria is duration of more than 6 weeks
- Occult infection (e.g., sinusitis, oral infection, cholecystitis, vaginitis, prostatitis, hepatitis, HIV, tinea manus or pedis)
- Malignancy
- Thyroid disease
- Drugs (e.g., radiocontrast media, penicillin, salicylates, benzoates, azo dyes)
  - May result in life-threatening episodes of urticaria and acute angioedema that can lead to anaphylaxis
- Urticaria secondary to physical stimuli [e.g., exercise (cholinergic), vibratory pressure, sun exposure (solar urticaria), cold exposure]
  - Dermographism occurs in 5% of the population; manifests as a physical urticaria that arises in the distribution line of a scratch or rubbed skin area
- Hereditary or acquired deficiency of complement factor C1
  - Generally appears as episodic angioedema in the absence of urticaria
  - Only in the absence of urticaria should hereditary or acquired complement deficiency be considered
- Angioedema-urticaria-eosinophilia syndrome
  - Associated with elevated serum IgE, fever, and fluid retention during an acute attack
- Urticarial vasculitis
  - Presents as urticaria that lasts longer than 12–24 hours
  - Associated with autoimmune disease (e.g., systemic lupus erythematosus)
- Cutaneous mastocytosis/urticaria pigmentosa

Workup and Diagnosis

- Complete history and physical examination
  - Family history of angioedema, anaphylaxis, etc.
  - Seasonal or activity-related (work/home) symptoms
  - Note whether urticaria occurs after ingestion of certain foods or with physical stimuli (e.g., exercise, pressure)
  - Physical exam should evaluate for underlying occult infections (e.g., UTI, vaginal yeast infection, tinea)
  - Firmly trace the blunt tip of a cotton applicator across the patient's back; patients with dermographism will develop a pruritic urticarial wheal within 5 minutes
- Determine whether the patient has isolated urticaria, urticaria with angioedema, or isolated angioedema
- Consider sinus X-rays, T_4, TSH, and thyroid antibodies
- In isolated angioedema without urticaria, check C2, C4, and/or C1 esterase inhibitor serum levels
- IgE level measurement is indicated if angioedema-urticaria-eosinophilia syndrome is suspected
- If urticarial lesions last longer than 12–24 hours, a punch biopsy of the involved skin is indicated to confirm the presence of vasculitis
- Perform age-appropriate malignancy screening
- If a cause cannot be found, consider referral to a dermatologist to rule out an occult etiology, although many cases will ultimately be deemed idiopathic

Treatment

- Identify and avoid physical or drug triggers
- Systemic antihistamines (e.g., hydroxyzine, doxepin, cimetidine) are helpful and may be used alone or in combination with each other or with nonsedating antihistamines (e.g., loratidine, cetirizine, fexofenadine)
- Severe attacks with associated angioedema may require administration of prednisone and epinephrine (consider pen-type epinephrine injector such as Epi-Pen^R)
- Danazol is used to treat only the rare, hereditary subset of angioedema (without urticaria); it stimulates hepatic production of the dysfunctional or absent C1 esterase inhibitor, thereby normalizing the complement cascade
- Treat yeast, tinea, or bacterial infections of the skin, mucosa, sinuses, or other locations with appropriate antifungal or antibacterial preparations
- Treat thyroid disease if found

172. Vaginal Discharge

Vaginal discharge is a common complaint that is often accompanied by concerns about the presence of a sexually transmitted disease. *Candida* may present with extremely intense, often unbearable itch. Whenever one sexually transmitted disease is identified, a search for all other STDs is indicated in an effort to treat the individual patient as well as to prevent spread to others in the community or beyond. If an STD is identified, the patient should be encouraged to inform all sexual partners of the diagnosis.

Differential Diagnosis

- Physiologic
  - Many women will have a consistent, slightly clear, non-odor-producing discharge, either midcycle or premenstrually, particularly if they are on oral contraceptives
  - A change in odor, consistency, or color of discharge may signify that evaluation is necessary
  - Increased discharge is associated with pregnancy
- Sexually transmitted disease
  - *Trichomonas vaginalis:* "Strawberry cervix" with punctate erythema, flagellated oval organisms on wet mount
  - Gonorrhea/*Chlamydia* may be associated with pelvic pain/dysmenorrhea and dyspareunia
- Bacterial vaginosis
  - Various organisms and changes in normal flora with a characteristic fishy odor
  - Not considered an STD
  - Increases the risk of preterm delivery in pregnant women
- Alteration of normal vaginal flora and/or inflammatory response
  - *Candida albicans* overgrowth is more common with recent antibiotic use, poorly controlled diabetes, and/or pregnancy; presents with intensely pruritic, inflamed, and erythematous introitus
  - Doderlein's cytolysis (caused by an overgrowth of lactobacilli)
- Atrophic vaginitis
  - Common in postmenopausal women, especially those not on HRT
  - Poor coital lubrication, dyspareunia
  - Dysuria due to atrophic urethral tissue
- Foreign body vaginitis (e.g., retained tampon)
- Noninfectious irritant/allergic contact vaginitis (e.g., soaps, feminine pads, perfumes)
- Cervicitis (usually due to gonorrhea or *Chlamydia*)
- Cervical dysplasia, cancer, or polyps
- Vaginal or vulvar trauma or cancer

Workup and Diagnosis

- A focused history and physical examination are crucial, including a complete sexual and exposure history, and full abdominal and pelvic examination
  - A wet mount and KOH of the discharge are imperative
  - pH of the discharge may aid in diagnosis
  - A whiff test is done by smelling the discharge after KOH is added; a positive test reveals a fishy odor characteristic of bacterial vaginosis
- Initial labs may include CBC, urinalysis, urine culture, β-hCG, and gonorrhea and *Chlamydia* cultures
- Test and treat for other STDs when one STD is found (HIV, hepatitis B and C, syphilis)

pH		Discharge	Odor	Wet Mount
Trich	>4.5	yellow-green, copious	present	motile, flagellated
BV	>4.5	white-grey	fishy	clue cells
Candida	<4.5	white, curd-like	none	pseudo-hyphae
GC/chlamydia		mucopurulent	varies	PMNs
Atrophic vaginitis		thin, gray, watery	none	few epithelial cells

Treatment

- See most recent CDC guidelines for all STDs
- Trichomonas
  - Metronidazole single dose or for 7 days (avoid alcohol with metronidazole use)
  - Intravaginal clotrimazole if pregnant or unable to use metronidazole
- Gonorrhea
  - Oral ciprofloxacin or IM ceftriaxone
- *Chlamydia*
  - Azithromycin or doxycycline orally
- Bacterial vaginosis
  - Metronidazole single dose or for 7 days
- *Candida*
  - Clotrimazole cream or intravaginal suppository
  - Fluconazole single dose
- Atrophic vaginitis
  - Topical or oral hormone replacement if appropriate
- Advise to avoid douching/perfumed hygiene products

173. Vesicular & Bullous Lesions

Vesicular and bullous rashes must be approached systematically so that serious causes are not missed. Initially, a determination as to whether the lesions are focal or diffuse is made, followed by a history of the lesions, a review of systems, and a focused physical examination. For lesions that do not have an obvious diagnosis, referral to a dermatologist can be invaluable.

Differential Diagnosis

Localized
- Allergic contact dermatitis (e.g. rhus)
  - Localized vesicular and bullous eruptions
- Herpes-zoster or shingles
  - Due to reactivation of latent virus
  - More common in adults
  - Presents as painful vesicles on an erythematous base in a dermatomal distribution, beginning with fever, dysesthesia, and/or malaise
- Herpes simplex virus
  - Herpetic lesions present as painful, recurrent vesicles on an erythematous base
  - Type 1 usually affects oral mucosa and vermilion border
  - Genital HSV (most commonly HSV-2) may manifest as nonspecific symptoms (e.g., dysuria, urethritis)
- Bullous impetigo
  - Most common in children
  - Presents as flaccid vesicles and bullae with honey-colored crust
- Bites from many insects
- Many viral infections of childhood can present with focal vesicles, especially hand-foot-and-mouth disease
- Burns and friction blisters
  - Common causes of bullae, especially on hands
- Diabetics can develop bullae on the legs
- Dyshidrotic eczema (pompholyx)
  - Causes itching, scaling, and erythema, and minute vesicles and painful fissures

Diffuse
- Polymorphous light eruption
  - Common reaction to ultraviolet light
  - Presents as itchy vesicles or erythematous papules on sun-exposed areas
- Varicella or "chicken pox"
  - Presents with vesicles in crops, and in many stages of evolution
- Stevens-Johnson syndrome and toxic epidermal necrolysis (TEN)
  - Most commonly caused by medications
  - TEN is life threatening
- Blistering diseases like bullous pemphigoid, pemphigus vulgaris, and porphyria cutanea tarda present with coalescing vesicles and bullae

Workup and Diagnosis

- History and physical examination
  - Determine whether the lesions are focal or diffuse
  - Thorough review of systems
- Culture from bullous lesions is not usually indicated, because most bullous reactions to bacteria are due to toxin production; thus, the bacteria are not commonly found within the bulla itself
- If HSV-2 (genital herpes) is the suspected etiology of a vesicular eruption, viral culture is the gold standard for diagnosis; obtain a culture by lancing an intact vesicle and swabbing the contents and floor of the erosion; serum IgM and IgG antibodies can also aid in the diagnosis
- Suspected orolabial HSV-1 infection is diagnosed on the basis of a history of similar recurrent episodes
- Consider a viral etiology if the patient has low-grade fevers, myalgias, pharyngitis, or other systemic symptoms
- Skin biopsy is indicated if an autoimmune blistering disease is suspected. PCT, pemphigus, and pemphigoid have distinct microscopic features
- In patients with widespread bullae, also consider incipient toxic epidermal necrolysis. Drugs such as sulfonamides, certain antibiotics, and several anticonvulsants are the most likely causative agents. Skin biopsy may also aid in this diagnosis, but frozen sections must be examined urgently, since this disease can quickly prove fatal

Treatment

- HSV-1, HSV-2, and HZV can be effectively treated with antiviral medication (e.g., acyclovir, famciclovir). Early antiviral therapy may decrease the risk of post-herpetic neuralgia. HSV is infectious until all cutaneous lesions have crusted over
- Bullous impetigo can be treated with topical mupirocin, or systemic antibiotics (e.g., erythromycin, cephalexin)
- Dyshidrotic eczema can be difficult to treat. It is not curable, but can be controlled with high-potency topical steroid ointments and heavy emollients
- PMLE is preventable with sun avoidance and zinc- or titanium-based sun blocks. Topical steroids can diminish the pruritus that accompanies an episode
- SJS/TEN treatment consists of supportive care and discontinuing the offending drug, often requiring a burn center; IVIG and systemic steroids are sometimes used.
- Systemic immunosuppressants (e.g., prednisone, cyclosporin, azathioprine) are often necessary to control autoimmune bullous diseases like pemphigus

174. Vision Loss

Vision loss may be unilateral or bilateral; transient or persistent; of sudden or gradual onset; and painless or painful. Vision loss in one eye may be followed quickly by ensuing vision loss of the other eye, rendering the patient completely blind (e.g., untreated giant cell arteritis). In some situations, vision loss may be reversible with timely intervention. Vision loss may be a harbinger of more serious, even life-threatening, conditions (e.g., brain tumor, meningitis, giant cell arteritis, cavernous sinus thrombosis, mucormycosis).

Differential Diagnosis

Transient vision loss (<24 hours)
• Papilledema: Lasts seconds, bilateral
• Amaurosis fugax: Lasts minutes, unilateral
• Vertebrobasilar artery insufficiency: Lasts minutes, bilateral
• Migraine: Lasts 10–60 minutes
• Impending central retinal vein occlusion
• Ocular ischemic syndrome (carotid occlusive disease)
• Sudden change in blood pressure; orthostatic hypotension
• Transient acute increase in intraocular pressure (e.g., acute angle closure glaucoma, retro- or peribulbar hemorrhage)

Vision loss >24 hours: Sudden, painless
• Retinal artery or vein occlusion
• Ischemic optic neuropathy (must rule out giant cell/temporal arteritis to prevent permanent bilateral vision loss)
• Vitreous or aqueous hemorrhage (hyphema)
• Retinal detachment
• Other retinal or CNS disease (e.g., cortical blindness due to occipital lobe CVA)
• Exposure ("Welder's flash") or prolonged exposure to intense sunlight

Vision loss >24 hours: Gradual, painless
• Cataract
• Refractive error
• Open angle glaucoma
• Chronic retinopathy (e.g., age-related macular degeneration, diabetic retinopathy)
• Chronic corneal disease (e.g., corneal dystrophy)
• Optic neuropathy/atrophy (e.g., compressive lesion, toxic-metabolic cause, dominant optic neuropathy, radiation)
• Retinitis pigmentosa
• Pseudotumor cerebri

Vision loss >24 hours: Painful
• Acute angle closure glaucoma
• Optic neuritis (pain with extraocular motion)
• Orbital apex/superior orbital fissure/ cavernous sinus syndrome
• Uveitis
• Corneal hydrops (keratoconus)
• Ocular onchocerciasis ("river blindness")
 –Common cause of blindness in developing nations due to *Onchocerca volvulus* worm
• Corneal abrasion or ulcer
• Herpes simplex or zoster infection

Workup and Diagnosis

• History should include age, onset, tempo of vision loss, history of trauma, associated headache, medications, past history (e.g., carotid or cardiac disease, HTN, diabetes, vertigo, migraine, syphilis, ocular, orbital, cranial radiation, keratoconus), family history of vision loss, alcohol and tobacco use
• Physical exam should include a thorough eye examination, vision acuity, refractive error, color vision, blood pressure, refractive error, cranial examination, cranial nerve innervation, intraocular pressure, ocular media opacity (corneal edema, dystrophy, anterior chamber or vitreous cells, cataracts), and fundus and optic disc exam
• Consider a visual field exam and fluorescein angiogram
• Initial laboratory evaluation may include ESR, CRP, fasting blood glucose, Hgb_{A1C}, PPD, RPR, FTA-ABS, ACE level, vitamin B_{12}, and folate
• Consider CT/MRI of orbits and head with contrast, carotid Doppler, echocardiogram, electroretinography, and VEP (retinal dystrophies, optic neuropathies, nonphysiologic)
• Consider ophthalmologic consultation

Treatment

• Treat underlying causes (e.g., brain tumor, carotid stenosis, cardiac valvular vegetations, hypotension)
• Temporal arteritis: Systemic steroids
• Nonarteritic ischemic optic neuropathy: Aspirin
• Optic neuritis: Systemic steroids
• Glaucoma: Topical antiglaucoma medications; peripheral iridotomy for angle closure
• Retinal detachment: Surgical repair
• Cataracts: Surgical removal
• AV fistula: Embolize
• Cavernous sinus thrombosis: Antibiotics, anticoagulation
• Mucormycosis: Amphotericin B, debridement
• Pituitary apoplexy: Systemic steroids, neurosurgical intervention
• Herpes zoster: Systemic acyclovir
• Tolosa-Hunt: Systemic steroid
• Keratoconus/corneal hydrops: Cycloplegic, hypertonic (5%) NaCl ointment, corneal transplant

175. Weight Gain

Weight gain is a very common complaint in adult medicine and has a vast differential diagnosis. The key to diagnosis is often a good history and physical examination. It is important to quantify the degree and rapidity of weight gain by comparing old weights in the chart and questioning the patient.

Differential Diagnosis

- Primary obesity due to overeating and a sedentary lifestyle
- Medication side effects (e.g., oral contraceptives, corticosteroids, antidepressants, benzodiazepines, hypoglycemics, and anticonvulsants)
- Overeating secondary to nicotine withdrawal, depression, binge phase of bulimia nervosa
- Pregnancy
- Pre-eclampsia/eclampsia
- Premenstrual syndrome
- Nephrotic syndrome
  - Renal loss of protein results in decreased intravascular oncotic pressure, leading to water "leakage" to extravascular compartments (e.g., edema, ascites)
  - Due to primary renal disease or secondary causes (e.g., diabetes mellitus)
- Acute or chronic liver disease
  - Decreased hepatic protein production results in decreased intravascular oncotic pressure, leading to water "leakage" to extravascular compartments (e.g., edema, ascites)
- Congestive heart failure
- Hypothyroidism
- Diabetes mellitus
- Polycystic ovarian syndrome
  - Associated with hirsutism, menstrual irregularities, insulin resistance, obesity
- Cushing's syndrome
  - Excess cortisol levels due to ACTH-secreting adrenal adenoma, adrenal hyperplasia, ACTH-secreting ectopic tumor, or ACTH-secreting pituitary adenoma (Cushing's disease)
- Less common etiologies ("zebras") include hypothalamic lesions (e.g., tumor, infection), hyperphagia due to hyperthyroidism, acromegaly (growth hormone excess, usually due to a pituitary tumor), or growth hormone deficiency

Workup and Diagnosis

- Complete history and physical examination
  - Baseline weight, rapidity of weight gain, food diary, medication list, tobacco and/or alcohol use, menstrual history, review of systems, and screen for depression
  - Note body habitus (e.g., Cushing's often presents with moon facies, buffalo hump, and thin extremities)
  - Note body hair distribution (scarce in hypothyroidism; hirsutism in PCOS and Cushing's syndrome)
  - Note skin appearance (abdominal striae and easy bruising in Cushing's; acanthosis nigricans in diabetes)
  - Check for peripheral edema and ascites (CHF, nephrotic syndrome, liver disease, pre-eclampsia)
- Initial labs include CBC (leukocytosis in Cushing's, thrombocytopenia in pre-eclampsia), fasting glucose (elevated in diabetes and Cushing's), BUN/creatinine (rule out renal failure), urinalysis (excessive proteinuria and lipiduria in nephrotic syndrome; proteinuria in pre-eclampsia and diabetes), TSH (hypothyroidism), lipid profile (hypercholesterolemia in nephrotic syndrome, Cushing's, diabetes), albumin (decreased in nephrotic syndrome and liver disease), and urine β-hCG
- Further studies may include 24-hour urine (if urinalysis reveals >3 g proteinuria), LFTs (elevated in liver disease and pre-eclampsia), dexamethasone suppression test (rule out Cushing's), chest X-ray and/or echocardiogram (rule out CHF if pulmonary edema suspected on exam), abdominal ultrasound and/or CT scan (rule out liver or renal disease), and/or pelvic ultrasound (rule out polycystic ovaries)

Treatment

- Weight loss by low-calorie diet and exercise
- Discontinue or change offending medications if possible
- Treat underlying medical disorders
  - CHF: Diuretics, digoxin, ACE inhibitor, nitrates, salt restriction
  - Liver disease: Diuretics, paracentesis, salt restriction
  - Nephrotic syndrome: Diuretics, anticoagulation, nephrology referral
  - Cushing's disease: Surgery to remove tumor
  - Cushing's syndrome: Search for and treat the underlying cause (e.g., resection of tumor); diet
  - Depression: Antidepressants, counseling
  - Hypothyroidism: Thyroid hormone replacement
  - Diabetes: Oral medications, insulin, diet, exercise
  - Polycystic ovarian syndrome: Diet, oral contraceptives
  - Pregnancy: Prenatal care
  - Pre-eclampsia: Bedrest, magnesium sulfate, antihypertensive meds, deliver baby if necessary
  - Bulimia: Psychiatry referral

176. Weight Loss

Unexplained, involuntary weight loss (defined as loss of 5% of baseline body weight over 6–12 months) is a common clinical presentation and is nearly always a sign of a serious medical or psychiatric illness. Numerous studies have independently associated unintentional weight loss with various adverse health outcomes, including decreased functional status and increased mortality.

Differential Diagnosis

- Malignancy
  - Mediated by enhanced production of cytokines (e.g., TNF-α, interleukin-6)
- Gastrointestinal and malabsorption disorders (e.g., celiac disease, Crohn's disease, cystic fibrosis, PUD)
  - Diarrhea is often present
- Depression
  - Weight loss is one diagnostic criterion
  - Most common cause of weight loss in outpatient populations
- HIV infection
- Hypercalcemia
  - Usually occurs in patients with cancer
- Advanced cardiac and pulmonary disease
  - CHF ("cardiac cachexia")
  - COPD
- Chronic drug use (e.g., alcohol, nicotine, lead, opiates, CNS stimulants)
- Hyperthyroidism
  - Increased appetite and increased energy expenditure
  - May present with tachycardia, hypertension, brisk reflexes, and ophthalmopathy
- Uncontrolled diabetes mellitus
- Hyperemesis gravidarum
  - Pathologic exaggeration of early-pregnancy nausea
  - Elevated β-hCG and estrogen levels
- Adrenal insufficiency
  - Anorexia, nausea, and fatigue are common
- Anorexia nervosa
  - May present with low albumin, parotid enlargement, lesions on knuckles and diminished tooth enamel from induced vomiting, and menstrual irregularities
- Failure to thrive (infants)
  - Parental neglect, emotional deprivation
  - Improper mixing of formula
  - Significant heart (shunts) or lung disease
  - Inborn errors of metabolism
- Intestinal parasites

Workup and Diagnosis

- Comprehensive history and physical examination, including assessment of diet and caloric intake
- In patients with adequate caloric intake, endocrine and malabsorptive disorders are more likely
- Initial tests may include CBC, serum chemistries, glucose (to rule out diabetes), thyroid function tests, ESR, and albumin and/or prealbumin
- HIV testing if risk factors are present
- Chest X-ray in smokers
- Age-appropriate cancer screening (e.g., mammography, fecal occult blood testing, flexible sigmoidoscopy or colonoscopy)
- Morning (AM) cortisol and ACTH stimulation test if suspect adrenal insufficiency
- Consider upper GI endoscopy, colonoscopy, and GI consult

Treatment

- Identify and address the underlying cause
- Appetite disturbance of depression may be reversed by antidepressant medications
- Pancreatic enzymes for pancreatic malabsorption
- Referral to nutritionist if necessary
- Referral to social services if necessary
- Anorexia of malignancy and AIDS can be treated with megestrol acetate or dronabinol
- Aggressive treatment of anorexia nervosa, including evaluation for electrolyte and cardiac disorders and consultation with psychiatrist or psychologist

177. Wide Pulse Pressure

Pulse pressure is the difference between systolic and diastolic blood pressures. Wide pulse pressure is a difference greater than 60–70 mmHg. This often results from conditions that produce an increase in stroke volume.

Differential Diagnosis

- Atherosclerosis
  - Large arteries stiffen with age, resulting in increased systolic blood pressure and, thus, increased pulse pressure
- Chronic aortic regurgitation (acute AR does not result in wide pulse pressure)
  - Results in heart failure, syncope, and/or angina
  - Exam may reveal early diastolic murmur
  - Corrigan's pulse: Rapid rise and rapid fall
  - Hill's sign: Systolic blood pressure of lower extremities >20 mmHg more than systolic blood pressure in arms
  - de Musset's sign: Head bobs with each heartbeat
  - Causes include rheumatic heart disease, idiopathic root dilatation, Marfan's disease, and endocarditis
- Thyrotoxicosis
  - Associated with nervousness, sweating, heat intolerance, tachycardia, weight loss
  - Thyroid nodule(s) may be present
- Increased cardiac output states
  - Fever
  - Anemia
  - Pregnancy
  - Anxiety
- Patent ductus arteriosus
  - "Bounding" pulses
  - Continuous murmur through diastole and systole
- Complete heart block
  - Often secondary to MI or CAD
- Sinus bradycardia
- Systemic AV fistula
- Aortic dissection
- Endocarditis
- Increased intracranial pressure

Workup and Diagnosis

- History and physical examination
- Initial labs may include CBC and TSH
- Consider blood cultures, lipid panel, free T_4, and free T_3
- Evaluate for cardiac causes, especially if murmurs or abnormal pulses are appreciated on exam
- ECG may reveal LVH, complete heart block (no relationship between P and QRS), irregularly irregular rhythm (atrial fibrillation), and evidence of CAD
- Echocardiogram (transesophageal and transthoracic) may reveal abnormal valves or regurgitation
  - Transesophageal echocardiography is more useful than transthoracic for evaluation of aortic regurgitation
  - Transesophageal echocardiography is very sensitive and specific for diagnosing aortic dissection because it can evaluate both anatomically (dissection flap) and physiologically (flow between true and false lumen)
- Chest X-ray will show widening of mediastinum and enlargement of the aortic knob with aortic dissection
- CT scan may be indicated to evaluate for aortic dissection
- MRI is as sensitive and specific as TEE for diagnosing aortic dissection
- Aortography is not as good as transesophageal echocardiography for quantifying the amount of aortic regurgitation and also may not reveal two aortic lumens in cases of aortic dissection
- If suspect atherosclerosis, evaluate CAD risk stratification, cholesterol screening, stress testing, and cardiac catheterization as necessary

Treatment

- Assess hemodynamic stability
- Treat emergent causes as necessary
  - Immediate medical or surgical management of aortic dissection
  - Immediate blood cultures and IV antibiotic therapy for endocarditis
- Chronic atrial regurgitation: Aortic valve replacement may be necessary, especially if patient has a low ejection fraction; medical therapy (e.g., diuretics, vasodilators, pressors) may improve cardiac function
- Evaluate and treat underlying causes of anemia, fever, hyperthyroidism, increased intracranial pressure, chronic disease
- Hyperthyroidism: β-blockers for symptoms, antithyroid medications (e.g., PTU), radioactive iodine ablation, or thyroidectomy

178. Wrist & Hand Pain/Swelling

The wrist is composed of eight carpal bones that are held in alignment by a series of ligaments and cartilaginous connective tissue. Wrist pain is fairly common in primary care. Although carpal tunnel syndrome is one of the most common etiologies of wrist pain, pain and numbness in the hand is a more common presentation.

Differential Diagnosis

- Carpal tunnel syndrome
  - Most common cause of significant wrist discomfort and morbidity
  - Associated with repetitive use activities (e.g., typing)
  - Pain and numbness symptoms result from entrapment of the median nerve under the transverse ligament
- Overuse injury
- Osteoarthritis
- Tenosynovitis (DeQuervain's) of the radial wrist
  - Results from inflammation of the tendon sheaths of the extensor pollicis brevis and abductor pollis longus
- Ganglion cysts
  - Common growths of tendons and ligaments in the wrist area occurring on both the dorsal and ventral surface
  - They are compressible, round, often tender, and mobile
- Trauma
  - The most common mechanism of injury is a fall on the outstretched hand
  - The most commonly fractured carpal bone is the scaphoid
  - Other mechanisms include direct blows, crush injuries, fall on an angulated wrist, and severe twisting motions
- Fibromyalgia
- Compartment syndrome
- Chest or shoulder masses, resulting in compression of lymphatic or venous systems
- Venous thrombosis of the subclavian or distal veins
- Flaccid paralysis following a CVA
- Angioedema secondary to hymenoptera sting
- Rheumatologic disease
- Peripheral neuropathy
- Insect or animal bite/sting
- Infection (e.g., staphylococcus aureus, streptococci)

Workup and Diagnosis

- History and physical examination of the hand, wrist, elbow, and shoulder
  - Tinel's sign is positive if pain is elicited by tapping the anterior wrist
  - Phalen's sign is positive if wrist flexion for >30 seconds elicits pain or numbness
- Lab investigation is usually unnecessary, but may include rheumatoid factor, ANA, ESR, CBC, uric acid, TSH, β-hCG (pregnancy test)
- Standard X-rays include PA, lateral, and oblique views
- EMG and nerve conduction studies are indicated if carpal tunnel syndrome or other neuropathy is suspected
- Arthrocentesis with crystal analysis may be indicated if warmth and redness are noted in the wrist and MCP joints
- Bone scan may be necessary to evaluate for avascular necrosis, occult fracture, or bone infection
- Rarely, CT or MRI is indicated
- Shoulder/chest CT may be indicated to evaluate for masses resulting in nerve entrapment or vascular compromise

Treatment

- Corticosteroid injection for carpal tunnel improves symptoms in more than half of patients; surgical intervention to release the transverse ligament and decompress the nerve entrapment may be indicated
- NSAIDs reduce inflammation and use of cock-up splints applied during activities and while sleeping reduces strain from repetitive use and reduces symptoms
- Corticosteroid injection along tendon sheaths and wearing a thumb spica splint treat tenosynovitis
- Ganglion cysts are treated by draining the thick fluid and injecting with steroid; surgical removal is occasionally necessary
- Casting of suspected fractures and repeat X-ray in 7–9 days prevents complications of occult fracture
- Antihistamines and steroids treat swelling from stings
- Treat rheumatologic and medical causes
- Biofeedback and relaxation may be beneficial in selected cases

Index

Congenital mydriasis, as differential dx, for
pupillary dilation, 141
Congenital neck masses, as differential dx, for
neck masses, 110
Congenital scoliosis, as differential dx, for
scoliosis, 151
Congested liver, as differential dx, for abdominal
pain in upper quadrants, 6
Congestive heart failure (CHF), as differential dx
for cardiomegaly, 30
for cyanosis, 39
for delirium, 40
for dizziness/lightheadedness, 47
for fatigue, 59
for hemoptysis, 74
for jugular venous distension, 100
for nonproductive cough, 36
for orthopnea, 116
for palpitations, 119
for paroxysmal nocturnal dyspnea, 124
for periorbital edema, 129
for peripheral edema, 130
for productive cough, 37
for splenomegaly, 157
for stridor, 159
Conjunctivitis, as differential dx
for blurred vision, 22
for periorbital edema, 129
for photophobia, 131
for red eye, 147
Connective tissue diseases, as differential dx
for hematemesis/upper GI bleeding, 64
for lymphadenopathy, 103
for pleural rubs, 133
for Raynaud's phenomenon, 144
for shoulder pain/swelling, 154
Constipation, 35
Constipation, as differential dx
for abdominal mass, 4
for pelvic masses, 125
for rectal pain, 146
for testicular pain, 164
Constitutional delay of puberty, as differential dx,
for amenorrhea, 11
Constrictive pericarditis, as differential dx, for
jugular venous distension, 100
Contact dermatitis, as differential dx
for periorbital edema, 129
for pruritis with rash, 137
for scalp rash, 150
Contact lens problems, as differential dx, for
red eye, 147
Conversion disorder, as differential dx, for
paraplegia, 122
Convulsions/seizures. *See* Seizures/convulsions
Corneal abrasion, as differential dx
for blurred vision, 22
for photophobia, 131
for red eye, 147
for vision loss, 174
Corneal hydrops, as differential dx, for vision
loss, 174
Corneal opacity, as differential dx, for diplopia, 45
Coronary arteriovenous fistula, as differential dx,
for diastolic murmur, 104
Coronary artery disease (CAD), as differential dx
for dyspnea, 53
for fatigue, 59

Cor pulmonale, as differential dx
for cardiomegaly, 30
for cyanosis, 39
Cortical lesions, as differential dx, for
hypesthesia, 86
Corynebacterium, 137
Costochondritis, as differential dx
for breast pain/discharge, 27
for chest pain, 32
Cough
with hemoptysis, 74
nonproductive, 36
productive, 37
Crackles/rales, 38
"Cradle cap," 150
Cranial nerve disorder, as differential dx
for diplopia, 45
for pupillary dilation, 141
Craniopharyngioma, as differential dx, for
amenorrhea, 11
Creutzfeldt-Jakob disease, as differential dx, for
dementia, 42
Croup, as differential dx
for decreased/absent breath sounds, 29
for stridor, 159
Cruveilhier-Baumgarten murmur, as differential dx,
for abdominal bruit, 1
Cryoglobulinemia, as differential dx, for Raynaud's
phenomenon, 144
Cryptogenic organizing pneumonia, as
differential dx
for crackles/rales, 38
for nonproductive cough, 36
Cryptosporidium, 43
Cushing's syndrome, as differential dx
for amenorrhea, 11
for hyperglycemia, 79
for hypokalemia, 89
for weight gain, 175
Cutaneous mastocytosis, as differential dx, for
urticaria, 171
Cutaneous vasculitis, as differential dx
for Janeway lesions, 97
for Osler nodes, 117
CVA tenderness/flank pain, 61
Cyanosis, 39
Cyclospora, 43
Cyst, as differential dx
for abdominal mass, 4
for breast mass, 26
for breast pain/discharge, 27
Cystic fibrosis, as differential dx
for hemoptysis, 74
for hyperglycemia, 79
Cystic mastitis, as differential dx, for breast
mass, 26
Cystitis, as differential dx, for abdominal pain in
lower quadrants, 5
Cystosarcoma phylloides, as differential dx, for
breast mass, 26

Dacryocystitis/dacryoadenitis, as differential dx,
for periorbital edema, 129
"Dandruff," 150
Deconditioning, as differential dx, for
palpitations, 119
Deep dyspareunia, as differential dx, for
dyspareunia, 51

Newborns, pelvic masses in, 125
Night sweats, 112
Nodular lesions, 113
Nodular melanomas, as differential dx, for nodular lesions, 113
Nodules, as differential dx, for hoarseness, 77
Noise-induced hearing loss, as differential dx
  for hearing loss, 70
  for tinnitus, 165
Nonalcoholic steatohepatitis (NASH), as differential dx
  for abdominal pain in upper quadrants, 6
  for jaundice, 98
Nonallergic rhinitis with eosinophilia (NARES), as differential dx, for nasal congestion, 108
Nonepileptic seizures, as differential dx, for seizures/convulsions, 153
Noninfectious cystitis, as differential dx, for dysuria, 54
Noninfectious irritant/allergic contact vaginitis, as differential dx, for vaginal discharge, 172
Nonpalpable purpura, as differential dx, for purpura, 142
Nonproductive cough, 36
Normal "athletic" heart, 30
Norwalk virus, as differential dx, for acute diarrhea, 43
Nosebleed, 57
Numbness, 86, 123
Nummular eczema, as differential dx, for papulosquamous lesions, 121
Nutcracker esophagus, as differential dx, for dysphagia, 52
Nutrition/diet. See Diet/nutrition
Nystagmus, 114
Nystagmus blocking syndrome, as differential dx, for nystagmus, 114

Obesity, as differential dx
  for abdominal distension, 2
  for decreased/absent breath sounds, 29
  for fatigue, 59
  for hyporeflexia, 91
  for paroxysmal nocturnal dyspnea (PND), 124
Obsessive-compulsive disorder (OCD), as differential dx, for anxiety, 16
Obstructive sleep apnea, as differential dx
  for fatigue, 59
  for night sweats, 112
  for paroxysmal nocturnal dyspnea (PND), 124
Occipital lobe injury, as differential dx, for hallucinations, 67
Occupational trauma, as differential dx, for Raynaud's phenomenon, 144
Ocular cicatricial pemphigoid, as differential dx, for periorbital edema, 129
Ocular ischemic syndrome, as differential dx, for vision loss, 174
Ocular media opacity, as differential dx, for blurred vision, 22
Ocular onchocerciasis, as differential dx, for vision loss, 174
Olgilvie's syndrome, as differential dx
  for abdominal distension, 2
  for abdominal masses, 4
  for nausea/vomiting, 109
Onychomycosis, as differential dx, for nail disorders, 107

Open-angle glaucoma, as differential dx, for vision loss, 174
Opening snap, as differential dx, for gallops/extra heart sounds, 62
Optic-disc vasculitis, as differential dx, for papilledema, 120
Optic neuritis, as differential dx, for vision loss, 174
Optic neuropathy, as differential dx, for vision loss, 174
Oral hypoglycemia medications, as differential dx, for hypoglycemia, 88
Oral lesions, 115
Orbital apex, as differential dx, for vision loss, 174
Orbital disease, as differential dx, for diplopia, 45
Orbital fat herniation, as differential dx, for periorbital edema, 129
Orbital optic-nerve tumors, as differential dx, for papilledema, 120
Orbital vasculitis, as differential dx, for proptosis/exophthalmos, 136
Orchiectomy, as differential dx, for night sweats, 112
Orchitis, as differential dx, for scrotal masses, 152
Organomegaly, as differential dx, for abdominal masses, 4
Orthodromic AV reentrant tachycardia, as differential dx, for tachycardia, 161
Orthopnea, 116
Orthostatic hypotension, as differential dx
  for hypotension, 92
  for syncope, 160
  for vision loss, 174
Osgood-Schlatter disease, as differential dx, for knee pain/swelling, 101
Osler nodes, 117
Osler-Weber-Rendu syndrome, as differential dx, for hemoptysis, 74
Osmotic diarrhea, as differential dx, for chronic diarrhea, 44
Osteoarthritis, as differential dx
  for elbow pain/swelling, 56
  for knee pain/swelling, 101
  for wrist and hand pain/swelling, 178
Osteochondritis dessicans (OCD), as differential dx, for knee pain/swelling, 101
Osteomyelitis, as differential dx
  for fever, 60
  for knee pain/swelling, 101
  for night sweats, 112
Ostium primum atrial septal defect, as differential dx, for pericardial rubs, 128
Otitis externa, as differential dx
  for ear pain, 55
  for otorrhea (ear discharge), 118
Otitis media, as differential dx
  for ear pain, 55
  for hearing loss, 70
  for otorrhea (ear discharge), 118
  for tinnitus, 165
  for toothache, 167
Otomycosis, as differential dx, for otorrhea (ear discharge), 118
Otorrhea, 118
Otosclerosis, as differential dx, for tinnitus, 165
Ototoxicity, as differential dx, for tinnitus, 165
Ovarian cancer, as differential dx, for abdominal distension, 2

decreased urinary stream, 170
dysuria in, 54
hematuria in, 72
incontinence in, 94
polyuria in, 134
Urinary tract infection (UTI), as differential dx
for abdominal guarding, 3
for abdominal pain with rebound tenderness, 7
for abnormal uterine bleeding, 8
for delirium, 40
for dysmenorrhea, 50
for dysuria, 54
for female pelvic pain, 126
for hematuria, 72
for testicular pain, 164
Urolithiasis, as differential dx
for dysuria, 54
for flank pain/CVA tenderness, 61
Urticaria, 171
Urticarial vasculitis, as differential dx, for
urticaria, 171
Urticaria pigmentosa, as differential dx, for
urticaria, 171
Urticaria secondary to physical stimuli, as
differential dx, for urticaria, 171
Uterine fibroids, as differential dx
for abdominal masses, 4
for abnormal uterine bleeding, 8
for dysmenorrhea, 50
for female pelvic pain, 126
for pelvic masses, 125
Uterine polyps, as differential dx, for abnormal
uterine bleeding, 8
Uveitis, as differential dx
for papilledema, 120
for red eye, 147
for vision loss, 174

Vaginal discharge, 172
Vaginal trauma, as differential dx, for abnormal
uterine bleeding, 8
Vaginitis, as differential dx
for dysuria, 54
for female pelvic pain, 126
Valvular disease, as differential dx
for cardiomegaly, 30
for fatigue, 59
for syncope, 160
Varicella, as differential dx
for ear pain, 55
for stomatitis, 158
for vesicular and bullous lesions, 173
Varicocele, as differential dx
for scrotal masses, 152
for testicular pain, 164
Vascular disease, as differential dx, for
tinnitus, 165
Vasculitis, as differential dx
for acute diarrhea, 43
for paresthesias, 123
for Raynaud's phenomenon, 144
Vasculopathy, as differential dx, for blurred
vision, 22
Vasomotor rhinitis, as differential dx, for nasal
congestion, 108
Vasovagal episode, as differential dx
for dizziness/lightheadedness, 47
for syncope, 160

Venous hypertension, as differential dx, for
cyanosis, 39
Venous insufficiency, as differential dx, for
peripheral edema, 130
Venous sinus thrombosis, as differential dx, for
Babinski's sign, 20
Venous stasis, as differential dx, for restless
legs, 148
Venous thrombosis, as differential dx, for wrist
and hand pain/swelling, 178
Ventral hernia, as differential dx, for abdominal
distension, 2
Ventricular septal defect (VSD), as differential dx
for pericardial rubs, 128
for systolic murmur, 105
Ventricular tachycardia (VT), as differential dx
for palpitations, 119
for tachycardia, 161
Vertebral disc disease, as differential dx, for
restless legs, 148
Vertebral fracture, as differential dx, for low back
pain, 102
Vertebrobasilar insufficiency, as differential dx
for diplopia, 45
for vertigo, 47
for vision loss, 174
Vertigo, as differential dx, for diplopia, 45
Vertigo/dizziness/lightheadedness, 47
Vesicular lesions, 173
Vestibular dysfunction, as differential dx
for Romberg's sign, 149
for vertigo, 47
Vestibular nystagmus, as differential dx, for
nystagmus, 114
Vinyl chloride poisoning, as differential dx, for
Raynaud's phenomenon, 144
Viral conjunctivitis, as differential dx, for red
eye, 147
Viral exanthems, as differential dx, for rash with
fever, 143
Viral hepatitis, as differential dx, for jaundice, 98
Viral infection, as differential dx
for oral lesions, 115
for pericardial rubs, 128
for pruritis, 137
for vesicular and bullous lesions, 173
Viral keratitis, as differential dx, for red
eye, 147
Viral pharyngitis/laryngitis, as differential dx, for
sore throat, 156
Viral pleurisy, as differential dx, for pleural
rubs, 133
Vision
blurred, 22
loss of, 174
See also Eye
Vitamin A intoxication, as differential dx, for
hypercalcemia, 78
Vitamin B$_{12}$ deficiency, as differential dx
for anemia, 13
for anosmia, 15
for dementia, 42
for paresthesias, 123
for Romberg's sign, 149
Vitamin C deficiency, as differential dx, for
stomatitis, 158
Vitamin D deficiency, as differential dx, for
hypocalcemia, 87

Vitamin D intoxication, as differential dx, for hypercalcemia, 78
Vitamin E deficiency, as differential dx, for Romberg's sign, 149
Vitamin K deficiency, as differential dx, for excessive bleeding, 21
Vitiligo, as differential dx, for decreased skin pigmentation, 155
Vitreous hemorrhage, as differential dx, for vision loss, 174
Vocal cord problems, as differential dx, for hoarseness, 77
Voice abuse, as differential dx
  for hoarseness, 77
  for sore throat, 156
Volume depletion, as differential dx, for hypotension, 92
Volvulus, as differential dx
  for abdominal guarding, 3
  for abdominal pain in lower quadrants, 5
  for constipation, 35
Vomiting, 109
Von Willebrand's disease, as differential dx, for excessive bleeding, 21
Vulvar vestibulitis, as differential dx, for dyspareunia, 51
Vulvodynia, as differential dx, for dyspareunia, 51

Wandering atrial pacemaker, as differential dx, for irregular heart rhythms, 96
Wardenberg's syndrome, as differential dx, for hearing loss, 70
Water loss/intake, as differential dx, in hypernatremia, 81
Wegener's granulomatosis, as differential dx, for hemoptysis, 74
Weight gain, 175
Weight loss, 176
"Welder's flash," as differential dx, for vision loss, 174
Wenckebach, as differential dx, for bradycardia, 25
Wernicke's aphasia, as differential dx, for aphasia, 17
Wheezing, 159
"White coat" hypertension, 85

Wide pulse pressure, 177
Wilms' tumor, as differential dx, for pelvic masses, 125
Wilson's disease, as differential dx
  for chorea, 33
  for dementia, 42
  for hepatomegaly, 76
  for tremors, 168
Withdrawal from drugs/substances, as differential dx
  for delirium, 40
  for fatigue, 59
  for hallucinations, 67
  for headache, 69
  for hyperreflexia, 83
  for paresthesias, 123
  for weight gain, 175
Wolff-Parkinson-White syndrome, as differential dx, for palpitations, 119
Wrist pain/swelling, 178

Xanthomas, as differential dx, for nodular lesions, 113
Xerosis, 48
Xerostomia, as differential dx, for halitosis, 66
Xyphodenia, as differential dx, for chest pain, 32

Yersinia enterocolitica, 43

"Zebras." See Differential dx for specific sign or symptom
Zenker's diverticulum, as differential dx, for halitosis, 66
Zoon's plasma cell balanitis, as differential dx, for genital skin lesions, 63
Zoster, as differential dx
  for abdominal guarding, 3
  for breast pain/discharge, 27
  for chest pain, 32
  for ear pain, 55
  for flank pain/CVA tenderness, 61
  for jaw pain/swelling, 61
  for periorbital edema, 129
  for vesicular and bullous lesions, 173
  for vision loss, 173